SECOND EDITION

Veterinary Laboratory Medicine

CLINICAL PATHOLOGY

SECOND EDITION

Veterinary Laboratory Medicine

CLINICAL PATHOLOGY

J. Robert Duncan, D.V.M., Ph.D.
Keith W. Prasse, D.V.M., Ph.D

DEPARTMENT OF VETERINARY PATHOLOGY
COLLEGE OF VETERINARY MEDICINE
UNIVERSITY OF GEORGIA, ATHENS, GEORGIA

Iowa State University Press, Ames, Iowa

Printed in the United States of America from camera-ready copy provided by the authors

First edition, 1977
Second printing, 1978
Third printing, 1979
Fourth printing, 1981
Fifth printing, 1982
Sixth printing, 1983
Seventh printing, 1984
Eighth printing, 1985
Second edition, 1986
Second printing, 1987
Third printing, 1988

Library of Congress Cataloging in Publication Data

Duncan, J. Robert
    Veterinary laboratory medicine.

    Includes index.
        1. Veterinary clinical pathology.   I. Prasse, Keith W.
II. Title.
SF772.6.D86   1986   636.089′607   85-19786
ISBN 0-8138-1916-4

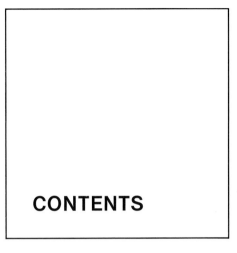

CONTENTS

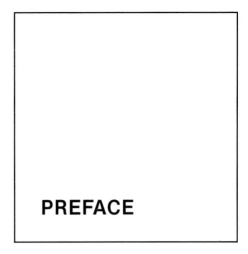

PREFACE

THE CLINICAL LABORATORY has an integral role in the practice of scientific medicine. The progressive diagnostic regimen includes identification of the patient's problems from history, clinical signs, physical examination, and laboratory findings. Certain laboratory tests are used and relied upon as frequently as the thermometer or stethoscope.

The discipline of laboratory medicine, in its broad definition, includes hematology, clinical chemistry, cytology, microbiology, parasitology, and toxicology. Our mission over the past nine years has involved teaching and diagnostic service in hematology, clinical chemistry, and cytology; this text is limited to these subjects.

The stimulus for this work originated with our desire to teach clinical pathology through an open discussion of laboratory data about selected clinical cases. We abandoned the classical lecture and provided our students with a set of notes from which to prepare for the case discussions that replaced the lecture hour. In 1973 the notes were compiled into a publication titled "A Syllabus of Veterinary Clinical Pathology." Its use by other veterinary schools encouraged us to revise the publication, add illustrations and case examples, and publish it in book form. It is written for students and practitioners of veterinary medicine.

The primary focus of the book is to relate abnormalities identified by laboratory procedures to organ dysfunctions or lesions, emphasizing the pathophysiologic basis for the development of the abnormal test result. General disease processes and their mechanisms are discussed; specific diseases are cited as examples and not described in detail. The interpretive aspects of laboratory medicine are stressed in a problem-oriented approach, with emphasis on the differential diagnosis created by an abnormal test value. Throughout the book reference is made to the cases listed in Appendix II, in which actual laboratory data serve to reinforce or illustrate the concept being described. This is not a laboratory manual, so detailed procedures of the various tests are not included.

The organization of the text represents the culmination of many trials and modifications of ways to present the subject of laboratory medicine to veterinary students. We hope that our years of teaching clinical pathology as a team are reflected in uniformity and singleness of purpose throughout the book.

In an attempt to provide a compendium of information in a fresh, palatable, and readily accessible form, we have strayed from the traditional type of scientific writing. Research data are not included, nor are citations of specific publications, although selected references are provided at the end of each chapter.

We gratefully acknowledge the many contributions made by students, fellow clinical pathologists, academic clinicians, medical technologists, and private practitioners with whom we have been associated. These contributions have come through interaction in the classroom, laboratory, and clinicopathologic conferences as well as in discussions about a particular case record, laboratory report, blood smear, or cytologic preparation. These interactions and discussions have been our stimulus to learn and a major source of the concepts and information in this book.

PREFACE TO THE SECOND EDITION

Since the publication of the first edition in 1977, the field of veterinary laboratory medicine has grown tremendously. This is obvious when one reviews the vast literature now available on the subject. Because of this expansion of knowledge, the second edition represents an almost total revision and a significant increase in subject matter. The goals, focus, and style, however, remain the same as those of the first edition.

We have tried to organize the text to facilitate the problemsolving approach to disease diagnosis through the interpretation of laboratory data. Again we have emphasized mechanisms and the pathophysiology of disease processes rather than individual diseases, and actual cases are used to illustrate these features. Material pertaining to plasma proteins, lipids, and carbohydrates has been presented in a separate chapter in this edition.

We again acknowledge those colleagues and students who daily provide our stimulus as clinical pathologists and help mold our methods of teaching the subject. We are happy to have Dr. Jeanne Wright George, a fellow teacher, contribute the chapter "Water, Electrolytes, and Acid Base." We thank the users of the first edition who provided us with constructive criticism, encouragement to proceed with updating the work, and the personal satisfaction of observing well-worn copies lying about the teaching hospital. We also acknowledge the support and guidance provided by the staff of the Iowa State University Press. A special thank you is extended to our typists, Linda Shapira, Cindy McElwee, and Diane Kistner King. And finally we sincerely thank each member of our two families for their support and encouragement in this endeavor.

SECOND EDITION

Veterinary Laboratory Medicine

CLINICAL PATHOLOGY

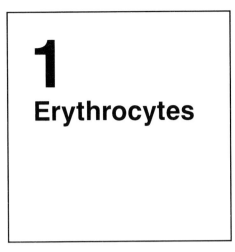

1

Erythrocytes

BASIC CONCEPTS OF ERYTHROCYTE PRODUCTION, METABOLISM, AND BREAKDOWN

I. Heme synthesis
    A. Heme synthesis is unidirectional and irreversible and
        controlled at the first step via the enzyme aminolevulinic
        acid synthetase whose formation is induced by a decrease in
        heme concentration.
    B. Certain enzyme excesses or deficiencies in the synthetic
        pathway can lead to porphyria (excessive production of
        porphyrins and their precursors). Lead inhibits several
        enzymatic steps, and chloramphenicol inhibits
        ferrochelatase.

II. Globin synthesis
    A. Each hemoglobin molecule is composed of four globin chains
        (two like pairs), each binding to a heme group.
        1. The hemoglobin type depends on the type of globin
            chains, which are determined by amino acid sequences.
        2. Heme and globin synthesis are balanced (increase in one
            results in an increase in the other).
    B. Abnormalities in globin synthesis (hemoglobinopathies) have
        not been described in domestic animals.

III. Iron metabolism
    A. Body iron content is regulated by rate of absorption rather
        than excretion. Absorption is regulated by the amount of
        storage iron (large stores decrease absorption) and rate of
        erythropoiesis (accelerated erythropoiesis increases
        absorption).
        1. Iron is transported in blood via a beta globulin,
            transferrin. Transferrin is measured as total iron-
            binding capacity; usually only one-third of transferrin
            binding sites are occupied by iron.
        2. Ceruloplasmin, a copper-containing protein synthesized
            in the liver, is necessary for transfer of iron from gut

3

epithelium and macrophages to transferrin.
3.   Iron is incorporated into hemoglobin during the latter
     stages of heme synthesis. Lack of intracellular iron
     causes an increase in erythrocyte protoporphyrin.
4.   Iron is stored in macrophages as ferritin and hemo-
     siderin. Serum ferritin is an indirect measurement of
     the storage iron pool.
  B.   Abnormalities are related to absorptive failures, nutri-
       tional deficiencies, iron loss via hemorrhage, and iron
       diversion to macrophages at the expense of hematopoietic
       cells (chronic disease processes).

IV.   Erythrocyte metabolism. Metabolism is limited after the
      reticulocyte stage because mature erythrocytes lack mitochondria
      for oxidative metabolism. Biochemical pathways found in mature
      erythrocytes are listed below with their function and associated
      abnormalities.
  A.   Embden–Meyerhof pathway
       1.   By this pathway glucose utilization generates adenosine
            triphosphate (ATP), which is essential for membrane
            function and integrity.
       2.   Enzyme deficiencies in this pathway can lead to anemia
            (e.g., pyruvate kinase deficiency anemia of dogs).
  B.   Hexose-monophosphate pathway
       1.   Glutathione is maintained in the reduced state by this
            pathway. Reduced glutathione neutralizes oxidants, which
            can denature hemoglobin.
       2.   Enzyme deficiency in this pathway or excess oxidant
            causes Heinz body formation and anemia.
  C.   Methemoglobin reductase pathway
       1.   Hemoglobin is maintained in the reduced state necessary
            for transport of oxygen by this pathway.
       2.   Enzyme deficiency results in methemoglobin formation.
            Methemoglobin cannot transport oxygen, and cyanosis
            results.
  D.   Luebering–Rapoport pathway
       1.   This pathway allows formation of 2,3 diphosphoglycerate
            (2,3 DPG), which has a regulatory role in oxygen
            transport. Increased 2,3 DPG favors oxygen release to
            tissues by lowering oxygen affinity of hemoglobin.
       2.   Anemic animals usually have increased 2,3 DPG
            concentrations and deliver more oxygen to tissues with a
            lesser amount of hemoglobin (a compensatory mechanism).

V.   Erythrokinetics (Fig. 1.1)
  A.   Hematopoietic stem cell characteristics
       1.   Multipotential stem cell
            a.   Its morphology is unknown, but it may appear similar
                 to a small lymphocyte.
            b.   This stem cell self-replicates or differentiates
                 into a unipotential (committed) stem cell; the type
                 is determined by the microenvironment. Unipotential
                 stem cells include erythrocytic, granulomonocytic,
                 and megakaryocytic types.
       2.   The erythrocytic unipotential stem cell is self-

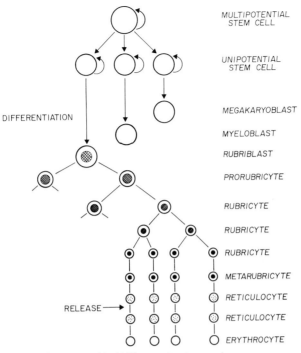

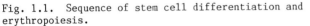

Fig. 1.1. Sequence of stem cell differentiation and erythropoiesis.

replicating and responsive to erythropoietin, which causes differentiation to a rubriblast.
B. Characteristics of erythropoiesis
  1. In mammals erythropoiesis occurs extravascularly in the bone marrow parenchyma.
  2. Characteristic morphologic changes take place during differentiation and maturation from rubriblast to mature erythrocyte.
    a. Cells become smaller.
    b. Nuclei become smaller and their chromatin more aggregated.
      (1) Division stops in the late rubricyte stage when a critical cytoplasmic concentration of hemoglobin is reached.
      (2) The nucleus is extruded at the end of the metarubricyte stage, and the cell becomes a reticulocyte.
    c. The color of the cytoplasm changes from blue to gray to orange as hemoglobin accumulates and RNA is lost; the nuclear/cytoplasmic ratio decreases. Cytoplasm of the anucleate reticulocyte contains blue aggregates of RNA after treatment with supravital stains.
  3. Reticulocytes and erythrocytes migrate into venous sinuses of the bone marrow and then into peripheral blood.

4. Approximately 5 days are required from stimulation of
    the erythropoietic stem cell by erythropoietin until
    reticulocyte release from the bone marrow. Four
    divisions usually produce 16 erythrocytes.
5. Reticulocytes normally remain in bone marrow 2 to 3
    days.
6. Bone marrow has the potential for increasing
    erythropoiesis.
    a. Erythrocyte production can be increased several
        times the normal rate if the necessary stimulation
        and nutrients are present, and the bone marrow is
        capable of responding. This capacity to increase
        production varies with the species, being greatest
        in the dog and least in the cow and horse.
    b. Increase in number of cells delivered to the blood
        occurs primarily by increased stem cell input;
        shortening of maturation time has minimal effect.
    c. Cells may be delivered to circulation faster by
        earlier release of reticulocytes and skipped cell
        divisions. These processes do not result in an
        increase in total number of cells produced.
7. Regulation of erythropoiesis
    a. Erythropoietin
        (1) Erythropoietin is produced by the kidney in an
             active form in response to hypoxia. An alter-
             nate theory is that the kidney produces an
             erythropoietic factor, which reacts with an
             alpha globulin produced by the liver to form
             the active erythropoietin.
        (2) It stimulates the stem cell differentiation to
             rubriblasts, early reticulocyte release, and
             hemoglobin synthesis.
    b. Other hormones
        (1) Androgens stimulate production of
             erythropoietin or potentiate its action.
        (2) Estrogens have an inhibitory effect on
             erythropoiesis.
        (3) Thyroid, pituitary, and adrenocortical hormones
             alter tissue demands for oxygen, thereby
             changing the requirement for erythropoiesis.
    c. T lymphocytes play a role in modulating
        erythropoiesis.

VI. Erythrocyte breakdown
    A. The average erythrocyte life span varies with the species:
        dog, 110 days; cat, 70 days; cow, 160 days; horse, 145 days;
        pig, 86 days; and sheep, 150 days.
    B. Aging of erythrocytes is accompanied by changes in enzyme
        content and cell membrane structure, causing a less
        deformable cell that is subject to removal by the spleen.
    C. In health, senescent erythrocytes are removed from
        circulation by two routes.
        1. Phagocytosis by macrophages is the major route
            (Fig. 1.2).

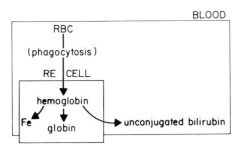

Fig. 1.2. Outline of phagocytic destruction of erythrocytes.

> 2. Intravascular lysis and release of free hemoglobin is a
>   minor route (Fig. 1.3).
> 3. Similar routes of destruction are followed in hemolytic
>   anemia.

MEANS OF EVALUATING ERYTHROCYTES

I. Hematocrit (Hct), hemoglobin (Hb) concentration, and red blood
    cell (RBC) count
    A. Hct is the percent of blood composed of erythrocytes.
        1. Centrifugal methods give a packed cell volume (PCV), a
            very accurate measurement ($\pm$ 1%).
            a. Plasma obtained by this method can be used for other
                routine determinations such as:
                (1) Plasma protein concentration by refractometry
                (2) Plasma fibrinogen concentration using heat
                     precipitation and refractometry
                (3) Plasma color and transparency
                     (a) Normal plasma is clear and colorless (dog
                          and cat) to light yellow (horse and cow).

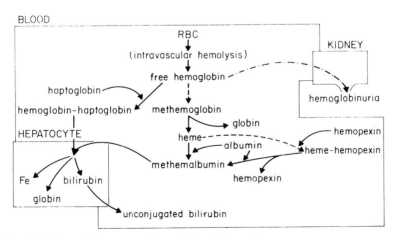

Fig. 1.3. Outline of intravascular destruction of
erythrocytes.

              (b)   Icteric plasma is yellow and clear.

              (c)   Hemoglobinemic plasma is pink to red and clear.

              (d)   Lipemic plasma is whitish and opaque.

    b. Microfilaria may be detected by microscopic examination of the plasma just above the buffy coat zone.

  2. Certain automated cell counters calculate the Hct after determining the RBC count and mean corpuscular volume (MCV). Potential for error is greater than the PCV method because of the complexity of the measurement and standardization of most instruments with human cells rather than animal cells.

B. Hb concentration

  1. Colorimetric determination by the cyanmethemoglobin method is used most frequently.

    a. Accuracy is approximately $\pm$ 5%.

    b. Erythrocyte refractile bodies may cause false high values in the cat.

  2. Some automated instruments directly measure optical density of oxyhemoglobin.

  3. Hb concentration provides the most direct indication of oxygen transport capacity of the blood and should be approximately one-third the PCV if erythrocytes are of normal size.

  4. It provides no clinical advantage over the PCV other than allowing the determination of mean corpuscular hemoglobin (MCH) and mean corpuscular hemoglobin concentration (MCHC) (see below).

C. RBC count

  1. Direct counting using a hemocytometer is of limited value because of the large error involved.

  2. Automatic counters, if standardized for animal blood, allow for more accurate counts.

  3. The main value of the RBC count is that it allows determination of MCV and MCH (see below).

D. Factors affecting Hct, Hb, and RBC count

  1. Change in circulating RBC mass affects all three parameters.

    a. Low values occur in anemia. Decreases in the three parameters may be disproportionate if cell size and/or Hb content per cell are also altered. Calculation and interpretation of RBC indices are helpful in these cases.

    b. Increased RBC mass (absolute polycythemia) causes high values.

    c. Splenic contraction causes transitory high values (spurious polycythemia) and is particularly common in excited horses.

  2. Change in plasma volume affects all three parameters; interpretation must always be made with knowledge of the hydration status (Cases 4, 6).

    a. Dehydration or fluid shifts to visceral organs cause increased values.

    b. Overhydration with parenteral fluids causes reduction in values, simulating anemia.

II. RBC indices. RBC indices are helpful in the classification of
     certain anemias.
     A. Mean corpuscular volume (MCV)
         1. (Hct × 10)/RBC (millions) = MCV (femtoliters).
         2. The MCV can be determined directly by automatic
             counters.
         3. Factors affecting MCV values
             a. MCV is increased in macrocytic anemias in which
                 interference with nucleic acid synthesis causes
                 inhibition of cell division and thereby larger
                 erythrocytes (e.g., B_{12} and folic acid
                 deficiencies).
             b. Reticulocytosis causes a transitory increase in MCV
                 (Cases 1, 2).
             c. Iron deficiency causes decreased MCV. An extra cell
                 division occurs before the critical level of
                 hemoglobin is reached that is necessary to stop
                 division; erythrocytes are smaller.
     B. Mean corpuscular hemoglobin (MCH)
         1. (Hb × 10)/RBC (millions) = MCH (picograms).
         2. Factors affecting MCH values
             a. Iron deficiency causes a decreased MCH.
             b. Reticulocytosis causes normal or slightly increased
                 values.
             c. In vivo and in vitro hemolysis increases the MCH
                 (Case 3); extracellular Hb is also measured, but the
                 formula assumes all Hb is intracellular.
     C. Mean corpuscular hemoglobin concentration (MCHC)
         1. (Hb × 100)/Hct = MCHC (g/dl).
         2. The MCHC is the most accurate of the indices because it
             does not require the RBC count.
         3. Factors affecting the MCHC
             a. Reticulocytosis and iron deficiency cause decreased
                 MCHC.
             b. In vivo and in vitro hemolysis increases the MCHC
                 (Case 3).
             c. The MCHC may be increased when significant
                 spherocytosis is present.

III. Peripheral blood smear
     A. Staining of the smear
         1. New methylene blue (NMB). A drop of NMB between a
             coverslip and an air-dried smear gives a rapid, mean-
             ingful stain but is a nonpermanent preparation. Acid
             groups stain blue (i.e., nuclear DNA and RNA, cyto-
             plasmic RNA, and basophil granules). Eosinophil granules
             are unstained. Reticulocytes are best stained by mixing
             equal parts of NMB and blood, holding at room tempera-
             ture for 10 minutes, and then making the smear.
         2. Romanowsky stains (Wright's stain). These polychromic
             preparations stain certain acid groups blue (RNA), basic
             groups orange (proteins, eosinophil granules), and
             metachromatic substances violet (mast cell and basophil
             granules and nuclear DNA).

B. Systematic evaluation of the smear
    1. Low magnification. Select a thin area of the smear where
        the cells are evenly distributed and observe for the
        following features:
        a. RBC rouleaux formation (described below)
        b. RBC agglutination (described below)
        c. Platelet aggregation (see Chapter 4)
        d. Relative number of leukocytes
    2. High-dry magnification. Confirm observations made at low
        magnification and:
        a. Note the concentration of leukocytes and obtain an
            impression as to whether the white blood cell (WBC)
            count is low, normal, or high.
        b. Calculate a differential leukocyte count. This can
            usually be done at high-dry magnification, but
            certain cells may require oil immersion for
            identification.
    3. Oil-immersion magnification
        a. Examine the erythrocyte morphology (described
            below).
        b. Conduct the differential leukocyte count at this
            magnification if difficulty is encountered at high-
            dry magnification.
        c. Examine leukocyte morphology (see Chapter 2).
        d. Estimate the adequacy of platelet number and
            evaluate their morphology (see Chapter 4).
C. Erythrocyte morphology (Fig. 1.4)
    1. Normal morphology
        a. Canine erythrocytes are large (7 μm), uniform in
            size, and have central pallor (biconcave disk).
            Crenation (an artifact characterized by pointed
            margins) does not readily occur.
        b. Feline erythrocytes average 5.8 μm in diameter and
            exhibit very slight central pallor and mild aniso-
            cytosis (variation in size); crenation is common.
            Howell-Jolly bodies (nuclear remnants) occur in up
            to 1% of the cells.
        c. Bovine erythrocytes average 5.5 μm in diameter.
            Anisocytosis is common, and central pallor is
            usually slight. Crenation is common.

Fig. 1.4. Erythrocyte and platelet morphology. A. Normal
canine erythrocytes and platelets; B. normal feline erythrocytes and platelets; C. normal bovine erythrocytes and platelets; D. normal equine erythrocytes in rouleaux; E. canine
reticulocytes and platelets (arrow) (wet NMB); F. canine
reticulocytes (dry NMB); G. feline reticulocytes (dry NMB);
H. polychromasia (dog); I. metarubricyte (dog); J. basophilic
stippling (cow); K. Howell-Jolly bodies, leptocyte (dog);
L. spherocytes, anisocytosis (dog); M. hypochromia, poikilocyte
(dog); N. poikilocytes, fragmented cell (dog); O. stomatocytes
(dog); P. autoagglutination (dog); Q. Heinz bodies (horse);
R. Heinz bodies (dry NMB) (horse); S. ER bodies (cat); T. ER
bodies (dry NMB) (cat); U. giant shift platelet (arrow) (dog);
V. Babesia caballi; W. Hemobartonella felis; X. H. felis;
Y. Anaplasma marginale. (All smears are Wright stained unless
indicated, ×1100.)

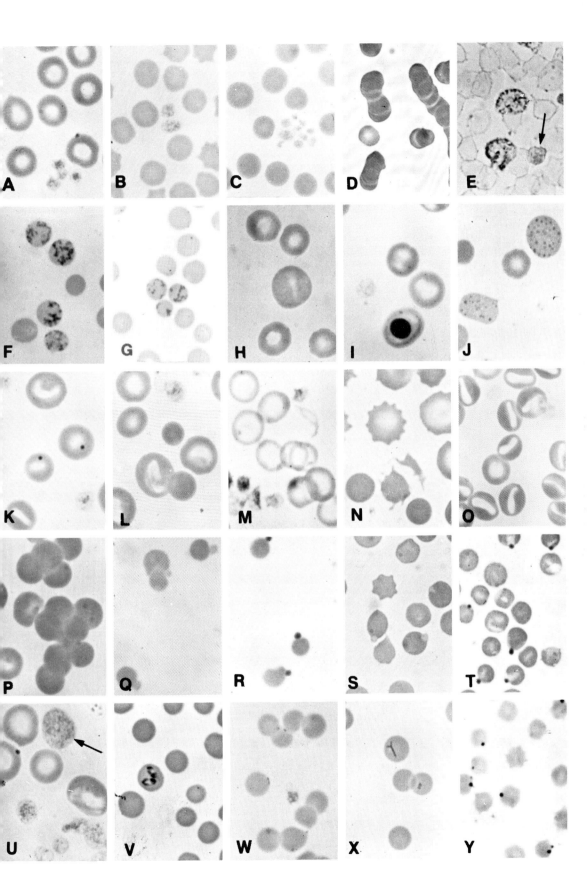

    d.   Equine erythrocytes average 5.7 μm in diameter and lack central pallor. Rouleaux formation is common.

    e.   Pig erythrocytes average 6.0 μm in diameter and lack central pallor.

    f.   Sheep erythrocytes are similar to those of the cow but smaller. The average diameter is 4.5 μm.

    g.   Goat erythrocytes are the smallest of the domestic animals, usually under 4 μm. Anisocytosis and poikilocytosis are common.

2. Rouleaux formation is a grouping of erythrocytes resembling a stack of coins. The degree tends to parallel the erythrocyte sedimentation rate and is associated with an increase in fibrinogen concentration or a qualitative change in serum globulins. Rouleaux disappears on dilution with saline.

    a.   Marked rouleaux formation is common in the horse in health but may not occur in severely anemic or cachectic horses.

    b.   In the dog and cat it may occur to a mild degree in health and may be marked during inflammatory and neoplastic disease.

    c.   Rouleaux formation is rare in ruminants in health and disease.

3. Agglutination is a grapelike aggregation of erythrocytes occurring in some cases of antibody-mediated anemia. It may be observed on the glass of the blood sample tube as well as microscopically in an unstained wet mount or on a stained smear. It can be differentiated from rouleaux by its failure to disappear on dilution with saline.

4. Anisocytosis is variation in the size of cells because of the presence of macrocytes and/or microcytes among normal cells.

5. Macrocytes are large cells with increased MCV. They may exhibit polychromasia and represent reticulocytes. Normochromic macrocytes may occur in certain other disease states (e.g., B_{12} or folic acid deficiency anemias).

6. Microcytes are small cells with decreased MCV, which may be observed in iron and pyridoxine deficiency anemias. They represent cell remnants in Heinz body and fragmentation anemias. Spherocytes associated with immune-mediated anemias are also a type of microcyte.

7. Polychromasia is variation in color among cells. Bluish (residual RNA) erythrocytes are generally large and represent reticulocytes. Increased numbers are associated with increased erythropoietic activity and a regenerative response to anemia. A few polychromic cells are normal in the dog and cat. Their number correlates with the reticulocyte count in these species.

8. Hypochromia is decreased staining intensity and increased central pallor of the erythrocyte caused by insufficient Hb in the cell. The most common cause is iron deficiency.

9. Poikilocytes are abnormally shaped cells commonly observed in chronic blood loss and diseases charac-

terized by erythrocyte fragmentation (Case 10). They may
be removed prematurely from the circulation, potentiat-
ing the anemic state. Schizocytes and acanthocytes are
types of poikilocytes.

10. Leptocytes are thin cells with increased membrane/volume
    ratio and are observed in chronic debilitating diseases
    and certain anemias. Polychromic cells (reticulocytes)
    may appear as leptocytes.

11. Spherocytes are small dark microcytes lacking central
    pallor and having a reduction in amount of membrane per
    cell. They are readily detected only in the dog and are
    observed in autoimmune (Case 2) and isoimmune hemolytic
    anemias and following transfusions. They are removed
    prematurely from circulation by splenic macrophages
    because of their reduced deformability and inability to
    traverse the splenic sinus pores.

12. Stomatocytes have oval-shaped areas of central pallor
    and are observed in hereditary stomatocytosis of Alaskan
    malamutes and certain liver diseases.

13. Basophilic stippling is sometimes observed in
    Romanowsky-stained cells containing residual RNA. This
    finding occurs often in sheep and cattle and occasion-
    ally in the cat during response to anemia. It can be a
    characteristic of lead poisoning.

14. Howell-Jolly bodies are basophilic nuclear remnants more
    frequently observed in responding anemia.

15. Heinz bodies are round structures on the internal
    erythrocyte membrane, representing denatured Hb caused
    by certain oxidant drugs or chemicals (Case 3). They do
    not stain well with Wright's stain but are visible with
    NMB staining. Heinz bodies disrupt the cell membrane and
    are associated with intravascular hemolysis, leaving a
    RBC ghost. Affected cells or only the Heinz body may be
    removed by phagocytosis.

16. Erythrocyte refractile bodies are similar to Heinz
    bodies and may be seen in up to 10% of feline erythro-
    cytes in health. They are increased in a variety of
    diseases in the cat and may or may not play a role in
    the development of anemia.

17. Nucleated erythrocytes, metarubricytes or earlier
    stages, can represent early release of immature cells
    during anemia (Cases 1, 2) but also may be observed in
    bone marrow disease when there is damage to the
    parenchyma-sinus barrier. Growing swine have significant
    metarubricytosis in health.

18. Parasites occur within the erythrocyte or on the cell
    surface. Hemobartonella felis, Anaplasma marginale,
    Babesia canis, B. equi, B. caballi, and Eperythrozoon
    suis are those most commonly encountered.

IV. Blood reticulocyte evaluation
    A. Species characteristics of reticulocytes
        1. The dog has small numbers of reticulocytes in health (up
           to 1%).

2. Two types of reticulocytes have been reported in the cat.
    a. The aggregate type is similar to those of other species and accounts for up to 0.4% of the erythrocytes in health. This is the type usually counted.
    b. The punctate type is more difficult to identify and occurs in large numbers in health (up to 10%). They are increased in regenerative anemia and remain increased for at least 2 weeks after the aggregate count has returned to normal. They can indicate a bone marrow response as much as 3 to 4 weeks previously.
3. Reticulocytes are absent in health in ruminants but are increased in responding anemias.
4. Reticulocytes are absent in the blood of horses in both health and responding anemias.
5. Reticulocytosis is a prominent feature of healthy suckling pigs, but the adult percentage is less than 1.0%; counts increase in responding anemias.

B. Means of enumeration
1. Reticulocyte percentage. This parameter can give a false high impression of bone marrow response because:
    a. In the blood of anemic animals there are fewer mature erythrocytes present to mix with reticu-locytes being released from the bone marrow, and a relative increase in reticulocytes is apparent.
    b. In response to anemia, reticulocytes are released earlier (shift reticulocytes). They persist as reticulocytes for longer periods in the blood because it takes longer for them to mature.
2. Absolute reticulocyte count (reticulocyte percentage × RBC count). This parameter corrects for 1a above but does not correct for the effect described in 1b.
3. Reticulocyte production index (RPI). This correction index is used in humans and is adaptable to the dog to correct for 1a and 1b above. RPI = [observed reticulocytes (%)] × [observed PCV (%)/45 (normal PCV)] × [1/blood maturation time (days)].
    a. Blood maturation times of reticulocytes at various PCVs are 45%, 1.0 days; 35%, 1.5 days; 25%, 2.0 days; 15%, 2.5 days.
    b. RPI values equal the increase in erythrocyte production (e.g., RPI of 3.0 equals 3 times normal erythrocyte production).

C. Interpretation of reticulocyte parameters
1. Absolute increases in reticulocytes indicate a responding bone marrow (hemorrhagic or hemolytic type of anemia).
2. Reticulocytosis does not become clearly evident until 48 to 72 hours following occurrence of the anemia; it should reach a maximum in 7 days after onset.
3. Reticulocytosis is more marked in hemolytic than hemor-rhagic (external) anemias because iron from disrupted cells is more readily available for erythropoiesis;

release of iron from macrophage stores is slower. RPI
greater than 3 usually indicates a hemolytic mechanism
(Case 2).
4. Dogs have greater reticulocyte responses than cats.
5. Significant reticulocytosis does not develop in cattle
in acute responding anemias until the PCV is very low.
6. Reticulocytosis does not occur in the horse in any type
of anemia.
7. Healthy suckling pigs have high reticulocyte counts.

V. Bone marrow examination
  A. Technique
    1. Aspiration can be made via the iliac crest, trochanteric
       fossa, sternum, or rib, employing special bone marrow or
       18-gauge cerebrospinal needles.
    2. Particle smears are preferred because they are least
       likely to be contaminated with blood.
  B. Examination of the stained smear (Fig. 1.5).
    1. Observe the relative number, size, and cellularity of
       the particles and proportion of fat cells. The number
       and cellularity of particles is an estimation of the
       overall cellularity of the bone marrow; however, low-
       cellularity aspirates may occur with hypercellular bone
       marrow. Histologic examination of a bone marrow core
       biopsy is a more accurate method of assessing marrow
       cellularity.
    2. Note the adequacy of megakaryocyte numbers and relative
       number of immature forms.
    3. The ratio of myeloid to nucleated erythroid cells (M/E
       ratio) may be estimated. Interpretation of the ratio is
       facilitated by a knowledge of the PCV and WBC count
       (e.g., high M/E ratio with a normal WBC count suggests
       erythroid hypoplasia).
    4. The relative percentages of the various stages of each
       series should be observed. In health approximately 80%
       of the myeloid series should be metamyelocytes, bands,
       and segmenters (nonproliferating maturation storage
       pool); 90% of the erythroid series should be rubricytes
       and metarubricytes. A high percentage of immature forms
       can suggest hyperplasia, neoplasia, or maturation abnor-
       mality of the respective series, or in the myeloid
       series, depletion of the storage pool.
    5. Abnormal cells should be identified.
    6. Staining for iron and observation of the amount in bone
       marrow macrophages may be useful when evaluating iron
       deficiency anemia (absence of iron) or anemia of chronic
       disease (increased iron).

VI. Antigen and antibody detection
  A. Blood cell antigen determination
    1. Agglutination and hemolytic tests with specific antisera
       for each antigen are used for identification. Some
       antigens are more important than others in hemolytic
       disorders (e.g., CEA-1 (A_1), CEA-2 (A_2), and CEA-7 (Tr)
       in the dog; Aa and Qa in the horse; A, F, and V in the

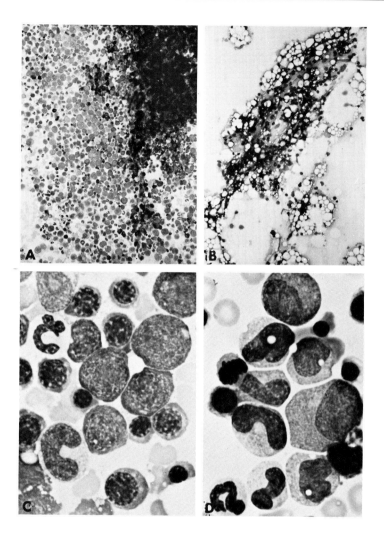

Fig. 1.5. Bone marrow cytology. A. Hypercellular bone marrow
particle from a cat with preleukemia (subleukemic granulocytic
leukemia). B. Hypocellular bone marrow particle from a cat with
infectious feline panleukopenia. Note the large amount of fat
and relatively few hematopoietic cells. C. Bone marrow aspiration smear from a cat illustrating erythroid series. All the
erythroid cells have round nuclei in which the chromatin
becomes more aggregated as the cells mature and become smaller.
Segmented and metamyelocyte neutrophils are present. D. Bone
marrow aspiration smear from a dog illustrating the myeloid
series. The large cell is a progranulocyte and the cell at the
top is a myeloblast. The remaining myeloid cells have progressive indentation of nuclei and aggregation of chromatin as they
mature. The small cells with dark round nuclei are rubricytes
and metarubricytes. (Wright's stain; A and B, ×110, C and D,
×1100.) (From Duncan JR and Prasse KW: Clinical examination of
bone marrow. Vet Clin North Am 6:597, 1976.)

cow; and A and B in the cat).
2. Antigen identification is helpful in parentage testing, identifying potentially compatible donors (e.g., CEA-1 negative dogs are best as blood donors), and identifying matings likely to lead to isoimmunization.
B. Blood cross matching
1. These tests are used to determine when blood may be safely transfused; antibodies are detected.
2. Incompatible cross matches usually indicate prior sensitization; naturally occurring antibodies usually are not present in significant amounts to cause incompatible reactions. Anti-A antibody has been demonstrated in cats without prior evidence of sensitization.
3. The major cross match tests erythrocytes of the donor against serum of the recipient, and the minor cross match tests serum of the donor against erythrocytes of the recipient. Incompatibilities in the major cross match are the most significant clinically.
4. Agglutination tests are used for most species, but the hemolytic test is best for the horse and cow.
C. Antiglobulin (Coombs') tests
1. The direct antiglobulin test detects antibody and/or complement attached to the patient's washed erythrocytes. The antiglobulin reagent (Coombs' serum) may be prepared against any antibody type or complement. A species-specific Coombs' serum must be used (e.g., rabbit anticanine IgG for the dog).
2. The indirect test detects antierythrocyte antibody in the serum of the patient by reacting with erythrocytes from the sire, offspring, or donor animal. Supernatant (whey) from colostral milk may be used instead of serum in postpartum mares to test for potential reaction against the foal's cells.

ANEMIA: DIAGNOSIS AND CLASSIFICATION
Anemia is an absolute decrease in the PCV, Hb concentration, and RBC count.

I. Diagnosis. As with any disease, the diagnosis rests on information gained from historical, physical, and laboratory findings.
A. History. The following may be significant.
1. Drug administration
2. Exposure to toxic chemicals or plants
3. Family or herd occurrence
4. Recent transfusions or colostral ingestion
5. Age at onset
B. Physical findings
1. Clinical signs suggesting the presence of anemia are related to decreased oxygen transport capacity and physiologic adjustments made to increase the efficiency of the erythron and reduce the work load on the heart.

They include the following.
    a. Pale mucous membranes
    b. Weakness, loss of stamina, and exercise intolerance
    c. Tachycardia and polypnea, particularly after exercise
    d. Hypersensitivity to cold
    e. Heart murmur caused by reduced viscosity and increased turbulence of the blood
    f. Shock if one-third of the blood volume is lost in a short period
    g. Icterus, hemoglobinuria, hemorrhage, or fever, depending on the pathophysiologic mechanism involved

2. Signs are less marked if onset is gradual and the animal can adapt to the decreased erythrocyte mass.

C. Laboratory findings. Laboratory confirmation is necessary because anemias do not always present diagnostic clinical signs. Anemia is often detected from the laboratory data of a sick animal when its presence was not previously suspected.

  1. The PCV is the easiest, most accurate method for detecting anemia. Its result should be interpreted with knowledge of the hydration status and any alteration by splenic contraction.

  2. Hb concentration and RBC count may be used to further classify the anemia but are not usually needed to confirm its presence.

  3. Other laboratory procedures are used to further characterize the anemia and arrive at a specific diagnosis; these procedures are discussed below and earlier in the chapter.

II. Classification. The etiology of all anemias should be identified where possible because the term "anemia" per se does not constitute a diagnosis. Classification schemes are an attempt to accomplish this, although no one classification is entirely satisfactory.

A. Classification according to size (MCV) and Hb concentration (MCHC) of the erythrocyte

  1. Anemias may be normocytic, macrocytic, or microcytic.

  2. Anemias may be normochromic or hypochromic; absolute increases in Hb concentration do not occur except in the case of marked spherocytosis.

  3. This classification is useful primarily in the detection of iron deficiency and megaloblastic anemias.

B. Classification according to bone marrow response

  1. Regenerative (or responsive) anemia

    a. The bone marrow is actively responding to the anemia by increasing its production of erythrocytes.

    b. Findings that denote regeneration are polychromasia, reticulocytosis, and hypercellular bone marrow with a low M/E ratio.

    c. The presence of regeneration suggests an extramarrow cause; it implies a blood loss or erythrocyte destruction mechanism that is of sufficient duration

(2 to 3 days) for a regenerative response to be evident in the blood.
    d. Bone marrow examination is rarely necessary to detect regeneration; however, erythropoietic hyperplasia should be evident. It is the best means of detecting regenerative anemia in horses, since reticulocytosis does not occur in this species.
  2. Nonregenerative anemia
    a. Its presence indicates an inadequate bone marrow response because of either a primary or secondary bone marrow disorder.
    b. Polychromasia and reticulocytosis are absent. Bone marrow examination is indicated; it may reveal the pathophysiologic mechanism.
    c. During the first 2 to 3 days after onset of peracute or acute hemorrhage or hemolysis, anemia may present a nonregenerative pattern.
C. Classification according to the pathophysiologic mechanism. The remainder of the chapter characterizes these types of anemia.
  1. Blood loss (hemorrhagic) anemias
  2. Anemias caused by accelerated erythrocyte destruction (hemolytic, decreased erythrocytic life span)
  3. Anemias caused by reduced or defective erythropoiesis

ANEMIA FROM BLOOD LOSS (HEMORRHAGIC ANEMIA) (Table 1.1)

I. Characteristics of acute blood loss (Cases 1, 24)
  A. Clinical findings
    1. Usually there is direct visual evidence of hemorrhage, but some cases may be occult. The evidence may be indirect (e.g., thrombocytopenia and clotting test abnormalities indicate the potential for hemorrhage).
    2. Clinical signs depend on the amount of blood lost, period of time during which bleeding occurred, and site of hemorrhage. Hemorrhage from multiple sites suggests clotting abnormalities.
  B. Laboratory findings
    1. Initially, the PCV will be normal because all blood

TABLE 1.1. Causes of Blood Loss

Acute Hemorrhage	Chronic Hemorrhage
Trauma	Parasitism
Surgery	Hookworms
Gastrointestinal ulcers (large)	Strongylosis
Hemostasis defects	Haemonchosis
Disseminated intravascular	Coccidiosis
coagulation	Fleas, ticks, mosquitoes
Sweet clover poisoning	Gastrointestinal ulcers
Warfarin poisoning	Hematuria
Bracken fern poisoning	Vascular neoplasia
Factor X deficiency in pups	Hemophilia
	Thrombocytopenia

             components (cells and plasma) are lost in similar
             proportions. The animal may be in hypovolemic shock.

    2. Splenic contraction delivers high–PCV blood (80%) to the
circulation, temporarily elevating the PCV.

    3. Starting at 2 to 3 hours after onset of hemorrhage and
proceeding for 48 to 72 hours, the blood volume is
restored by the addition of interstitial fluid. This
causes dilution of the erythrocyte mass, and laboratory
signs of anemia (reduced PCV, RBC, and Hb) become
evident. Plasma protein concentration is also decreased.

    4. Platelet numbers usually increase during the first few
hours; they may be decreased if their consumption is
extensive because of excessive coagulation. Persistent
thrombocytosis may suggest continued bleeding.

    5. Neutrophilic leukocytosis commonly occurs by approxi-
mately 3 hours posthemorrhage.

    6. Signs of increased erythrocyte production (poly-
chromasia, reticulocytosis) become evident by 48 to 72
hours and reach a maximum approximately 7 days after the
onset of hemorrhage. Erythroid hyperplasia is evident in
the bone marrow and precedes the changes in the
peripheral blood.

    7. The hemogram returns to normal in 1 to 2 weeks following
a single acute hemorrhagic episode. If reticulocytosis
persists longer than 2 to 3 weeks, continuous bleeding
should be suspected.

    8. Thrombocytopenia and hemorrhage may occur with primary
bone marrow failure; the anemia in these cases is
nonregenerative in its presentation.

II. Characteristics of chronic blood loss
    A. Clinical findings
        1. Anemia develops slowly and hypovolemia does not occur.
        2. PCV can reach low values before clinical signs of anemia
become obvious because slow onset allows for physiologic
adaptation.
    B. Laboratory findings
        1. Regenerative response (usually less intense than in
acute blood loss) and hypoproteinemia are usually
observed.
        2. Persistent thrombocytosis may be evident.
        3. Body stores of iron may become depleted, and an iron-
lack anemia characterized by low serum iron, low percent
saturation of transferrin, absence of bone marrow
macrophage iron, and often microcytosis and hypochromia
develops. Regenerative signs become less pronounced;
poikilocytosis is commonly present at this stage.
        4. The bone marrow response may end abruptly in prolonged
cases of chronic hemorrhage and iron loss, causing a
nonregenerative, iron–lack anemia.
        5. Iron–lack anemia occurs more readily in young, rapidly
growing animals because they have less storage iron and
are usually on a milk diet low in iron.

III. Differential features between anemias caused by external and
internal hemorrhage

A. External blood loss prevents reutilization of certain
    components (iron, plasma protein). These may be reabsorbed
    following internal hemorrhage (gastrointestinal bleeding is
    considered external hemorrhage).
B. In internal hemorrhage (blood loss into body cavities)
    approximately two-thirds of the erythrocytes are reabsorbed
    into lymphatics (completed in 24 to 72 hours) and one-third
    are lysed or phagocytized; iron and plasma proteins are
    reutilized. Therefore, the anemia is usually not severe.

ANEMIA FROM ACCELERATED ERYTHROCYTE DESTRUCTION (HEMOLYTIC ANEMIA)
(Table 1.2)

I. Characteristics of hemolytic anemia
    A. Clinical findings
        1. Clinical signs of hemorrhage are absent.
        2. Clinical signs, in relation to severity of anemia, may
            be dramatic in acute cases because certain compensatory
            mechanisms develop slowly (e.g., increased 2,3 DPG).
        3. Icterus and/or hemoglobinuria may be seen in severe
            cases.
    B. Laboratory findings
        1. Reticulocyte counts are higher in hemolytic anemias than

TABLE 1.2. Causes of Accelerated Erythrocyte Destruction

Intravascular Hemolysis	Phagocytosis Hemolysis
Bacteria	RBC parasites
Leptospira spp.	Anaplasma spp.
Clostridium perfringens,	Hemobartonella spp.
Type A	Eperythrozoon spp.
C. hemolyticum	Cytauxzoon sp.
RBC parasites	Immune-mediated
Babesia spp.	Autoimmune hemolytic anemia
Chemicals and plants	Lupus erythematosus
Heinz body-type	Equine infectious anemia
Phenothiazine	Feline leukemia virus
Onions	Ehrlichia spp.
Red maple	RBC parasites
Rye grass	Hematopoietic neoplasia
Brassicaceae family	Hemangiosarcoma
Benzocaine	Intrinsic erythrocytic defect
Acetaminophen	Pyruvate kinase deficiency
Phenazopyridine	Porphyria
Copper	Hereditary stomatocytosis
Ricin (castor bean)	Fragmentation
Snake venoms	Disseminated intravascular
Immune-mediated	coagulation
Neonatal isoerythrolysis	Vasculitis
Incompatible transfusions	Hemangiosarcoma
Autoimmune hemolytic anemia	
Hypo-osmolality	
Cold hemoglobinuria	
Hypotonic fluids	
Fragmentation	
Vena caval syndrome	
Hypophosphatemia	
Postparturient hemoglobinuria	
Hyperalimentation	

hemorrhagic anemias because iron from destroyed
erythrocytes is more readily available for erythropoiesis than is storage iron.
2. Plasma protein concentration is normal or elevated.
3. Neutrophilic leukocytosis and monocytosis may occur.
4. Evidence of Hb degradation (e.g., hyperbilirubinemia)
   may not be readily apparent when anemia is of gradual
   onset.
5. Abnormal erythrocyte morphology (e.g., Heinz bodies,
   erythrocytic parasites, spherocytes, or poikilocytes)
   associated with anemia may suggest a hemolytic
   mechanism.

II. Differentiation of hemolytic anemias. A helpful approach in
determining the cause of a hemolytic anemia is identification of
the mechanism of destruction. Location of the site of hemolysis
(intravascular or extravascular) is the first step. Destruction
can occur at both sites but one will usually predominate.
  A. Intravascular hemolysis (Fig. 1.2) (Case 3)
     1. Mechanisms. The erythrocyte membrane must be
        significantly disrupted to allow escape of the Hb
        molecule into the plasma.
        a. Complement-mediate lysis. Complement attached to the
           membrane by antibody, if activated to C9, can create
           large enough membrane defects for Hb to escape
           (e.g., certain types of immune-mediated anemia).
        b. Physical injury. Traumatic disruption of the
           membrane can occur from the shearing effect of
           fibrin (e.g., microangiopathic anemia of
           disseminated intravascular coagulation).
        c. Oxidative injury. Oxidants denature Hb into Heinz
           bodies, which attach to the inner surface of the
           erythrocyte membrane with resultant lysis (e.g.,
           phenothiazine toxicity).
        d. Osmotic lysis. Membrane alterations insufficient to
           allow leakage of Hb may alter permeability to the
           extent that excess water is drawn into the normally
           hypertonic cell and lysis occurs. Hypotonic intra-
           venous fluids have the same effect. Many of the
           causes listed under extravascular hemolysis (Table
           1.2) may alter the membrane of some cells to the
           degree that osmotic lysis occurs before
           phagocytosis.
     2. Characteristics
        a. Most cases present as peracute or acute episodes.
        b. History may reveal exposure to causative drugs or
           plants, recent transfusion of incompatible blood, or
           recent ingestion of colostrum by a neonate.
        c. A regenerative response may not be evident in
           peracute and early acute stages because 2 to 3 days
           are required before significant reticulocytosis.
        d. Free Hb in the plasma (hemoglobinemia) is the
           principal feature in detection of intravascular
           hemolysis. Hemoglobinemia may be indicated by any of
           the following findings: red discoloration of plasma,

increased MCHC, decreased serum haptoglobin
concentration, increased serum methemalbumin
concentration, decreased serum hemopexin
concentration, hemoglobinuria, and hemosiderinuria.

   e. Hyperbilirubinemia will be observed if:
     (1) Hemolysis has been of sufficient duration for
        bilirubin to be formed. It may not be evident
        for 8 to 10 hours after the initial hemolytic
        episode.
     (2) Bilirubin formation is of sufficient magnitude
        to exceed the capacity of the liver to remove
        it from circulation and conjugate it.

   f. Additional laboratory findings may include
fragmented erythrocytes, Heinz bodies (Case 3),
erythrocytic parasites, positive Coombs' test on
patient's erythrocytes, or antibody titer to or
culture of potentially causative organisms.

B. Extravascular hemolysis (phagocytosis) (Fig. 1.2) (Case 2)
  1. Mechanisms
    a. Decreased erythrocyte deformability from changes in
the erythrocyte membrane, increase in internal
viscosity, or decrease in surface area/volume ratio
predisposes to splenic sequestration and phagocytosis by macrophages (e.g., schizocytes of
microangiopathic anemia, spherocytes of immune-
mediate anemia, and parasitized erythrocytes).
    b. Reduced glycolysis and ATP content of the cell leads
to early removal of erythrocytes (e.g., pyruvate
kinase deficiency anemia).
    c. Antibody and/or the third component of complement
attached to the erythrocyte membrane are recognized
by receptors of macrophages, and the erythrocyte is
phagocytized (partially or completely) (e.g.,
immune-mediated anemias).
    d. Increased macrophage activity may result in
phagocytosis of normal erythrocytes (e.g.,
hypersplenism).
  2. Characteristics
    a. The clinical course is usually chronic with an
insidious onset.
    b. A regenerative response is associated with normal or
increased plasma protein concentration.
    c. Hb is not evident in plasma and/or urine.
    d. Hyperbilirubinemia does not occur except in a
minority of the cases. The magnitude of the
hemolysis is usually insufficient to exceed the
conjugating capacity of the liver.
    e. The bone marrow response may compensate for the
destruction of erythrocytes in cases of low-grade
hemolysis (PCV is in the normal range). This is
referred to as a compensated hemolytic anemia.
    f. Neutrophilia and monocytosis are common.
    g. Splenomegaly may result from increased macrophage
activity and extramedullary hematopoiesis.
    h. Low-grade extravascular hemolysis occurs in many

anemias that are primarily nonhemolytic (e.g., anemia of chronic renal disease). This is referred to as the "hemolytic component" in other types of anemia.

3. Aids in identification of the specific cause of extravascular hemolysis

   a. History of a particular breed and/or littermates affected may suggest hereditary causes.

   b. Additional laboratory findings may include a positive direct Coombs' test on patient's erythrocytes in immune-mediated anemia and abnormal erythrocyte morphology in a variety of anemias. Erythrocytic parasites, spherocytes, and fragmented erythrocytes suggest the possibility of excessive erythrocyte phagocytosis.

ANEMIA FROM REDUCED OR DEFECTIVE ERYTHROPOIESIS (Table 1.3)

Anemias caused by reduced or defective erythropoiesis are nonregenerative and characterized by an abnormal bone marrow that cannot maintain effective erythropoiesis. The clinical course is usually long and the onset insidious.

I. General considerations

   A. Mechanisms

      1. Proper function of the bone marrow in the maintenance of normal erythrocytic mass requires adequate precursor

TABLE 1.3. Causes of Reduced or Defective Erythropoiesis

Reduced Erythropoiesis	Defective Erythropoiesis
Erythropoietin lack	Disorders of nucleic acid
Chronic renal disease	synthesis
Hypopituitarism	B_{12} deficiency
Hypoadrenocorticism	Folic acid deficiency
Hypothyroidism	Disorders of heme synthesis
Hypoandrogenism	Iron deficiency
Anemia of chronic disease	Pyridoxine deficiency
Chronic inflammation	Copper deficiency
Neoplasia	Molybdenum poisoning
Cytotoxic bone marrow damage	Lead poisoning
Radiation	Chloramphenicol toxicity
Estrogen	Disorders of globin synthesis
Phenylbutazone	Abnormal maturation
Cytotoxic cancer drugs	Erythremic myelosis
Bracken fern	Erythroleukemia
Immune-mediated	
Pure red cell aplasia	
Myelophthisis	
Granulocytic leukemia	
Lymphocytic leukemia	
Metastatic neoplasia	
Myelofibrosis, osteosclerosis	
Osteopetrosis	
Infections	
Feline leukemia virus	
Infectious panleukopenia virus	
Ehrlichia spp.	
Trichostrongyles (nonbloodsucking)	

cells (multi- and unipotential stem cells), nutrients (iron and B vitamins), and stimulation (erythropoietin).

2. Bone marrow failure may be primary (intramarrow disease resulting in inadequate stem cells) or secondary (extramarrow causes, e.g., nutrient or erythropoietin lack).

3. Bone marrow failure may be selective for the erythroid series or may also affect the other cell lines, in which case granulocytopenia and/or thrombocytopenia occur.

B. Bone marrow response

1. When the number of precursor cells or erythropoietic stimulation is inadequate, the erythroid marrow is hypocellular.

2. Maturation abnormalities that characterize the nutritional deficiencies are associated with a hypercellular marrow and ineffective erythropoiesis (failure of the erythrocytes produced to be delivered to the blood).

3. All degrees of bone marrow failure can occur, from complete aplasia to a suboptimal response of the erythroid marrow following hemorrhage or hemolysis.

II. Differentiation of anemias caused by reduced or defective erythropoiesis. A practical approach to the differentiation of nonregenerative anemias in an attempt to elucidate the pathogenic mechanism is based on erythrocyte morphology, blood neutrophil and platelet numbers, and bone marrow cellularity. These anemias can be divided into the following hematologic patterns.

A. Normocytic, normochromic anemia; normal neutrophil and platelet numbers; increased M/E ratio caused by hypocellular erythroid marrow. The general types include:

1. Anemia of erythropoietin lack. The causes are:
    a. Chronic renal disease (Cases 14, 15)
    b. Endocrine disorders (e.g., hypoadrenocorticism, hypoandrogenism)

2. Anemia of chronic inflammatory or neoplastic disease (Cases 9, 10, 11)
    a. Iron is diverted to the storage pool where it is not available for erythropoiesis.
    b. Findings include low serum iron concentration, low total iron-binding capacity, and a large amount of macrophage iron (identified by iron stains of bone marrow smears). The anemia is moderate and usually nonprogressive. Rarely, microcytosis and hypochromia occur.
    c. Alleviation of the primary disease process is associated with recovery.

3. Feline leukemia virus (FeLV)-associated nonregenerative anemia

4. Pure red cell aplasia. This type of anemia is thought to be immune-mediated.

B. Normocytic, normochromic anemia; neutropenia and thrombocytopenia; M/E ratio difficult to determine because of generalized bone marrow hypocellularity. Types include:

1. Aplastic anemia

        a.   Certain chemicals and radiation are cytotoxic to the multipotential stem cell.

        b.   The disease is characterized by pancytopenia with concomitant deficiency in erythropoiesis, granulopoiesis, and thrombopoiesis. Leukopenia and thrombocytopenia usually precede anemia because of the shorter life span of these cells.

        c.   Bone marrow particles are small, acellular, and fatty.

   2.   Myelophthisic anemia

        a.   Physical replacement of bone marrow by abnormal proliferation of cells occurs. Neoplastic cells may be evident on aspiration, or the cells replacing the normal bone marrow may be impossible to aspirate (e.g., myelofibrosis). Metarubricytosis without reticulocytosis may occur because of disruption of marrow architecture.

        b.   In early stages of this type of anemia, some regenerative response caused by isolated viable foci of hematopoiesis may be evident.

   3.   Anemia caused by infectious agents

        a.   Feline infectious panleukopenia virus causes granulocytopenia with or without a decrease in megakaryocytes and thrombocytopenia; anemia is a late finding.

        b.   Ehrlichiosis may present as pancytopenia.

        c.   FeLV infection may cause a concomitant anemia and leukopenia. These anemias may be macrocytic.

C.   Normocytic, normochromic anemia; neutrophilia with immature cells and variable platelet number; very high M/E ratio caused by increased granulopoiesis and erythroid hypoplasia. Causes include:

   1.   Granulocytic leukemia (Case 8)

   2.   Feline infectious panleukopenia in recovery

   3.   Early stage of estrogen toxicity

D.   Microcytic, hypochromic anemia; variable neutrophil and platelet number; usually a hypercellular marrow with a variable M/E ratio. Causes include:

   1.   Iron deficiency, late stages

        a.   Iron deficiency resulting from hemorrhage has been discussed under chronic hemorrhagic anemia.

        b.   A transient dietary iron deficiency that can lead to a mild anemia occurs primarily in the rapidly growing young of many species.

   2.   Pyridoxine deficiency

   3.   Copper deficiency

E.   Macrocytic, normochromic anemia; variable neutrophil and platelet number; M/E ratio usually low because of hypercellular erythroid marrow. Causes include:

   1.   Vitamin B_{12} and folic acid deficiency and ruminant cobalt deficiency

        a.   This type of anemia is rare in domestic animals.

        b.   Megaloblastic erythroid precursors are observed in the bone marrow.

        c.   Large, hypersegmented neutrophils may be observed.

2. Erythremic myelosis or erythroleukemia (see Chapter 3)
3. Macrocytosis without anemia occasionally observed in poodles

POLYCYTHEMIA

Polycythemia is an increase in the PCV, RBC count, and Hb concentration.

I. Spurious or relative polycythemia. The total RBC mass is normal. Causes include:
   A. Hemoconcentration. A decrease in plasma volume causes a relative increase in the PCV and plasma protein concentration. Mechanisms are:
      1. Dehydration. Water loss is caused by vomiting, diarrhea, excessive diuresis, water deprivation, and febrile dehydration (Case 6).
      2. Fluid shifts from the intravascular to the extravascular compartment.
   B. Redistribution of erythrocytes
      1. Excitement causes epinephrine release, and splenic contraction delivers high–PCV blood into the general circulation.
      2. This occurrence is common in the horse and cat.

II. Absolute polycythemia. The total RBC mass is increased because of increased erythropoiesis. Plasma volume and plasma protein concentration are normal.
   A. Secondary absolute polycythemia is caused by increased erythropoietin secretion.
      1. Appropriate compensatory erythropoietin secretion occurs during chronic hypoxia (low PO_2). Causes include high altitude, chronic pulmonary disease, and cardiovascular shunting (right to left).
      2. Inappropriate erythropoietin secretion (normal PO_2, no hypoxia) is found in some cases of hydronephrosis or renal cysts, erythropoietin–secreting tumors (embryonal nephroma), and certain endocrine diseases (hyperadrenocorticism).
   B. Primary absolute polycythemia (polycythemia vera) is a myeloproliferative disorder of unknown etiology characterized by decreased erythropoietin levels, normal PO_2, thrombocytosis, and leukocytosis (the latter two are inconsistent findings).

REFERENCES

Alsaker RD, Laber J, Stevens J, et al: A comparison of polychromasia and reticulocyte counts in assessing erythrocytic regenerative response in the cat. J Am Vet Med Assoc 170:39, 1977.
Auer L, Bell K: Transfusion reactions in cats due to AB blood group incompatibility. Res Vet Sci 35:145, 1983.
Auer LA, Bell K, Coates S: Blood transfusion reactions in the cat. J Am Vet Med Assoc 180:729, 1980.
Badylak SF: A pathophysiologic approach to the diagnosis of hemolytic anemia in the dog. Compend Contin Educ Pract Vet 3:827, 1981.
Bessis M: Blood smears reinterpreted. Berlin, Springer International, 1977.
Breitswerdt EG, Malone JB, McWilliams P, et al: Babesiosis in the greyhound. J Am Vet Med Assoc 182:978, 1983.

Brown RV, Teng Y: Studies of inherited pyruvate kinase deficiency in the basenji. J Am
    Anim Hosp Assoc 11:362, 1975.
Bull RW: New knowledge about blood groups in dogs. Proc 22nd Gaines Vet Symp, 1972.
Bundza A, Lumsden JH, McSherry BJ, et al: Haemobartonellosis in a dog in association with
    Coombs' positive anemia. Can Vet J 17:267, 1976.
Cotter SM: Anemia associated with feline leukemia virus infection. J Am Vet Med Assoc
    175:1191, 1979.
Cramer DV, Lewis RM: Reticulocyte response in the cat. J Am Vet Med Assoc 160:61, 1972.
Dennis RA, O'Hara PJ, Young MF, et al: Neonatal immunohemolytic anemia and icterus of
    calves. J Am Vet Med Assoc 156:1861, 1970.
Divers TJ, George LW, George JW: Hemolytic anemia in horses after the ingestion of red
    maple leaves. J Am Vet Med Assoc 180:300, 1982.
Dixon PM, MacPherson EA, Muir A: Familial methaemoglobinaemia and hemolytic anemia in the
    horse associated with decreased erythrocytic glutathione reductase and glutathione.
    Equine Vet J 9:198, 1977.
Easley JR: The anemia of chronic renal failure revisited. Vet Clin Pathol 10(1):17, 1981.
Edwards DF: Bone marrow hypoplasia in a feminized dog with a Sertoli cell tumor. J Am Vet
    Med Assoc 178:494, 1981.
Ewing GO: Familiar nonspherocytic hemolytic anemia of basenji dogs. J Am Vet Med Assoc
    154:503, 1969.
Faircloth JC, Montgomery JK: Systemic lupus erythematosus in a cat presenting with
    autoimmune hemolytic anemia. Feline Pract 11(2):22, 1981.
Fan LC, Dorner JL, Hoffmann WE: Reticulocyte response and maturation in experimental acute
    blood loss anemia in the cat. J Am Anim Hosp Assoc 14:219, 1978.
Farwell GE, LeGrand EK, Cobb CC: Clinical observations on Babesia gibsoni and Babesia
    canis infections in dogs. J Am Vet Med Assoc 180:507, 1982.
Feldman BF: The anemia of inflammatory disease in the dog. Vet Clin Pathol 9(1):44, 1980.
Feldman BF: Anemia of inflammatory disease in the dog: Clinical characterization. Am J
    Vet Res 42:1108, 1981.
Feldman BF: Anemias associated with blood loss and hemolysis. Vet Clin North Am 11:265,
    1981.
Feldman BF: Hypoproliferative anemias and anemias caused by ineffective erythropoiesis:
    Depression or nonresponsive anemias. Vet Clin North Am 11:277, 1981.
Fletch SM, Pinkerton PH: An inherited anemia associated with hereditary chondrodysplasia
    in the Alaskan malamute. Can Vet J 13:270, 1972.
Gelberg H, Stackhouse LL: Three cases of canine acanthocytosis associated with splenic
    neoplasia. Vet Med Small Anim Clin 72:1182, 1977.
George JW, Duncan JR: The hematology of lead poisoning in man and animals. Vet Clin Pathol
    8:23, 1979.
Giddens WE, Labbe RF, Swango LJ, et al: Feline congenital erythropoietic porphyria
    associated with severe anemia and renal disease. Am J Pathol 80:367, 1975.
Glenn BL: Feline porphyria. Comp Pathol Bull 2(2):2, 1970.
Greene CE, Kristensen F, Hoff EJ, et al: Cold hemagglutinin disease in a dog. J Am Vet Med
    Assoc 170:505, 1977.
Halliwell REW: Autoimmune disease in the dog. Adv Vet Sci Comp Med 22:221, 1978.
Harvey JW: Canine hemolytic anemias. J Am Vet Med Assoc 176:970, 1980.
Harvey JW: Feline hemobartonellosis. In Kirk RW (ed): Current veterinary therapy VII.
    Philadelphia, WB Saunders Co, 1980.
Harvey JW, French TW, Meyer DJ: Chronic iron deficiency anemia in dogs. J Am Anim Hosp
    Assoc 18:946, 1982.
Harvey JW, Gaskin JM: Experimental feline haemobartonellosis. J Am Anim Hosp Assoc 13:28,
    1977.
Harvey JW, Gaskin JM: Feline haemobartonellosis: Attempts to induce relapse of clinical
    disease in chronically infected cats. J Am Anim Hosp Assoc 14:453, 1978.
Harvey JW, Kornick HP: Phenazopyridine toxicosis in the cat. J Am Vet Med Assoc 169:327,
    1976.
Harvey JW; Ling GV, Kaneko JJ: Methemoglobin reductase deficiency in a dog. J Am Vet Med
    Assoc 164:1030, 1974.
Harvey JW, Sameck JH, Burgard FJ: Benzocaine-induced methemoglobinemia in dogs. J Am Vet
    Med Assoc 175:1171, 1979.
Hauck WN, Snider TG: Cytauxzoonosis in a native Louisiana cat. J Am Vet Med Assoc
    180:1472, 1982.
Henson JB, McGuire TC: Immunopathology of equine infectious anemia. Am J Clin Pathol
    56:306, 1971.
Hirsch, VM: A retrospective study of canine hemangiosarcoma and its association with
    acanthocytosis. Can Vet J 22:152, 1981.
Hirsch V, Dunn J: Megaloblastic anemia in the cat. J Am Anim Hosp Assoc 19:873, 1983.
Hoover EA, Kociba GJ, Hardy WD Jr, et al: Erythroid hypoplasia in cats inoculated with
    feline leukemia virus. J Natl Cancer Inst 53:1271, 1974.

Huxsoll DL, Amyx HL, Hemelt IE, et al: Laboratory studies on tropical canine pancytopenia. Exp Parasitol 31:53, 1972.

Ishihara K, Kitagawa H, Ojima M: Clinopathological studies on canine dirofilarial hemoglobinuria. Jpn J Vet Sci 40:525, 1978.

Kaneko JJ: Iron metabolism. In Kaneko JJ (ed): Clinical biochemistry of domestic animals, 3rd ed. New York, Academic Press, 1980.

Kobayashi K: Onion poisoning in the cat. Feline Pract 11(1):22, 1981.

Kujala C, Randall JW: Iatrogenic acetaminophen poisoning. Feline Pract 11(5):12, 1981.

Laber J, Perman V, Stevens JB: Polychromasia or reticulocytes: An assessment of the dog. J Am Anim Hosp Assoc 10:399, 1974.

Lane VM, Anderson BL, Bulgin MS: Polycythemia and cyanosis associated with hypoplastic main pulmonary segment in the bovine heart. J Am Vet Med Assoc 183:460, 1983.

Lees GE, Polzin DJ, Perman V, et al: Idiopathic Heinz body hemolytic anemia in three dogs. J Am Vet Med Assoc 15:143, 1979.

Legendre AM: Estrogen-induced bone marrow hypoplasia in a dog. J Am Anim Hosp Assoc 12:525, 1976.

Legendre AM, Appleford MD, Eyster GE, et al: Secondary polycythemia and seizures due to right and left shunting patent ductus arteriosus in a dog. J Am Vet Med Assoc 164:1198, 1974.

Lewis HB: Management of anemia in the dog and cat. In Kirk RW (ed): Current veterinary therapy VI. Philadelphia, WB Saunders Co, 1977.

Lewis HB, Rebar AH: Bone marrow evaluation in veterinary practice. St. Louis, Ralston Purina Co, 1979.

Madewell BR, Feldman BF: Characterization of anemias associated with neoplasia in small animals. J Am Vet Med Assoc 176:419, 1980.

Mahaffey EA, Smith JE: Depression anemia in cats. Feline Pract 8(5):19, 1978.

McGrath CJ: Polycythemia vera in dogs. J Am Vet Med Assoc 164:1117, 1974.

McSherry BJ, Roe CK, Milne FJ: The hematology of phenothiazine poisoning in horses. Can Vet J 7:3, 1966.

Nelson RW, Hager D, Zanjani ED: Renal lymphosarcoma with inappropriate erythropoietin production in a dog. J Am Vet Med Assoc 182:1396, 1983.

North DC: Fatal haemobartonellosis in a non-splenectomized dog: A case report. J Small Anim Pract 19:769, 1978.

Penny RHC, Carlisle CH, Prescott CW, et al: Further observations on the effect of chloramphenicol on the haemopoietic system of the cat. Br Vet J 126:153, 1970.

Perman V, Schall WD: Disease of the red blood cells. In Ettinger SJ (ed): Textbook of veterinary internal medicine, Vol 2, 2nd ed. Philadelphia, WB Saunders Co, 1983.

Peterson ME, Zanjani ED: Inappropriate erythropoietin production from a renal carcinoma in a dog with polycythemia. J Am Vet Med Assoc 179:995, 1981.

Pierce KR, Joyce JR, England RB, et al: Acute hemolytic anemia caused by wild onion poisoning in horses. J Am Vet Med Assoc 160:323, 1972.

Pinkerton PH, Fletch SM, Brueckner PJ, et al: Hereditary stomatocytosis with hemolytic anemia in the dog. Blood 44:557, 1974.

Prasse KW, Crouser D, Beutler E, et al: Pyruvate kinase deficiency anemia with terminal myelofibrosis and osteosclerosis in a beagle. J Am Vet Med Assoc 166:1170, 1975.

Rebar AH: Red cell fragmentation in the dog: An editorial review. Vet Pathol 18:415, 1981.

Rebar AH, Hahn FF, Halliwell WH, et al: Microangiopathic hemolytic anemia associated with radiation induced hemangiosarcomas. Vet Pathol 17:443, 1980.

Reef VB, Dyson SS, Beech J: Lymphosarcoma and associated immune mediated hemolytic anemia and thrombocytopenia in horses. J Am Vet Med Assoc 184:313, 1984.

Ristic M: Studies in anaplasmosis. III. An autoantibody and symptomatic macrocytic anemia. Am J Vet Res 22:871, 1961.

Ross CE: Chronic copper poisoning in a lamb. Compend Contin Educ Pract Vet 5:559, 1983.

Schalm OW: Differential diagnosis of anemia in cattle. J Am Vet Med Assoc 161:1269, 1972.

Schalm OW: Exogenous estrogen toxicity in the dog. Canine Pract 5(5):57, 1978.

Schalm OW: Phenylbutazone toxicity in two dogs. Canine Pract 6(4):47, 1979.

Schalm OW: Differential diagnosis of anemias in cattle. Part III. Hemolytic anemias: Leptospirosis and onion poisoning. Bovine Pract 1(3):16, 1980.

Schalm OW: Manual of feline and canine hematology. Santa Barbara, Veterinary Practice Publishing Co, 1980.

Schalm OW, Jain NC, Carroll EJ: Veterinary hematology, 3rd ed. Philadelphia, Lea and Febiger, 1975.

Schechter RD, Schalm OW, Kaneko JJ: Heinz body hemolytic anemia associated with the use of urinary antiseptics containing methylene blue in the cat. J Am Vet Med Assoc 162:37, 1973.

Scott AM, Jeffcott LB: Haemolytic disease of the newborn foal. Vet Rec 103:71, 1978.

Scott DW, Schultz RD, Post JE, et al: Autoimmune hemolytic anemia in the cat. J Am Anim Hosp Assoc 9:530, 1973.

Searcy GP: The differential diagnosis of anemia. Vet Clin North Am 6:567, 1976.

Searcy GP, Miller DR, Tasker JB: Congenital hemolytic anemia in the basenji dog due to erythrocyte pyruvate kinase deficiency. Can J Comp Med 35:67, 1971.

Sherding RG, Wilson GP, Kociba GJ: Bone marrow hypoplasia in eight dogs with Sertoli cell tumor. J Am Vet Med Assoc 178:497, 1981.

Shull RM: Inappropriate marrow release of hematopoietic precursors in three dogs. Vet Pathol 18:569, 1981.

Shull RM, Bunch SE, Maribei J, et al: Spur cell anemia in a dog. J Am Vet Med Assoc 173:978, 1978.

Stockham SL, Ford RB, Weiss DJ: Canine autoimmune hemolytic disease with a delayed erythroid regeneration. J Am Anim Hosp Assoc 16:927, 1980.

Stormont C: Neonatal isoerythrolysis in domestic animals: A comparative review. Adv Vet Sci Comp Med 19:23, 1975.

Stormont CJ: Blood groups in animals. J Am Vet Med Assoc 181:1120, 1982.

Tasker JB, Severin GA, Young S, et al: Familial anemia in the basenji dog. J Am Vet Med Assoc 154:158, 1969.

Tennant B, Asbury AC, Laben RC, et al: Familial polycythemia in cattle. J Am Vet Med Assoc 150:1493, 1967.

Tennant B, Dill SG, Glickman LT, et al: Acute hemolytic anemia, methemoglobinemia, and Heinz body formation associated with ingestion of red maple leaves by horses. J Am Vet Med Assoc 179:143, 1981.

Thenen SW, Rasmussen KM: Megaloblastic erythropoiesis and tissue depletion of folic acid in the cat. J Am Vet Med Assoc 161:1418, 1972.

Wagner JE: A fatal cytauxzoonosis-like disease in cats. J Am Vet Med Assoc 168:585, 1976.

Watson ADJ: Chloramphenicol toxicity in dogs. Res Vet Sci 23:66, 1977.

Watson ADJ, Middleton DJ: Chloramphenicol toxicosis in cats. Am J Vet Res 39:1199, 1978.

Weiser MG: Correlative approach to anemia in dogs and cats. J Am Anim Hosp Assoc 17:286, 1981.

Weiser MG, Kociba GJ: Sequential changes in erythrocyte volume distribution and microcytosis associated with iron deficiency in kittens. Vet Pathol 20:1, 1983.

Weiser MG, Kociba GJ: Erythrocyte macrocytosis in feline leukemia virus associated anemia. Vet Pathol 20:687, 1983.

Weiser G, O'Grady M: Erythrocyte volume distribution analysis and hematologic changes in dogs with iron deficiency anemia. Vet Pathol 20:230, 1983.

Werner LL: Coombs' positive anemias in the dog and cat. Compend Contin Educ Pract Vet 2:96, 1980.

Williams WJ, Beutler E, Erslev AJ: Hematology, 2nd ed. New York, McGraw-Hill Book Co, 1977.

Wintrobe MM: Clinical hematology, 8th ed. Philadelphia, Lea and Febiger, 1981.

Zook BC, Carpenter JL, Leeds EB: Lead poisoning in dogs. J Am Vet Med Assoc 155:1329, 1969.

Zook BC, McConnell G, Gilmore CE: Basophilic stippling of erythrocytes in dogs with special reference to lead poisoning. J Am Vet Med Assoc 157:, 1970.

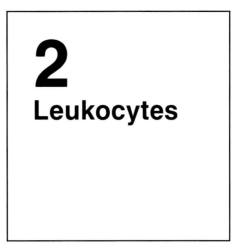

2
Leukocytes

ESSENTIAL CONCEPTS OF LEUKOCYTE FUNCTION, PRODUCTION, AND KINETICS
Leukocytes include the neutrophil, monocyte, eosinophil, basophil, and lymphocyte. All participate in body defense, but each is kinetically and functionally independent.

I.   Neutrophils
    A.   Neutrophil function
        1.   Phagocytosis and microbiocidal action are primary functions. This activity is efficiently conducted in tissue but not in blood.
            a.   Metabolically active processes for these functions include stickiness and emigration through the vessel wall; chemotaxis, a motile response toward an attractant (including components of complement and bacterial products) in the tissue; ingestion and degranulation; and microbiocidal action.
            b.   These functions may be compromised by deficiency of various humoral or cellular components, drugs, or toxic bacterial products, making the animal more susceptible to disease.
        2.   Neutrophils secrete various substances when exposed to bacteria or their products. These neutrophilic substances may function in extracellular digestion of fibrinogen and complement components and in stimulation of the generation of mediators of inflammation.
        3.   Neutrophils contribute to pathologic events of certain conditions (e.g., immune complex glomerulonephritis and rheumatoid arthritis).
    B.   Neutrophil production
        1.   Morphologic cellular compartments of granulopoiesis are the proliferation and maturation compartment and the maturation and storage compartment (Figs. 2.1, 2.2).
        2.   Cell stages and kinetics in the proliferation and maturation compartment

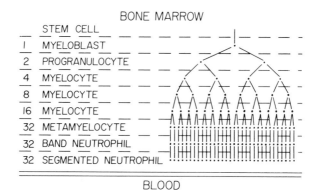

Fig. 2.1. Schema of granulopoiesis. (From Prasse KW: Disorders
of leukocytes. In A Textbook of Veterinary Internal Medicine,
Ettinger SJ (ed), Philadelphia, WB Saunders Co, 1975.)

    a. Myeloblast
       (1) It is derived from the bipotential stem cell
           specific for monocytes and neutrophils but
           cannot be morphologically distinguished from
           its counterpart in the other granulocytic
           series.
       (2) Myeloblasts are believed to divide once
           whereby maturation has then proceeded to the
           progranulocyte stage.
    b. Progranulocyte
       (1) It is identified by the presence of purple-
           staining cytoplasmic granules (primary
           granules) but cannot be morphologically
           distinguished from its counterpart in the
           other granulocytic series.
       (2) Progranulocytes are believed to divide once,

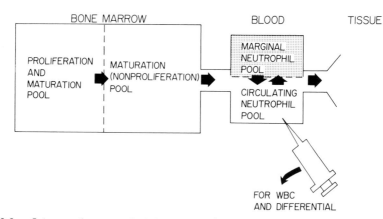

Fig. 2.2. Schema of neutrophil kinetics. (From Prasse KW:
Disorders of leukocytes. In A Textbook of Veterinary Internal
Medicine, Ettinger SJ (ed), Philadelphia, WB Saunders Co,
1975.)

whereby daughter cells are morphologically identified as myelocytes.

    c. Myelocyte

        (1) It is identified by the presence of specific granules in the cytoplasm (i.e., neutrophilic, eosinophilic, or basophilic). Each specific type of myelocyte is distinguishable by routine staining. Nuclei are round or oval with minimal indentation.

        (2) In health, approximately three myelocyte generations (three divisions) occur. Daughter cells of the third generation are morphologically identified as metamyelocytes, in which nuclear indentation and elongation are marked.

        (3) The approximate maturation time from myeloblast to metamyelocyte is 60 hours.

3. Cell stages and kinetics in the maturation and storage compartment

    a. Neutrophil maturation continues through three more morphologic stages (metamyelocyte, band, and segmenter). These cell stages make up approximately 80% of the bone marrow granulocyte population.

    b. These cells cannot divide and are functionally mature. The maturation process is principally nuclear; i.e., chromatin condensation and nuclear elongation, thinning, and segmentation occur.

    c. The transit time through this compartment is approximately 50 to 70 hours and varies with the length of storage time.

    d. An estimated 5-day supply of neutrophils exists in the storage compartment in health.

    e. Release of cells from the bone marrow to the blood is age related; the oldest cells are released first.

4. Mechanisms for increased neutrophil production

    a. Increased stem cell input

        (1) It probably occurs at the earliest demand for neutrophils.

        (2) Approximately 4 to 5 days are required to influence the blood neutrophil number.

        (3) Input into granulocyte and erythrocyte production may be competitive.

    b. Increased effective granulopoiesis in the proliferation and maturation compartment

        (1) Additional divisions may occur within the compartment, which has a transit time fixed by maturation; each additional division doubles the output of cells.

        (2) Increased output from the proliferation and maturation compartment may occur by reducing myelocyte attrition, which normally occurs in health in the dog.

5. Control of neutrophil production. Regulation is by a

granulopoietin that is referred to as the colony-stimulating factor (CSF).

    a. CSF is secreted by T lymphocytes, fibroblasts, and endothelial cells after stimulation by a monokine from bone marrow macrophages. As the storage pool of neutrophils is depleted, CSF synthesis increases, followed by increased stem cell input and increased mitotic activity among the early granulocytes. Replenishment of the storage pool diminishes the stimulation.

    b. CSF synthesis also is stimulated by bacterial products.

    c. CSF is an absolute requirement for stimulation of mitosis of bipotential stem cells, and the concentration of CSF determines differentiation into neutrophilic or monocytic cell lines.

    d. It affects the number of divisions of any cell in the proliferation and maturation compartment.

6. Neutrophil release from the bone marrow. Release may be promoted by a plasma factor, leukocytosis-inducing or neutrophil-releasing factor (LIF or NRF), of unknown origin.

    a. LIF concentration is increased by bacterial products and in certain neutropenic disorders.

    b. Increased rate of release from the storage compartment is the reason for rapid neutrophilia (earlier than 2 days), which follows the initial stimulus of a tissue demand for neutrophils. This response decreases the proportion of cells in the storage compartment and increases the proportion of cells in the proliferation compartment.

    c. As the peripheral demand for neutrophils intensifies and the storage reserve of mature cells diminishes, band neutrophils appear in the blood (a "left shift" of neutrophils); they may be followed by neutrophilic metamyelocytes or even more immature cells in severe situations.

C. Neutrophil kinetics in health

1. Neutrophils move more slowly than erythrocytes and plasma within postcapillary venules, causing an uneven distribution of the cells within the blood vasculature. The concentration of neutrophils in postcapillary venules is greater than that in large-vessel blood.

    a. Neutrophils that are hesitatingly adherent to the vascular endothelium make up the marginal neutrophil pool (MNP). They are not included in the routine white blood cell (WBC) count (Fig. 2.2).

    b. Cells moving as fast as erythrocytes and plasma within arteries and veins make up the circulating neutrophil pool (CNP).

        (1) Neutrophil number, derived from routine WBC and differential counts, represents the approximate size of the CNP.

(2) CNP plus MNP equals the total blood
neutrophil pool.
   c. The size of the MNP is equal to that of the CNP in
the dog, horse, and calf. Feline MNP is
approximately three times larger than the CNP
(other animals have not been studied).
  2. The average transit time for a neutrophil in blood in
health is about 10 hours; all blood neutrophils are
replaced about two and one-half times each day.
  3. Neutrophils move from the blood into tissue spaces
randomly, unaffected by cell age. They do not return
to circulation.
  4. In health, effete neutrophils are destroyed by
macrophages of the spleen, liver, and bone marrow.
Some also are lost in secretions and excretions and
through mucous membranes.

II. Monocytes
  A. Monocyte function and distribution
    1. Monocytes are derived from bone marrow, circulate for
a brief blood sojourn, and transform to macrophages in
tissues.
      a. Macrophages contain more granules and proteolytic
enzymes than the precursor monocyte.
      b. Macrophages may survive long periods in tissue,
are capable of division, and are functional
phagocytes.
    2. Monocyte-derived macrophages include:
      a. Macrophages or histiocytes of exudates
      b. Pleural and peritoneal macrophages
      c. Pulmonary alveolar macrophages
      d. Connective tissue histiocytes
      e. Macrophages of the spleen, lymph nodes, and bone
marrow
      f. Kupffer cells of the liver
    3. The monocyte-macrophage population makes up the so-
called "reticuloendothelial system," although none
produce reticulin fibers, and none are endothelial
cells.
    4. Macrophage functions include:
      a. Phagocytosis and digestion of foreign particulate
material and dead or effete cells. Although they
are responsive to infection, macrophages are less
responsive than neutrophils in the defense of
bloodborne pyogenic bacteria.
      b. Synthesis of certain complement components,
transferrin, interleuken I, and lysozyme. They may
be the major source of interferon.
      c. Expression of immune responses. Macrophages
process foreign substances to a more antigenic
form for lymphocytes; they secrete substances that
stimulate T and B lymphocytes; and in reciprocal
interaction they are activated by lymphocytes to
become suppressors (tumoricidal or microbiocidal).

B. Monocytopoiesis
1. Monocyte precursors are derived from a bipotential stem cell, which is shared by the neutrophilic series.
2. Monocytes are released to blood directly from a promonocyte proliferation pool in the bone marrow (equivalent in age to the first-generation neutrophil myelocyte).
C. Monocyte kinetics
1. Monocytes may be unevenly distributed in blood as the neutrophil (i.e., in humans, the circulating monocyte pool/marginated monocyte pool ratio is 1:3.5).
2. The average blood transit time is reported to be 12 hours in humans and somewhat longer in cattle. Data are unavailable for most animals.

III. Eosinophils
A. Eosinophil function
1. Eosinophils are attracted by and inhibit chemical mediators released from mast cells of immediate (allergic or anaphylactic) or delayed hypersensitivity.
2. Eosinophils have parasiticidal properties, which are antibody and/or complement dependent.
3. Eosinophil granules contain plasminogen activator.
4. Phagocytic and bacteriocidal capabilities are similar to those of neutrophils, but eosinophils are not protective against bacterial infection.
B. Eosinophil production and kinetics
1. Eosinophil production in the bone marrow parallels that of neutrophils.
2. Eosinophilic unipotential stem cells are responsive to eosinophilopoietin. This response is dependent on sensitized T lymphocytes.
3. Bone marrow storage of eosinophils is minimal, and emergence time following increased stem cell input is shorter than that of neutrophils.
4. The blood transit time is short (minutes to hours) but may be longer during eosinophilia. Evidence for a marginal pool is reported.
5. Eosinophils are long-lived in subepithelial sites, and minimal recirculation has been noted.

IV. Basophils
A. Basophil function
1. Basophils and mast cells degranulate when antigen complexes with IgE (or equivalent antibody) on their surfaces. Other physical and chemical agents also can cause degranulation.
2. Basophils and mast cells are the source of mediators of inflammation. Such mediators include histamine, eosinophil chemotactic factor of anaphylaxis, platelet-activating factor, slow reactive substance of anaphylaxis, and other substances.
3. Basophils and mast cells are the only sources of

heparin and an activator of plasma lipoprotein lipase
(plasma lipemia clearing agent).
  B. Basophil production and kinetics
      1. Basophils are sparse in most animals; species having
          few tissue mast cells have more basophils. (Mast cells
          are not derived from basophils, but their origin is
          believed to be from the so-called "persisting" cell in
          bone marrow.)
      2. Production parallels that of neutrophils, but bone
          marrow storage is minimal.

V. Lymphocytes
    A. Lymphocyte distribution, circulation, and function
        1. Lymphocytes are distributed in lymph nodes, spleen,
            thymus, tonsils, gastrointestinal lymphoid tissue,
            bronchial lymphoid tissue, bone marrow, and blood.
        2. Differentiation of lymphocyte types is marked by
            acquisition of surface receptors and markers rather
            than by dramatic morphologic changes. Most lymphocytes
            are morphologically indistinct.
            a. T lymphocytes are embryologically derived from
                bone marrow, mature in the thymus, and function in
                cell-mediated immunity.
            b. B lymphocytes are embryologically derived from
                bone marrow and function in humoral (antibody)
                immunity.
        3. All lymphocytes are long-lived compared with other
            leukocytes and are capable of division and/or
            transformation to more functionally active forms.
            a. The life span of lymphocytes is defined by either
                the time interval between cell divisions or the
                interval between the last division and cell death.
            b. Some cells are believed to be short-lived (about 2
                weeks), and others are long-lived with inter-
                mitotic intervals of weeks, months, or years.
        4. Among the leukocytes, lymphocytes are unique because
            they recirculate.
            a. The majority of T cells recirculate; most of the B
                cells found in blood are thought to be transient
                members of the recirculating population. The
                majority of B cells remain in the lymphoid tissue.
            b. Estimates based on surface marker analyses of the
                proportions of T and B cells in blood indicate
                that T cells predominate in most species. Most of
                these cells are memory cells. Some are antigenic-
                ally naive. A very few are effector cells derived
                primarily from gastrointestinal or bronchial
                lymphoid tissues.
            c. The average blood transit time for a given
                lymphocyte is about 30 minutes.
            d. The primary route of recirculating lymphocytes is
                efferent ducts of lymph nodes, thoracic duct and
                right lymphatic duct, blood, emigration from blood
                through venules of the cortex of lymph nodes, and

eventually return to efferent lymph again.
  (1) The recirculation of splenic lymphocytes is
       more direct, from blood to spleen to blood
       again.
  (2) Cells from gastrointestinal and bronchial
       lymphoid tissues enter afferent lymph.
B. Lymphocytic production
  1. Lymphopoiesis (i.e., division and transformation)
      occurs in the lymphoid tissues and is entirely
      dependent on the degree and type of antigenic
      stimulation.
    a. Certain antigens stimulate B lymphocytes to
        divide and/or transform into effector cells, which
        produce immunoglobulin (i.e., IgG, IgA, IgM, IgE,
        or IgD); plasma cells are so derived.
    b. Certain antigens stimulate T lymphocytes to divide
        and/or transform into effector cells, which
        produce lymphokines, mediators of cellular
        immunity.
  2. Although morphologically defined, lymphoblasts are not
      to be considered precursor or poorly differentiated
      cells; instead, they are a morphologic manifestation
      representing a pre- or postmitotic stage in the
      lymphocyte cell cycle.

LABORATORY EVALUATION OF LEUKOCYTES

  I. WBC count
    A. Methods of determination
      1. Manual dilution (glass pipettes or disposable plastic
          chambers) coupled with a hemocytometer and microscopy
          is a common method. Inherent error is approximately
          20% even when technical skills are excellent.
      2. Automated cell counters
        a. Results are more reproducible than by manual
            counting. Inherent error is approximately 5%, but
            it may be greater if the counts are extremely low
            or high.
        b. Several counting errors may be introduced by blood
            abnormalities.
          (1) Clumping of leukocytes or fragile leukocytes
               will give erroneously low counts.
          (2) Neoplastic lymphocytes, especially in cattle,
               may be lysed by the red blood cell (RBC)
               lysing agents, and the WBC count will be
               erroneously low.
          (3) Abnormally large or clumped platelets will
               contribute to the automated WBC count.
          (4) In cats with large numbers of erythrocyte
               refractile bodies (ER or Heinz bodies), the
               bodies do not lyse; they clump together and
               may cause false high WBC counts.
        c. Normal feline platelets may be large and contrib-
            ute to the automated WBC count.

          d. In addition to correct standardization and quality control practices, the best check on the automated WBC count is microscopic examination of the stained blood smear.

  B. Pathophysiologic factors affecting the WBC count

    1. All nucleated cells in the blood are counted by manual or automated methods; this includes nucleated erythrocytes if they are present (Case 2).

        a. Detection of nucleated erythrocytes requires examination of a stained blood smear; the number per 100 leukocytes is recorded (nRBC).

        b. The WBC count is then corrected by the following formula: Corrected WBC count = (initial WBC count × 100)/(100 + nRBC).

    2. Leukocytosis is indicated by a WBC count that exceeds the upper limit of normal values for the species in question.

        a. Neutrophilia is the usual cause of leukocytosis.

        b. Lymphocytosis and eosinophilia are rarely of sufficient magnitude to cause leukocytosis.

    3. Leukopenia is a WBC count below the lower limit of the reference value range.

        a. In monogastric animals, leukopenia is essentially synonymous with neutropenia. Lymphopenia and eosinopenia usually will not cause leukopenia if neutrophil number is adequate.

        b. In ruminants, leukopenia may be caused by neutropenia or lymphopenia.

II. Blood smear evaluation

  A. A systematic approach to microscopic evaluation of the blood smear is described in Chapter 1. Automatic differential leukocyte counters programmed for human cells may give erroneous counts on domestic animal blood smears.

  B. Microscopic examination of leukocytes

    1. Neutrophil morphology (Figs. 1.5, 2.3)

        a. Normal neutrophils, species differences

            (1) Canine neutrophils usually have narrowing between nuclear lobes without filament formation. Cytoplasm is pale pink with dustlike granulation.

            (2) Feline neutrophils are similar to those of the dog.

            (3) Bovine neutrophilic nuclear membranes present one or more points of constriction without filament formation. Granules are usually faintly visible and impart an orange color to the cytoplasm.

            (4) Equine neutrophilic nuclear membranes are extremely irregular, and nuclei may appear to be multilobulated.

        b. Immature neutrophils in significant numbers in the blood are referred to as a "left shift."

            (1) The nucleus of a band neutrophil is thicker and the chromatin is less aggregated than

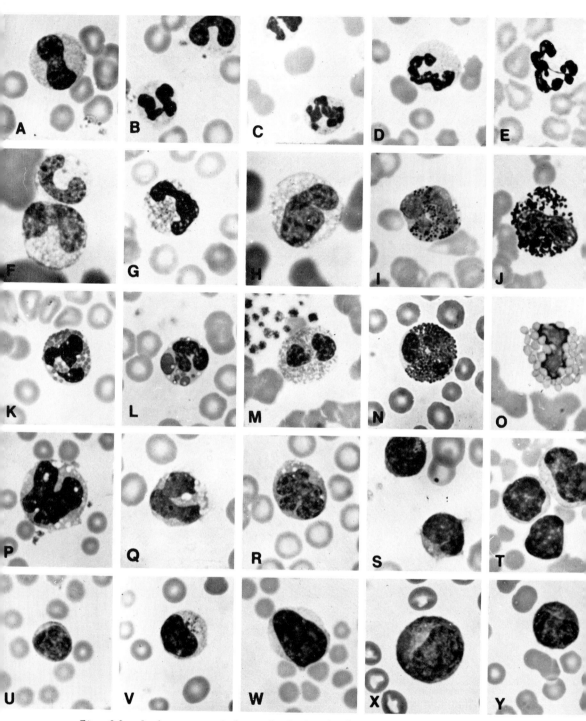

Fig. 2.3. Leukocyte morphology. A. Canine band neutrophil,
B. canine segmented and band neutrophils, C. equine neutrophils, D. feline neutrophil, E. hypersegmented neutrophil
(dog), F. toxic band (Doehle bodies) and metamyelocyte neutrophils (dog), G. toxic segmented neutrophil (dog), H. toxic band
neutrophil (dog), I. canine basophil, J. equine basophil,
K. canine eosinophil, L. canine eosinophil, M. feline
eosinophil, N. bovine eosinophil, O. equine eosinophil,
P. feline monocyte, Q. canine monocyte, R. canine monocyte,
S. canine monocytes, T. bovine lymphocytes and a monocyte,
U. feline lymphocyte, V. feline lymphocyte with granules,
W. bovine large lymphocyte, X. immunocyte (dog), Y. immunocyte
(cat). (Wright's stain, ×1100.)

that of the mature segmented form. A commonly
used criterion is to classify as a band any
cell in which the nuclear membrane is smooth
without indentations and has parallel sides.
Equine band neutrophils have rougher nuclear
membranes than other species.

    (2)   Progressively more immature neutrophils
(metamyelocytes, myelocytes, or progranulo-
cytes) may be encountered in blood in certain
circumstances. The nucleus is less elongated
and more rounded, the chromatin is less
clumped, and the cytoplasm more basophilic in
these cells (Fig. 1.5).

  c. Toxemia may disturb neutrophil maturation, and
cytoplasmic changes may be observed in neutrophils
(Cases 4, 5, 6, 19).

    (1)   Doehle bodies are bluish, angular cytoplasmic
inclusions. They are very common in cats but
in any species are a mild toxemic
manifestation.

    (2)   Diffuse cytoplasmic basophilia and concomi-
tant cytoplasmic vacuolization (foamy appearance) is a more severe manifestation of toxic
change. It occurs during severe bacterial
infections in most species but is not
specific for infection.

    (3)   Toxic granulation is characterized by
prominent purplish cytoplasmic granules and
indicates severe toxemia. It is most common
in the horse.

  d. Nuclear hypersegmentation is five or more distinct
nuclear lobes.

    (1)   Hypersegmentation may indicate a prolonged
blood transit time as occurs during corticosteroid therapy, hyperadrenocorticism, or
late stages of chronic inflammatory disease.

    (2)   Giant hypersegmented neutrophils are a
manifestation of vitamin B_{12}, folic acid, or
ruminant cobalt deficiency.

  e. Nuclear hyposegmentation and condensed chromatin
may occur in dogs or cats as an anomaly (Pelger-
Huet anomaly), and it may be acquired and
transient (pseudo-Pelger-Huet)on rare occasions.
Differentiation of this change from hyposegmentation associated with the left shift is the most
important consideration.

  f. Asynchronous maturation of the nucleus and cytoplasm may be observed during resurgent granulopoiesis and granulocytic leukemia. It is
recognized by observing lobes with immature
chromatin separated by filaments.

2. Monocyte morphology (Fig. 2.3)

  a. Monocytes are large cells that must be
differentiated from neutrophilic metamyelocytes
and large lymphocytes.

      b. Criteria for monocyte identification include:
- (1) Oval, bilobed, or trilobed nucleus with lacelike chromatin and sharply angular contours on the nuclear envelope
- (2) Gray-blue cytoplasm (darker than any stage of neutrophil)
- (3) Cytoplasmic vacuoles, which may be very prominent features. On fresh blood smears, vacuoles in monocytes may indicate infection; whereas on smears made from EDTA anticoagulated blood 30 to 60 minutes after collection, monocyte vacuoles are artifacts of in vitro storage.
- (4) Short hairlike pseudopodia

      c. Monocytes transformed into macrophages are rarely encountered in blood but may be observed in capillary blood smears in disorders such as ehrlichiosis, histoplasmosis, or leishmaniasis. Macrophages are very large with abundant granular, vacuolated cytoplasm.

3. Eosinophil morphology (Fig. 2.3)
   - a. Species differences are quite prominent.
     - (1) Canine eosinophilic granules are variable in shape, size, and number and do not fill the cytoplasm; they stain dull orange. Cytoplasmic vacuoles may be observed.
     - (2) Feline eosinophilic granules are very small and ellipsoid or rod shaped; they fill the cell and stain dull orange.
     - (3) Bovine eosinophilic granules are small and round, fill the cell, and stain bright orange. Porcine granules are similar in size and shape but stain dull orange.
     - (4) Equine eosinophilic granules are large, round, and brilliant orange.
   - b. Eosinophils are difficult to identify in new methylene blue-stained smears; the granules do not stain and appear as greenish refractile bodies.

4. Basophil morphology (Fig. 2.3)
   - a. Canine basophilic granules are purple and usually quite sparse compared to mast cells in which granules fill the cytoplasm.
   - b. Feline basophil granules are biochemically altered so that they stain gray-blue, and the cell appears somewhat larger than a neutrophil. Feline basophilic myelocytes have purple granules.
   - c. Bovine and equine basophils have numerous purple granules.

5. Lymphocyte morphology (Fig. 2.3)
   - a. Lymphocytes vary in size according to the degree of flattening on smears rather than any specific classification.
     - (1) Canine lymphocytes are small with scanty amounts of bluish cytoplasm; rare cells contain a few dark red cytoplasmic granules.

The nucleus is round with clumped chromatin; nucleoli are usually not visible with routine stains.

    (2) Feline lymphocytes are similar to those of the dog. The nucleus is occasionally slightly indented, and cytoplasmic granules are rare.

    (3) Lymphocytes are the predominant bovine leukocyte. Morphologic features of small lymphocytes are similar to those in dogs. Larger lymphocytes have more abundant cytoplasm, indented nuclei, and lighter-staining chromatin. Cytoplasmic granules are common.

    (4) Equine lymphocytes are similar to those in the dog.

    (5) Storage of EDTA anticoagulated blood for 30 to 60 minutes causes lobulation of nuclei, cytoplasmic vacuolization, and smudging of lymphocytes on stained smears.

  b. Transformed lymphocytes (immunocytes or reactive lymphocytes) are occasionally encountered in low numbers in blood during periods of antigenic stimulation (Fig. 2.3) (Case 7).

    (1) These are probably T cells but could be B cells.

    (2) Immunocyte morphology is characterized by intense cytoplasmic basophilia and occasionally a pale Golgi zone. Nuclei appear like those of small lymphocytes or have gently scalloped edges. Nuclear chromatin is aggregated.

    (3) Plasma cells are a specific immunocyte occurring in lymph nodes and bone marrow and only rarely in blood. Nuclear and staining characteristics are the same as other immunocytes, but the cell is identifiable by an eccentrically placed nucleus and a pale perinuclear zone in the cytoplasm.

  c. Lymphoblasts are pre- or post-mitotic lymphocytes. They are larger, more basophilic, and have finer chromatin than lymphocytes. Their nucleoli are usually visible. They occur only rarely in blood.

C. Differential leukocyte count

  1. The stained smear is examined with high or oil magnification, and leukocytes are identified until 100 (preferably 200 to reduce error) cells are classified by type. The number of nucleated erythrocytes encountered during the classification of 100 leukocytes should be tallied.

  2. The percentage of each leukocyte multiplied by the WBC count gives the absolute number of each leukocyte type/μl of blood.

  3. Interpretations should always be made using the number of cells/μl and not the percentage.

III. Bone marrow examination. The systematic approach to examine
      bone marrow smears is described in Chapter 1.

INTERPRETATION OF LEUKOCYTE RESPONSES

  I. Physiologic leukocytosis
      A. Presumptive findings
          1. The leukogram is characterized by mild neutrophilia
              without a left shift; normal lymphocyte number; or,
              more often, lymphocytosis and normal numbers of
              eosinophils, basophils, and monocytes.
          2. The animal is usually young, excited or fearful but
              healthy and is in strange surroundings at the time of
              sample collection. Often the response occurs when a
              struggle develops during restraint for sample
              collection.
      B. Mechanisms
          1. Neutrophilia (increased CNP) occurs because marginal
              pool cells are decreased. Total blood neutrophil
              number (CNP + MNP) is unchanged (Fig. 2.4).
              a. Epinephrine released in response to fear,
                  excitement, or sudden strenuous exercise is the
                  mediator.
              b. Mobilization of marginated neutrophils is probably
                  secondary to increased muscular activity, heart
                  rate, and blood pressure.
          2. Lymphocytosis, more dramatic than neutrophilia, is
              unexplained. Two theories are:
              a. Epinephrine may block receptors on endothelial
                  cells of postcapillary venules in lymph nodes,
                  preventing blood lymphocytes from reentering
                  lymphoid tissue.
              b. Arrival of recirculating lymphocytes into blood
                  from the thoracic duct may be facilitated by the
                  muscular activity.
      C. Species characteristics
          1. The response is uncommon in dogs.
          2. The response is common in young healthy cats, where
              WBC counts typically reach 20,000/μl and lymphocyte
              counts range from 6,000 to 15,000/μl.
          3. The response may occur in healthy cattle during
              parturition and strenuous exercise. WBC counts are
              15,000 to 27,000/μl, and neutrophilia and
              lymphocytosis occur; but unlike other species,
              eosinopenia is expected.
          4. The response is common in young healthy horses. WBC
              counts are 12,000 to 25,000/μl, and lymphocyte counts
              are 6,000 to 14,000/μl.
          5. Physiologic leukocytosis, especially lymphocytosis,
              accompanies lactation in sows and occurs 3 to 5 hours
              after feeding in healthy pigs.
 II. Leukocyte response to corticosteroids
      A. Presumptive findings
          1. The leukogram is characterized by neutrophilia,

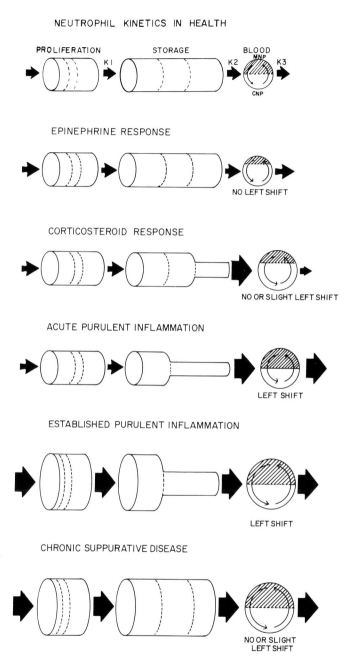

Fig. 2.4. Mechanisms of neutrophilia. Sizes of arrows represent rates of movement of cells through the compartments of granulopoiesis, marrow storage, and blood. The sizes of the tubes, circles, and shaded areas represent bone marrow proliferation and storage pools, blood total neutrophil pools, and blood marginal pools, respectively. (From Prasse KW: White blood cell disorders. In A Textbook of Veterinary Internal Medicine, 2nd ed, Ettinger SJ (ed), Philadelphia, WB Saunders Co, 1983.)

usually without a left shift; lymphopenia; eosinopenia; and in some animals, monocytosis.

2. The response follows therapeutic use of corticosteroids and ACTH. The type of corticosteroid, route of administration, and dose affect the magnitude of the response.

3. The response occurs in animals with endogenous release of corticosteroid, most often stimulated by pain or extremely high or low body temperature (Case 16).

4. Animals with hyperadrenocorticism have this leukocyte response (Case 20). The magnitude of neutrophilia diminishes with longevity of the disease, but the other leukocyte changes persist.

B. Mechanisms

1. Corticosteroid-induced neutrophilia (Cases 16, 21) (Fig. 2.4)

   a. Transit time in circulation and neutrophil number (CNP) are increased because corticosteroids reduce neutrophil stickiness and random emigration from blood.

   b. Bone marrow release rate, the major neutrophilic effect, is increased, but usually the storage pool is adequate and immature neutrophils are not released.

   c. The peak of the response occurs within 4 to 8 hours after the onset of corticosteroid stimulation. Pretreatment leukocyte values are expected to return within 24 hours after single treatments and within 48 to 72 hours after cessation of longer therapeutic use of the drugs. The magnitude of neutrophilia diminishes with long-term treatment, but the other changes persist.

2. Corticosteroid-induced lymphopenia

   a. The lowest count occurs within 4 to 8 hours after the onset of corticosteroid stimulation.

   b. The principal, immediate effect is redistribution of recirculating lymphocytes; they remain transiently sequestered in the lymphoid tissues or bone marrow rather than entering efferent lymph and blood.

   c. A long-term effect is lysis of lymphocytes in the thymic cortex and uncommitted lymphocytes in the lymph nodes. Thymic medullary and bone marrow lymphocytes resist corticosteroid-induced lysis, and effector T and B cells do not lyse.

   d. Transient lymphopenia follows dosing during alternate-day corticosteroid therapy.

3. Corticosteroid-induced monocytosis may be caused by an effect similar to that on neutrophils (i.e., mobilization of marginated cells within the blood vasculature).

4. Corticosteroid-induced eosinopenia

   a. An immediate effect is sequestration within the blood vasculature; cells do not emigrate from blood and recirculate after cessation of the corticosteroid stimulation.

        b. Release of eosinophils from bone marrow is
          inhibited, but eosinophilopoiesis continues. Total
          number of marrow eosinophils increases during
          corticosteroid stimulation.

C. Species characteristics
   1. Dog
      a. WBC counts are typically 15,000 to 25,000/μl, but
         they may reach 40,000/μl on rare occasions.
      b. Neutrophilia without a left shift is typical, but
         immature neutrophils up to 1,000/μl may occur if
         the storage pool is depleted at the time of
         corticosteroid stimulation.
      c. Low normal lymphocyte number (or less than
         1,000/μl) is common.
      d. Monocytosis and eosinopenia are typical.
   2. Cat
      a. The response is less frequently observed than in
         dogs.
      b. The leukogram pattern is similar to that of dogs;
         the most extreme leukocytosis is about 30,000/μl.
   3. Cattle
      a. In addition to the general causes of the
         corticosteroid release (pain and temperature
         extremes), the response may be seen with displaced
         abomasum, milk fever, ketosis, dystocia, feed
         overload, and indigestion.
      b. WBC counts are 8,000 to 18,000/μl.
      c. Eosinopenia caused by corticosteroids always
         occurs; but even in healthy cattle, transportation
         or placement in strange surroundings may induce
         eosinopenia without other steroidal leukocyte
         changes.
   4. Horse
      a. This response may occur with sustained muscular
         exercise in healthy horses as well as with the
         usual causes of corticosteroid release.
      b. WBC counts range up to 20,000/μl.
      c. Lymphopenia is seldom dramatic. Low normal
         lymphocyte count is observed (2,000/μl in young
         horses and 1,500/μl in older horses).
   5. Swine
      a. The typical corticosteroid-induced changes are
         expected, but swine WBC, neutrophil, and lympho-
         cyte reference values are much wider than other
         species; the response may be missed by casual
         inspection of data.
      b. The corticosteroid-induced leukogram in swine may
         be seen during parturition, following strenuous
         exercise, or immediately after transportation as
         well as with the usual causes (i.e., pain and
         temperature extremes).

III. Neutrophil response in inflammatory disease
   A. General considerations and causes
      1. Inflammation characterized by neutrophilic exudate
         (purulent inflammation) represents a tissue demand for

TABLE 2.1.   Causes of Purulent Inflammation or Increased Utilization
             of Neutrophils
Bacteria
  <u>Actinobacillus</u> spp., <u>Actinomyces</u> spp., <u>Brucella</u> spp., <u>Coryne-</u>
  <u>bacterium</u> spp., <u>Escherichia</u> <u>coli</u>, <u>Klebsiella</u> spp., <u>Nocardia</u> sp.,
  <u>Pasteurella</u> spp., <u>Proteus</u> spp., <u>Pseudomonas</u> sp., <u>Salmonella</u> spp.,
  <u>Spherophorus</u> sp., <u>Staphylococcus</u> spp., <u>Streptococcus</u> spp.,
  <u>Yersinia</u> spp.
Virus
  Canine distemper, equine herpesvirus (foals), feline rhinotracheitis, infectious bovine rhinotracheitis, poxvirus
Fungi
  <u>Aspergillus</u> spp., <u>Blastomyces</u> sp., <u>Candida</u> sp., chromoblastomycosis
  (several genera), <u>Coccidioides</u> sp., mycetoma (several genera),
  phaeohyphomycosis (several genera), <u>Sporothrix</u> sp., zygomycosis
  (several genera)
Parasite
  <u>Fasciola</u> sp., <u>Paragonimus</u> sp., <u>Stephanurus</u> sp., <u>Toxoplasma</u> sp.
Immune-mediated
  Autoimmune hemolytic anemia, lupus erythematosus, polymyositis,
  polyserositis, rheumatoid arthritis
Necrosis
  Burns, infarction, infection, malignancy, thrombosis, uremia
Others
  Canine idiopathic polyarthritis, endotoxin, estrogen toxicity (early
  stages), foreign body, hemolysis, hemorrhage, Rocky Mountain spotted
  fever (late stages)

cells. Neutrophilia with a left shift is the classical response (Cases 10, 19, 22).

2. Certain types of inflammation lack significant neutrophilic exudation (e.g., hemorrhagic cystitis, seborrheic dermatitis, catarrhal enteritis, certain granulomatous reactions). Neutrophilia may or may not develop.

3. Causes of purulent inflammation are listed in Table 2.1.

4. Localized purulent diseases such as pyometra or empyema stimulate greater neutrophilic responses than generalized infections or septicemia.

5. Occasionally a neutrophilic leukocytosis and left shift are observed, but the site of purulent inflammation is obscure by clinical or even gross necropsy inspection.
   a. Example conditions are purulent dermatitis and purulent enteritis. In these conditions neutrophils emigrate to the body surface or gut lumen and are immediately lost without visible accumulation.
   b. These tissues represent "local" sites of inflammation, and the neutrophilia may be very dramatic compared to the unimpressive tissue reaction.

6. Hemolytic diseases are characterized by neutrophilia, but the site of neutrophilic accumulation or loss remains obscure (Cases 2, 3).

7. If a localized site of purulent inflammation is surgically extirpated, an exacerbation of neutrophilia during the immediate postsurgical period should be

anticipated until granulopoiesis subsides and the
sudden excessive blood supply of neutrophils is
consumed by normal processes of cellular demise.

B. Kinetic mechanisms. The mechanisms of neutrophilia are
    illustrated in Fig. 2.4.
    1. When tissue injury stimulates body defense culminating
        in purulent inflammation, neutrophil release from
        marrow stores and bone marrow granulopoiesis increase
        immediately.
    2. The number of neutrophils in blood during purulent
        inflammation reflects the balance between the rate of
        utilization (tissue demand) and the rate of bone
        marrow production and release of cells into blood.
        a. If production and release are greater than the
            tissue demand, neutrophilic leukocytosis occurs
            (Cases 10, 19, 22).
        b. If the tissue demand is greater than production
            and release from the bone marrow, neutropenia oc-
            curs (reduced survival neutropenia) (Cases 5, 6).
        c. During purulent inflammation, nearly any WBC count
            from very low to very high can be expected.
    3. As a tissue demand for cells and increased rate of
        bone marrow release occurs, the marrow storage pool
        becomes depleted of segmenters. Band neutrophils, or
        under severe situations neutrophilic metamyelocytes
        and earlier cells, appear in blood (Cases 2, 5, 6, 10,
        11, 13, 19, 22, 23).
        a. When the total neutrophil count is normal or high,
            greater than 1,000 immature neutrophils/μl in dogs
            and cats and greater than 300/μl in large animals
            are clear indications that the animal has purulent
            inflammation.
        b. When the animal has neutropenia and more than 10%
            of the total blood neutrophil number are immature
            cells, high tissue demand for neutrophils is
            indicated.
        c. The magnitude of left shift tends to parallel the
            intensity of the purulent inflammation.
        d. In certain severe purulent diseases, the intense
            response and left shift may include myelocytes,
            progranulocytes, or myeloblasts in blood, a
            situation called the "leukemoid" response.
    4. During chronic suppurative diseases, the rate of gran-
        ulopoiesis eventually exceeds the rate of tissue
        demand and bone marrow release. As marrow storage is
        replenished, the left shift diminishes and may dis-
        appear in spite of continued tissue demand (Fig. 2.5).
C. Species characteristics
    1. Dog
        a. WBC counts between 10,000 and 30,000/μl are
            common. A few cases have counts that exceed
            50,000/μl, and in rare cases counts may exceed
            100,000/μl.
        b. Gram-negative bacteria infecting the lung, thorax,
            peritoneum, or uterus may induce neutropenia

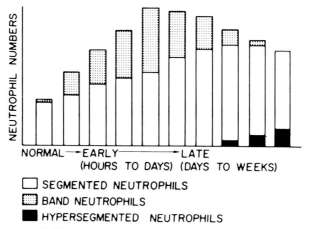

SEGMENTED NEUTROPHILS
BAND NEUTROPHILS
HYPERSEGMENTED NEUTROPHILS

Fig. 2.5. Course of blood neutrophil response in chronic
suppurative disorders. Intense suppuration may be indicated
when the number of immature neutrophils nearly equals or
exceeds the number of mature neutrophils. Repetitive
examination is necessary to establish if the left shift is
increasing or decreasing during continued suppuration. The
occurrence of hypersegmented neutrophils may reflect the
existence of a long-standing suppuration. (From Prasse KW:
White blood cell disorders. In A Textbook of Veterinary
Internal Medicine, 2nd ed, Ettinger SJ (ed), Philadelphia,
WB Saunders Co, 1983.)

         caused by overwhelming sepsis and endotoxemia.
         Salmonellosis causes similar response.

2. Cat
   a. WBC counts between 10,000 and 30,000/µl are
      common. A few cases have counts that exceed
      30,000/µl, and in rare cases counts may exceed
      75,000/µl.
   b. Gram-negative sepsis and endotoxemia cause
      neutropenia in cats as described for dogs.

3. Cattle
   a. Inflammatory leukograms in calves up to 3 or 4
      months old may be similar to those described for
      dogs and cats.
   b. Fibrinous, nonpurulent inflammation in cattle
      (e.g., early stages of shipping fever pneumonia)
      elicit little or no neutrophil response. High
      plasma fibrinogen concentration may be the only
      laboratory sign of inflammatory disease.
   c. In adult cattle acute purulent inflammation caused
      by streptococci, staphylococci, or coliforms
      typically induces leukopenia, neutropenia, and
      severe left shift with toxic neutrophils (Case 5).
      This pattern lasts 24 to 48 hours; later, if the
      animal survives, counts return toward normal
      limits with persisting left shift. Diseases
      causing this pattern include mastitis, metritis,
      traumatic reticulopericarditis, peritonitis, and
      salmonellosis.

        d. Persisting purulent inflammation commonly causes WBC counts from 4,000 to 15,000/μl. A few cases have counts that exceed 30,000/μl, and in rare cases counts may exceed 60,000/μl (especially pulmonary abscessation).

    4. Horse

        a. WBC counts are typically 7,000 to 20,000/μl. Rare cases may exceed 30,000/μl.

        b. Left shift of neutrophils associated with neutrophilia is seldom dramatic in the horse, but diseases of the gastrointestinal tract usually have severe left shifts with normal or low total WBC counts (Case 6).

    5. Swine

        a. Because the reference range of WBC count values is broad in swine, leukocytosis is seldom seen.

        b. Purulent inflammatory diseases typically cause dramatic left shifts (i.e., immature neutrophils back to myelocytes are commonly observed).

        c. As in cattle, plasma fibrinogen concentration may be the only laboratory sign of nonpurulent inflammation. Erythrocyte sedimentation rate also may be indicative of nonpurulent inflammation in swine concomitant with normal neutrophil patterns.

IV. Neutropenia. Causes of neutropenia listed by known or suspected type are given in Table 2.2. The kinetic patterns for each type of neutropenia are shown in Fig. 2.6 and described below.

    A. Reduced survival of circulating neutrophils (Cases 5, 6)

        1. Destruction of mature neutrophils or tissue utilization is massive, and the rate of cell loss exceeds the rate of granulopoiesis and release from the bone marrow.

        2. If the animal survives and the process continues for

TABLE 2.2. Causes of Neutropenia Listed by Mechanism

Reduced survival neutropenia
  Acute coliform diseases, bovine acute purulent diseases, caprine streptococcal mastitis, endotoxemia, immune-mediated neutropenia, overwhelming sepsis, porcine coliform mastitis, salmonellosis

Reduced production neutropenia
  Bracken fern poisoning, cancer chemotherapy, canine cyclic hematopoiesis, canine ehrlichiosis, canine parvovirus, estrogen toxicity (late stages), feline infectious panleukopenia, feline leukovirus, hog cholera, infectious canine hepatitis, irradiation, myelophthisis

Increased ineffective granulopoiesis
  Diphenylhydantoin, feline leukovirus, myelophthisis

Unknown mechanism (many are transient early in infection)
  Bovine enterovirus (calves), bovine parainfluenza-3, bovine virus diarrhea-mucosal disease complex, canine distemper, equine ehrlichiosis, equine infectious anemia, equine viral arteritis, equine viral rhinopneumonitis, malignant catarrhal fever, Rocky Mountain spotted fever, sporadic bovine encephalomyelitis, swine influenza, swine transmissible gastroenteritis, Venezuelan equine encephalomyelitis

NEUTROPHIL KINETICS IN HEALTH

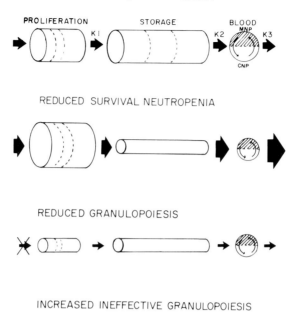

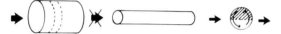

Fig. 2.6. Mechanisms of neutropenia. Sizes of arrows represent rates of movement of cells through the compartments of granulopoiesis, marrow storage, and blood. The sizes of the tubes, circles, and shaded areas represent bone marrow proliferation and storage pools, blood total neutrophil pools, and blood marginal pools, respectively. (From Prasse KW: White blood cell disorders. In A Textbook of Veterinary Internal Medicine, 2nd ed, Ettinger SJ (ed), Philadelphia, WB Saunders Co, 1983.)

        24 to 48 hours, the bone marrow exhibits granulopoietic hyperplasia (i.e., the myeloid/erythroid ratio increases, and the proportion of granulocytes in the proliferation and maturation compartment is increased).
    3. If the animal survives, neutrophilic leukocytosis should develop over the following 72 to 96 hours.
  B. Reduced production of neutrophils
    1. Diminished bone marrow production of granulocytes may be transient during acute or even preclinical stages of certain infectious diseases (Case 4). By 5 to 7 days following this transient insult to marrow stem cells and proliferating granulocytes, the resultant neutropenia is likewise transient. Granulopoietic hyperplasia reflecting recovery may be encountered in bone marrow by the time neutropenia is observed.
    2. In other diseases the onset is more insidious, the defect in granulopoiesis is more lasting, and the

neutropenia is more persistent. Pancytopenia or
aplastic anemia is the hematologic pattern, and bone
marrow exhibits hematopoietic hypoplasia.

  C. Excessive ineffective granulopoiesis

      1. Ineffective granulopoiesis resulting in neutropenia
may occur by:

          a. Failure in bone marrow release of cells (e.g.,
myelofibrosis)

          b. Intramedullary death of cells (e.g., bone marrow
necrosis)

          c. Arrest of granulocyte maturation (Case 8)

      2. Bone marrow examination reveals granulocytic hyper-
plasia concomitant with neutropenia; therefore, the
findings by routine technique may not be distinguished
from certain clinical stages of reduced survival
neutropenia and the transient types of granulopoietic
hypoplasia.

V. Monocyte responses

  A. Monocytosis

      1. Monocytosis can occur any time neutrophilia occurs,
including the response to physiologic events in health
and the response to corticosteroids (Case 20).

      2. Its occurrence is related to disorders characterized
by suppuration, necrosis, malignancy, hemolysis,
hemorrhage, immune injury, and certain pyogranulo-
matous diseases (Cases 2, 3, 4, 6, 9, 10, 24).

      3. Monocytosis may be observed during both acute and
chronic stages of disease.

  B. Monocytopenia is not a clinically useful feature of
leukograms.

VI. Eosinophil responses

  A. Eosinophilia

      1. Eosinophilia generally is associated with parasitic
infection or hypersensitivity (Case 7). Causes and

TABLE 2.3. Predictable and Infrequent Causes of Eosinophilia

Parasitisms*
  Predictable eosinophilia: aelurostrongylosis, ancylostomiasis,
  bovine lungworms, dirofilariasis, equine lungworms, feline
  trichinosis, Filaroides osleri, paragonimiasis, Spirocerca lupi,
  strongyloidosis
  Unpredictable eosinophilia: ascariasis, coccidiosis, demodicosis,
  fascioliasis, fleas, stephanuriasis, trichuriasis
  No eosinophilia: cestodiasis, Dipetalonema recunditum,
  habronemiasis, bovine trichostrongylosis
Hypersensitivities
  Predictable eosinophilia: eosinophilic pneumonitis, flea allergy
  Unpredictable eosinophilia: canine eosinophilic myositis and muscle
  atrophy, canine and feline eosinophilic granuloma complex, canine
  eosinophilic gastroenteritis, canine panosteitis, milk hypersensitivity in cattle
Other causes
  Unpredictable eosinophilia: feline staphylococcal or streptococcal
  infections, mast cell neoplasia
    *Listings refer to natural rather than experimental infections.

diseases that yield predictable and infrequent eosinophilia are listed in Table 2.3.

2. Animals with eosinophilic disorders may have a response tempered by a concomitant corticosteroid effect (an eosinopenic effect).

3. Frequently, localized lesions that contain significant numbers of eosinophils in the exudate are not accompanied by eosinophilia (e.g., eosinophilic granuloma).

4. Antigens that stimulate eosinophilia mediate the response via sensitized T lymphocytes. The second exposure to antigen yields more marked eosinophilia more quickly.

    a. The tissues most commonly affected in eosinophilic hypersensitivity conditions are skin, lung, gastrointestinal tract, and reproductive tract.

    b. Parasites with prolonged host-tissue contact promote the most dramatic eosinophilia.

B. Eosinopenia is a response to corticosteroids as previously described, but it also occurs with acute infection by a mechanism independent of corticosteroid action.

VII. Basophil responses. Basophilia (basocytophilia) is seldom numerically dramatic, but observing even a few cells on the blood smear usually attracts attention.

A. Basophilia occurring with eosinophilia (Case 7)

1. Those IgE-generating disorders (Table 2.3) that cause predictable eosinophilia often have concomitant basophilia.

2. Microfilaria-negative dirofilariasis may have basophilia more often than microfilaria-positive dirofilariasis.

3. This response occurs in cats, but it may be overlooked because the granules of mature basophils fail to stain.

B. Basophilia occurring without eosinophilia is rare; when observed, consideration should be given to altered plasma lipoprotein metabolism secondary to endocrine diseases, nephrotic syndrome, chronic liver disease, or genetic hyperlipoproteinemias.

VIII. Lymphocyte responses. The blood lymphocyte number is most often influenced by effects on cell recirculation and to a lesser extent by effects on cell function or production. The number tends to be quite constant in health and decreases slightly with age in most species.

A. Lymphocytosis

1. The epinephrine effect causing lymphocytosis in physiologic leukocytosis in healthy animals was described earlier in the chapter.

2. Enlarged lymph nodes caused by antigenic stimulation (lymphoid hyperplasia) are encountered commonly in all species, but blood lymphocyte numbers correlate poorly with functional reactivity.

    a. The blood lymphocyte number may be normal or low in association with enlarged lymph nodes, espe-

cially during acute stages of infection (see following discussion on lymphopenia).
b. Occasionally during chronic stages of infection, lymphocytosis may be seen (e.g., Rocky Mountain spotted fever in the dog).
3. Persistent lymphocytosis in cattle is a subclinical, nonneoplastic manifestation of bovine leukovirus infection (see Chapter 3). It is a B lymphocyte hyperplasia, and lymphocyte counts are typically 7,000 to 15,000/μl.
4. Lymphocyte counts in healthy growing swine are higher than other species, typically 13,000 to 26,000/μl. Lymphocyte counts rarely exceed reference values in swine.

B. Lymphopenia
1. Lymphopenia is a common abnormality in the leukogram of sick animals. The mechanism leading to lymphopenia is seldom differentiated before final diagnosis is made; it may be postulated only in retrospect.
2. Mechanisms that cause lymphopenia include:
a. Corticosteroid-induced redistribution of recirculating lymphocytes (see earlier discussion in this chapter) (Cases 2, 10, 16, 19, 20, 23).
b. Acute systemic infection (Cases 4, 6). Generalized disbursement of infectious antigen causes entrapment of recirculating lymphocytes in lymph nodes. Lymph nodes may be enlarged concomitant with lymphopenia. The lymphopenia tends to disappear with time.
(1) Viral infections are more likely to cause lymphopenia than bacterial infections.
(2) Local infections may cause entrapment of lymphocytes in the regional lymph nodes, but lymphopenia is unlikely.
c. Acquired T lymphocyte deficiency. Most recirculating lymphocytes are T cells. Certain infections in neonates cause thymic necrosis or atrophy; if the animal survives, persistent lymphopenia occurs.
d. Immunosuppressive therapy or irradiation. These agents suppress clonal proliferation, and lymphopenia slowly develops.
e. Loss of lymphocyte-rich, efferent lymph. This mechanism primarily occurs with loss of thoracic duct lymph.
f. Loss of lymphocyte-rich, afferent lymph (Case 18). The only afferent lymph that is rich in cells comes from gastrointestinal- or bronchial-associated lymphoid tissue.
g. Disruption of lymph node architecture by inflammation or neoplasia that replaces recirculating lymphocytes.
h. Hereditary immunodeficiency. T lymphocyte deficiency or combined T and B lymphocyte deficiency disorders show lymphopenia. Animals

TABLE 2.4. Causes of Lymphopenia Listed by Mechanism
Corticosteroid-induced
  Exogenous corticosteroids or ACTH, extremes in body temperature,
  hyperadrenocorticism, painful diseases
Acute systemic infection
  Bovine enzootic abortion, canine coronavirus, canine distemper,
  canine parvovirus, endotoxemia, equine herpesvirus, equine
  influenza, feline infectious panleukopenia, infectious canine
  hepatitis, mycoplasma infections, ovine bluetongue, septicemia
Acquired T lymphocyte deficiency (neonatal infections)
  Canine distemper, equine herpesvirus, feline infectious
  panleukopenia, feline leukovirus (fading kitten syndrome)
Immunosuppressive drugs or irradiation
  Azothioprine
Loss of lymphocyte-rich, efferent lymph
  Chylous thoracic effusion secondary to feline cardiovascular
  diseases, ruptured thoracic duct
Loss of lymphocyte-rich, afferent lymph
  Alimentary lymphosarcoma, enteric neoplasms, granulomatous
  enteritis, Johne's disease, protein-losing enteropathy
  (lymphangiectasia), ulcerative enteritis
Disruption of lymph node architecture
  Generalized granulomatous diseases, multicentric lymphosarcoma
Hereditary T lymphocyte deficiency
  Black-Pied Danish cattle thymic aplasia, combined T and B cell
  immunodeficiency of Arabian foals
  Note: Only infections found documented in the literature as
characterized by lymphopenia are listed.

with only B lymphocyte deficiency are not
lymphopenic.
3. Diseases associated with lymphopenia are listed by
   mechanism in Table 2.4.
4. Because the number varies widely among species,
   reference values for blood lymphocyte number should be
   consulted before lymphopenia is interpreted.

IX. Prognosis and leukocyte responses
  A. Favorable prognosis
    1. If sequential leukograms exhibit return toward normal
       values, the change obviously reflects a favorable
       prognosis when accompanied by convalescence in the
       animal.
    2. Specifically, disappearance of a neutrophilic left
       shift, lymphopenia, or eosinopenia may denote recovery
       and may precede clinical signs of remission.
  B. Guarded or poor prognosis
    1. Neutrophil changes
      a. When the number of immature neutrophils approach,
         equal, or exceed the number of segmenters in blood
         (a "degenerative left shift") regardless of the
         WBC count, the finding implies an intense tissue
         demand for neutrophils, which at the moment is
         exceeding the granulopoietic effort (Cases 5, 6).
      b. Neutropenia, regardless of type, is serious
         because of the nature of the causative disorders
         and the added risk of secondary infection.

      c. Extreme neutrophilic leukocytosis with left shift back to myelocytes or earlier cells (leukemoid response) is generally associated with intense suppurative diseases.

   2. Lymphocyte changes

      a. Declining lymphocyte count while the animal appears clinically healthy may indicate impending illness.

      b. Persisting lymphopenia implies persistence of the cause.

REFERENCES

Alexander JW, Jones JB, Michel RL: Recurrent neutropenia in a pomeranian: A case report. J Am Anim Hosp Assoc 17:841, 1981.

Allen BV, Powell DG, Singleton WB: Value and limitations of haematology in viral infections in horses. Vet Rec 110:348, 1982.

Andresen HA: Evaluation of leukopenia in cattle. J Am Vet Med Assoc 156:858, 1970.

Appel MJG, Cooper BJ, Greisen H, et al: Canine viral enteritis. I. Status report on corona- and parvo-like viral enteritides. Cornell Vet 69:123, 1979.

Appel MJG, Meunier P, Greisen H, et al: Enteric viral infections of dogs. Proc 29th Gaines Vet Symp, 1979.

Athens JW, Haab OP, Raab SO, et al: Leukokinetic studies. IV. The total blood, circulating and marginal granulocyte pools and the granulocytic turnover rate in normal subjects. J Clin Invest 40:989, 1961.

Athens JW, Raab SO, Haab OP, et al: Leukokinetic studies. III. The distribution of granulocytes in the blood of normal subjects. J Clin Invest 40:159, 1961.

Baggiolini M: The neutrophil. In Glynn LE, Houck JC, Weissmann G (eds): Handbook of inflammation, Vol 2. The cell biology of inflammation. New York, Elsevier/North Holland Biomedical Press, 1980.

Bainton DF: The cells of inflammation: A general review. In Glynn LE, Houck JC, Weissman G (eds): Handbook of inflammation, Vol 2. The cell biology of inflammation. New York, Elsevier/North Holland Biomedical Press, 1980.

Beeson PB, Bass DA: The eosinophil. Philadelphia, WB Saunders Co, 1977.

Biggs R, MacMillan RL: The errors of some hematological methods as they are used in a routine laboratory. J Clin Pathol 1:269, 1948.

Bishop CR, Athens JW, Boggs DR, et al: Leukokinetic studies. XIII. A nonsteady state kinetic evaluation of the mechanism of cortisone-granulocytosis. J Clin Invest 47:249, 1968.

Boggs DR: White cell manual. Philadelphia, FA Davis Co, 1983.

Braun JP, Guelfi JF, Thouvenot JP, et al: Haematological and biochemical effects of a single intramuscular dose of 6,alpha-methylprednisolone acetate in the dog. Res Vet Sci 31:236, 1981.

Burguez PN, Ousey J, Cash RSG, et al: Changes in blood neutrophil and lymphocyte counts following administration of cortisol to horses and foals. Equine Vet J 15:58, 1983.

Carakostas MC, Moore WE, Smith JE: Intravascular neutrophilic granulocyte kinetics in horses. Am J Vet Res 42:623, 1981.

Carlson GP, Kaneko JJ: Influence of prednisolone on intravascular granulocyte kinetics of calves under nonsteady state conditions. Am J Vet Res 37:149, 1976.

Chickering WR, Prasse KW: Immune mediated neutropenia in man and animals: A review. Vet Clin Pathol 10(1):6, 1981.

Chiu T: Studies on estrogen-induced proliferative disorders of hemopoietic tissue in dogs. PhD thesis, University of Minnesota, Minneapolis, 1974.

Coffman JR, Hammond LS, Garner HE, et al: Haematology as an aid to prognosis of chronic laminitis. Equine Vet J 12:30, 1980.

Cohen ZA: The structure and function of monocytes and macrophages. Adv Immunol 9:163, 1968.

Craddock CG: Corticosteroid-induced lymphopenia, immunosuppression, and body defense. Ann Intern Med 88:564, 1978.

Crafts RC: The effects of estrogens on the bone marrow of adult female dogs. Blood 3:276, 1948.

Cronkite EP: Kinetics of granulopoiesis. Clin Haematol 8:351, 1979.

Dannenberg AM: Macrophages in inflammation and infection. N Engl J Med 293:489, 1975.

DeSousa M: Lymphocyte circulation, experimental and clinical aspects. New York, Wiley, 1981.

Deubelbeiss KA, Dancey JT, Harker LA, et al: Neutrophil kinetics in the dog. J Clin Invest 55:833, 1975.

DiGiacomo RF, Hammond WP, Kunz LL, et al: Clinical and pathologic features of cyclic hematopoiesis in grey collie dogs. Am J Pathol 111:224, 1983.

Dorn CR, Coffman JR, Schmidt DA, et al: Neutropenia and salmonellosis in hospitalized horses. J Am Vet Med Assoc 166:65, 1975.

Dvorak AM, Dvorak HF: The basophil. Its morphology, biochemistry, motility, release reactions, recovery, and role in the inflammatory responses of IgE-mediated and cell-mediated origin. Arch Pathol 103:551, 1979.

Edwards DF: Bone marrow hypoplasia in eight dogs with Sertoli cell tumor. J Am Vet Med Assoc 178:497, 1981.

Fauci AS, Dole DC: The effect of hydrocortisone on the kinetics of normal human lymphocytes. Blood 46:235, 1975.

Faulkner M, Dixon JB, Green JR: Discrepancy between haemocytometer and electronic leukocyte counts in neutrophilic dogs. Vet Rec 110:202, 1982.

Ferrer JF, Marshak RR, Abt DA, et al: Relationship between lymphosarcoma and persistent lymphocytosis in cattle: A review. J Am Vet Med Assoc 175:705, 1979.

Fessler JF, Bottoms GD, Roesel OF, et al: Endotoxin-induced change in hemograms, plasma enzymes, and blood chemical values in anesthetized ponies: Effects of flunixen meglumine. Am J Vet Res 43:140, 1982.

Gossett KA, MacWilliams PS: Ultrastructure of canine toxic neutrophils. Am J Vet Res 43:1634, 1982.

Greaves MF, Owen JJT, Raff MC: T and B lymphocytes: Origins, properties and roles in immune responses. New York, American Elsevier Publishing Co, 1973.

Gwazdauskas FC, Paape MJ, Peery DA, et al: Plasma glucocorticoid and circulating blood leucocyte responses in cattle after sequential intramuscular injections of ACTH. Am J Vet Res 41:1052, 1980.

Hammer RF, Weber AF: Ultrastructure of agranular leukocytes in peripheral blood of normal cows. Am J Vet Res 35:527, 1974.

Hardy WD: Feline leukemia virus non-neoplastic diseases. J Am Anim Hosp Assoc 17:941, 1981.

Hendrick M: A spectrum of hypereosinophilic syndromes exemplified by six cats with eosinophilic enteritis. Vet Pathol 18:188, 1981.

Jacobs RM, Weiser MG, Hall RL, et al: Clinicopathologic features of canine parvoviral enteritis. J Am Anim Hosp Assoc 16:809, 1980.

Jain NC, Lasmanis J: Leukocytic changes in cows given intravenous injections of Escherichia coli endotoxin. Res Vet Sci 24:386, 1978.

Jain NC, Schalm OW, Lasmanis J: Neutrophil kinetics in endotoxin-induced mastitis. Am J Vet Res 39:1662, 1978.

Jones JB, Jones ES, Lange RD: Early-life hematologic values of dogs affected with cyclic neutropenia. Am J Vet Res 35:849, 1974.

Kay AB: Functions of the eosinophil leukocyte: Annotation. Br J Haematol 33:313, 1976.

Koepke JA: A delineation of performance criteria for the differentiation of leukocytes. Am J Clin Pathol 68:202, 1977.

Krammer JW, Davis WC, Prieur DJ: The Chediak-Higashi syndrome of cats. Lab Invest 36:554, 1977.

Kurtz HJ, Quast J: Effects of continuous intravenous infusion of Escherichia coli endotoxin into swine. Am J Vet Res 43:262, 1982.

Larsen S, Flagstad A, Aalbek B: Experimental feline panleukopenia in the conventional cat. Vet Pathol 13:216, 1976.

Lester SJ, Searcy GP: Hematologic abnormalities preceding apparent recovery from feline leukemia virus infection. J Am Vet Med Assoc 178:471, 1981.

Lew AM, Hosking CS, Studdert MJ: Immunologic aspects of combined immunodeficiency disease in Arabian foals. Am J Vet Res 41:1161, 1980.

Lewis HB, Rebar AH: Bone marrow evaluation in veterinary practice. St. Louis, Ralston Purina Co, 1979.

Lewis PA, Shope RE: The study of the cells of blood as an aid to the diagnosis of hog cholera. J Am Vet Med Assoc 74:145, 1929.

Luke D: The effect of adrenocorticotrophic hormone and adrenal cortical extract on the differential white cell count in the pig. Br Vet J 109:434, 1953.

Lund JE, Padgett GA, Ott RL: Cyclic neutropenia in grey collie dogs. Blood 29:452, 1967.

Maddison JE, Hoff B, Johnson RP: Steroid responsive neutropenia in a dog. J Am Anim Hosp Assoc 19:881, 1983.

Magnuson NS, McGuire TC, Banks KL, et al: In vitro and in vivo effects of corticosteroids on peripheral blood lymphoctyes from ponies. Am J Vet Res 39:393, 1978.

Maloney MA, Patt HM: Granulocyte transit from bone marrow to blood. Blood 31:195, 1968.

Malone MA, Patt HM, Lund JE: Granulocyte dynamics and the question of ineffective granulopoiesis. Cell Tissue Kinet 4:201, 1971.

Marsh JC, Boggs DR, Cartwright GE, et al: Neutrophil kinetics in acute infection. J Clin Invest 46:1943, 1967.

Moore TC, Lachmann PJ: Cyclic AMP reduces and cyclic GMP increases the traffic of lymphocytes through peripheral lymph nodes of sheep in vivo. Immunology 47:423, 1982.

Nathan CF, Murray HW, Cohn ZA: The macrophage as an effector cell. N Engl J Med 303:622, 1980.

Osbaldiston GW, Johnson JH: Effect of ACTH on selected circulating blood cells in horses. J Am Vet Med Assoc 161:53, 1972.

Patt HM, Lund JE, Maloney MA: A model of granulocyte kinetics. Ann NY Acad Sci 113:515, 1965.

Pattengale PK, Sahl WM, Thorbecke GJ: Fate of autogenous canine lymphocytes after injection into an afferent lymphatic of the popliteal lymph node. Am J Pathol 67:527, 1972.

Prasse KW: Disorders of the leukocytes. In Ettinger SJ (ed): Textbook of veterinary internal medicine, Vol 2. Philadelphia, WB Saunders Co, 1975.

Prasse KW, Duncan JR: Clinical interpretation of leucocyte abnormalities. Vet Clin North Am 6:581, 1976.

Prasse KW, Kaeberle ML, Ramsey FK: Blood neutrophilic granulocyte kinetics in cats. Am J Vet Res 34:1021, 1973.

Prasse KW, Seagrave RC, Kaeberle ML, et al: A model of granulopoiesis in cats. Lab Invest 28:292, 1973.

Prieur DJ, Collier LL, Bryan GM, et al: The diagnosis of feline Chediak-Higashi syndrome. Feline Pract 9(5):26, 1979.

Raab SO, Athens JW, Haab OP, et al: Granulokinetics in normal dogs. Am J Physiol 206:83, 1964.

Rausch PG, Moore TG: Granule enzymes of polymorphonuclear neutrophils: A phylogenetic comparison. Blood 46:913, 1975.

Rawlings CA: Clinical laboratory evaluations of seven heartworm infected beagles: During disease development and following treatment. Cornell Vet 72:49, 1982.

Reardon MJ, Pierce KR: Acute experimental canine ehrlichiosis. I. Sequential reaction of the hemic and lymphoreticular systems. Vet Pathol 18:48, 1981.

Renshaw HW, Davis WC: Canine granulocytopathy syndrome. Am J Pathol 95:731, 1979.

Reynolds J, Heron I, Dudler L, et al: T-cell recirculation in the sheep: Migratory properties of cells from lymph nodes. Immunology 47:415, 1982.

Ross RF, Orning AP, Woods RD, et al: Bacteriologic study of sow agalactia. Am J Vet Res 42:949, 1981.

Roth JA, Kaeberle ML: Effect of glucocorticoids on the bovine immune system. J Am Vet Med Assoc 180:894, 1982.

Schalm OW: Leukocyte responses to disease in various domestic animals. J Am Vet Med Assoc 142:147, 1962.

Schalm OW: Eosinophilia in canine diseases. Calif Vet 20(4):11, 1966.

Schalm OW: Interpretation of leukocyte responses in the dog. J Am Vet Med Assoc 142:147, 1963.

Schalm OW: Some observations on physiologic leukocytosis in the cat and horse. Calif Vet 18(5):23, 1964.

Schalm OW: Leukopenia and resurgence of granulopoiesis in the cat. Calif Vet 23(2):16, 1969.

Schalm OW: Equine hematology as an aid to diagnosis. In Kitchen H and Krehbiel JD (eds): Proc 1st Int Symp Equine Hematol, East Lansing, Mich, 1975.

Schalm OW: Granulopoiesis. 1. Leukemoid reaction in blood. Canine Pract 2(3):18, 1975.

Schalm OW: Granulopoiesis. 2. Regenerative and beginning degenerative left shifts in blood. Canine Pract 2(4):27, 1975.

Schalm OW: Granulopoiesis. 3. Degenerative left shift with toxic neutrophils. Canine Pract 2(5):22, 1975.

Schalm OW: Mucopolysaccharidosis. Canine Pract 4(6):29, 1977.

Schalm OW: Exogenous estrogen toxicity in the dog. Canine Pract 5(5)57, 1978.

Schalm OW: Special characteristics of lymphocytes and monocytes in infectious canine hepatitis. Canine Pract 6(1):51, 1979.

Schalm OW: Phenylbutazone toxicity in two dogs. Canine Pract 6(4):47, 1979.

Schalm OW: The bovine leukocytes. Part I. General comments. Bovine Pract 1(6):8, 1980.

Schalm OW: The bovine leukocytes. Part II. The neutrophil as a barrier to coliform mastitis. Bovine Pract 2(1):28, 1981.

Schalm OW: The bovine leukocytes. Part III. Neutropenia and gangrenous mastitis. Bovine Pract 2(2):32, 1981.

Schalm OW, Jain NC, Carroll EJ: Veterinary Hematology, 3rd ed. Philadelphia, Lea and Febiger, 1975.

Schalm OW, Lasmanis J: Cytologic features of bone marrow in normal and mastitic cows. Am J Vet Res 37:359, 1976.

Schnuda ND: Circulation and migration of small blood lymphocytes in the rat. Am J Pathol 93:623, 1978.

Scott DW, Kirk RW, Bentinck-Smith J: Some effects of short-term methylprednisolone therapy in normal cats. Cornell Vet 69:104, 1978.

Smith VD, Blackwell LH, Overman RR: Evidence for bone marrow cell attrition as a mechanism for granulocyte regulation in the canine. Fed Proc 31:342, 1972.

Straub OC: Bovine hematology. Berlin, Paul Parey, 1981.

Straub OC, Schalm OW, Hughes JP, et al: Bovine hematology. II. Effect of parturition and retention of fetal membranes on blood morphology. J Am Vet Med Assoc 135:618, 1959.

Tennant B, Harrold D, Reina-Guerra M: Hematology of the neonatal calf. II. Response associated with acute enteric infections, Gram-negative septicemia, and experimental endotoxemia. Cornell Vet 65:457, 1975.

Tumbleson ME, Scholl E: Hematology and clinical chemistry. In Leman AD, Glock RD, Mengeling WL, et al (eds): Diseases of swine, 5th ed, Ames, Iowa State University Press, 1981.

Tyler DE, Ramsey FK: Comparative pathologic, immunologic, and clinical responses produced by selected agents of the bovine mucosal disease-virus diarrhea complex. Am J Vet Res 26:903, 1965.

Watson ADJ, Wilson JT, Turner DM, et al: Phenylbutazone-induced blood dyscrasias suspected in three dogs. Vet Rec 107:239, 1980.

Weller PF, Goetzl EJ: The human eosinophil: Roles in host defense and tissue injury. Am J Pathol 100:793, 1980.

Wilkins RJ: Morphologic features of feline peripheral blood lymphocytes. J Am Anim Hosp Assoc 10:362, 1974.

Yu DTY, Clements PJ, Paulus HE, et al: Human lymphocyte subpopulations: Effect of corticosteroids. J Clin Invest 53:565, 1974.

Zatz MM, Lance EM: The distribution of ^{51}Cr-labelled lymphocytes into antigen-stimulated mice: Lymphocyte trapping. J Exp Med 134:224, 1971.

3
Hematopoietic Neoplasia

LYMPHOPROLIFERATIVE DISORDERS

This group of neoplastic disorders originates from lymphocytes or plasma cells in a variety of tissues.

   I. Lymphosarcoma

      A. Definitions

          1. Lymphosarcoma (malignant lymphoma) is a neoplasm of lymphocytes arising as sarcomatous masses in lymphoid organs other than bone marrow.

          2. Lymphosarcoma (lymphoid leukemia) is a neoplasm of lymphocytes arising from bone marrow and involving the blood.

          3. A leukemic blood profile is the presence of neoplastic cells (lymphocytes) in the peripheral blood. This may occur in some cases of lymphosarcoma (malignant lymphoma) and always occurs in lymphosarcoma (lymphoid leukemia).

          4. In the past the following terms have been used as synonyms: lymphosarcoma, malignant lymphoma, lymphoid leukemia, lymphocytic leukemia, lymphatic leukemia, leukosis, lymphomatosis, and lymphocytoma.

      B. Classification. Classification of these tumors into various subtypes may facilitate diagnosis and aid in predicting the clinical course, prognosis, and response to therapy of the disease. Different types of classification have been used based on the following:

          1. Anatomic distribution

             a. Multicentric. Widespread involvement of lymph nodes occurs as well as infiltration of a variety of organs.

             b. Thymic. The thymus is usually the only organ involved; therefore, this form occurs primarily in young animals.

             c. Alimentary. The gastrointestinal tract and its regional lymph nodes are affected. Other abdominal

viscera may be infiltrated, but superficial lymph
nodes are not usually involved.

    d. Skin. Lesions are usually multiple in this form,
which may progress into a multicentric form in the
later stages.

    e. Solitary. Isolated tumors may occur in a single
lymph node or organ.

    f. Leukemic. The neoplastic cells originate in the
bone marrow. Discrete tumorous masses are uncommon
except late in the disease in protracted cases.
Many classifications separate this form from those
characterized by tumorous masses (malignant
lymphoma) and call it lymphoid leukemia. Acute and
chronic forms may occur.

2. Histologic architecture of affected lymph node

    a. Nodular. This is a rare form in animals and may be
associated with a longer life expectancy.

    b. Diffuse. The great majority of cases are of this
type in domestic animals.

3. Cytology of neoplastic cell

    a. Attempts have been made to fit the various cell
types predominating in the lymphoid neoplasms of
animals into cytologic classification schemes used
for human neoplasms.

        (1) Lymphocytic, well-differentiated

        (2) Lymphocytic, poorly-differentiated

        (3) Lymphoblastic

        (4) Histiocytic

        (5) Mixed lymphocytic-histiocytic

    b. A simplified scheme is used by some, classifying
the lymphocytes as small, medium, and large.

    c. A functional classification in humans is based on
identification of lymphocytes by immunologic
techniques. Lymphoid tumors have been subdivided
into null cell, T cell, B cell, and mixed cell
types. Some attempts have been made to similarly
classify animal tumors.

    d. Neoplastic lymphocytes in humans are now being
classified by analyzing cell surface markers by
biochemical and immunologic techniques and
detecting certain chromosomal abnormalities.

C. Clinical staging

1. Classification into one of five stages has been used in
dogs as a means of determining prognosis. The higher
the stage, the poorer the prognosis.

    a. Stage I. Only a single lymph node or lymphoid
tissue in a single organ (excluding bone marrow)
is involved.

    b. Stage II. Several lymph nodes in a regional area
are involved.

    c. Stage III. Generalized lymph node involvement is
evident.

    d. Stage IV. Liver and spleen are infiltrated (+ Stage
III).

    e. Stage V. Neoplastic cells are demonstrated in the
blood, bone marrow, and/or other organs.

2. Each stage may be further subdivided according to the absence (A) or presence (B) of systemic signs.

D. Bovine lymphosarcoma

1. Leukosis is a term sometimes used for a proliferation of lymphocytes induced by the bovine leukemia virus (BLV) and includes both lymphosarcoma and persistent lymphocytosis, a nonneoplastic condition.

2. Several clinical forms are recognized.

   a. The adult, multicentric, or enzootic form is the most common and is caused by BLV.

   b. The other forms (calf, thymic, and skin) are sporadic and not caused by BLV.

3. Laboratory features of the adult form include the following.

   a. The WBC count is variable, ranging from leukopenia to counts greater than $100,000/\mu l$.

   b. A leukemic blood profile with a high percentage of atypical cells occurs in approximately 30% of the cases. Neoplastic cells are B cells.

   c. Anemia is uncommon except in protracted cases because of the usual rapid course of the disease, long life span of bovine erythrocytes (160 days), and infrequency of bone marrow involvement.

   d. The presence of BLV antibody is synonymous with infection but does not indicate lymphosarcoma. Less than 5% of infected animals will develop lymphosarcoma even if the animal lives to an advanced age.

4. Persistent lymphocytosis (PL), a nonneoplastic condition caused by BLV, occurs in approximately 30% of infected animals.

   a. PL is defined as a definite increase in the absolute lymphocyte count greater than the normal value for that particular age of animal for a 3-month period.

   b. PL does not indicate lymphosarcoma. It precedes lymphosarcoma in approximately 65% of the cases, but only a small percentage of cows with PL develop lymphosarcoma.

   c. The lymphocytes involved are B cells, but they are different from the malignant cells of lymphosarcoma.

   d. PL is not pathognomic for BLV infection.

E. Canine lymphosarcoma (Fig. 3.1)

1. Anatomic forms include the multicentric, alimentary, thymic, skin, and leukemic forms.

2. Laboratory features may include the following.

   a. A leukemic blood profile is present in approximately 50% of the cases on initial examination; the incidence is higher in advanced disease. Neoplastic cells are fragile and may be disrupted on the blood smear.

   b. Granulocytic leukemoid blood pictures may occur in some cases.

   c. Lymphocyte counts vary from absolute lymphopenia to lymphocytosis.

    d. A mild nonregenerative anemia is common.
    e. Bone marrow involvement occurs in advanced cases.
    f. Thrombocytopenia is common.
    g. Dysproteinemias have been reported.
    h. Hypercalcemia from pseudohyperparathyroidism occurs
        in some cases (Case 9).
F. Feline lymphosarcoma (Fig. 3.1)
    1. The disease is caused by the feline leukemia virus
        (FeLV), but some animals may be negative for the virus
        at the time of diagnosis. The FeLV test detects
        infection with the virus and indicates viremia. A
        positive test does not signify lymphosarcoma. Only
        approximately one-third of infected cats will develop
        lymphosarcoma. Neoplastic cells carry the feline
        oncornavirus-associated cell membrane antigen (FOCMA).
    2. Anatomic forms include the multicentric, alimentary,
        and thymic forms. Other forms involve the bone marrow
        (lymphoid leukemia), skin, central nervous system,
        kidney, and eye.
    3. Laboratory features include the following.
        a. Approximately 70% of the cases are FeLV-positive;
            all have low (less than 1:32) or no FOCMA antibody
            titer.
        b. A leukemic blood profile occurs in approximately
            30% of the cases. Neoplastic cells are B cells.
        c. Anemia is common; it is usually nonregenerative,
            but regenerative anemias do occur. Anemia may
            be caused by a variety of mechanisms; some are
            related directly to FeLV infection, and others are
            secondary to lymphosarcoma.
        d. FeLV-negative lymphosarcomas are less likely to be
            associated with anemia and leukemic blood profiles.
            Alimentary forms are more likely to be FeLV-
            negative.
        e. Normal white blood cell counts or leukopenia are
            more common than leukocytosis.
        f. Bone marrow findings are variable, depending on the
            type of anemia and/or leukopenia and the presence
            of neoplastic cells.
G. Equine lymphosarcoma. The disease is uncommon in the horse.
    Visceral involvement is the usual pattern (visceral lymph
    nodes, liver, spleen, gastrointestinal tract, and kidney),
    although peripheral lymph nodes may be affected in some
    cases. A leukemic blood profile, usually composed of small
    lymphocytes, and anemia can occur.

II. Plasma cell myeloma (Fig. 3.1)
    A. This neoplasm of plasma cells is a single clone that
        produces a homogeneous immunoglobulin or immunoglobulin
        subunit in excess.
    B. Clinical and anatomic features include the following.
        1. The tumor usually occurs in bones engaged in
            hematopoiesis.
        2. Multiple focal osteolytic lesions leading to pain and
            pathologic fractures may occur.

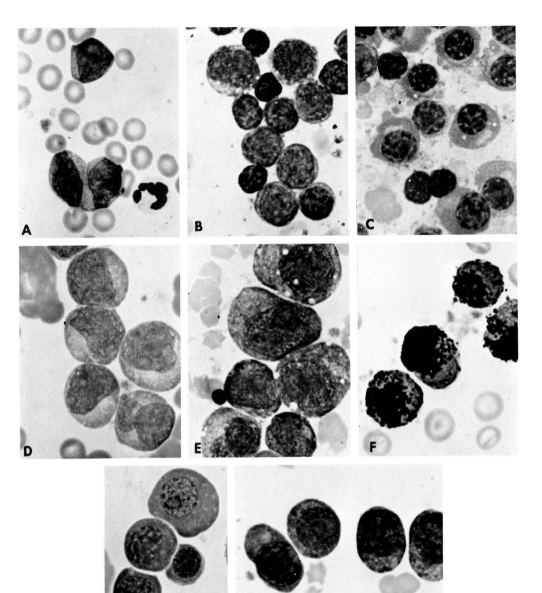

Fig. 3.1. Neoplastic hematopoietic cells. A. Immature lymphocytes in the blood of a dog with lymphosarcoma, B. immature
lymphocytes in the bone marrow of a cat with lymphocytic
leukemia, C. plasma cells predominating in the bone marrow in a
case of plasma cell myeloma in a dog, D. immature granulocytes
in the blood of a dog with granulocytic leukemia, E. large
granulocyte precursors in the bone marrow of a cat with preleukemia (subleukemic granulocytic leukemia), F. mast cells
infiltrating the bone marrow of a dog with a malignant mast
cell tumor of the skin, G. megaloblastoid rubricytes in the
bone marrow from a case of erythremic myelosis in a cat,
H. primitive cells characteristic of the blast form of
erythremic myelosis (reticuloendotheliosis) in the bone marrow
of a cat. (Wright's stain, ×1100.) (B, C, E, F, G, H from
Duncan JR, Prasse KW: Clinical examination of bone marrow.
Vet Clin North Am 6:597, 1976.)

3. Extramarrow origin is uncommon; metastasis can occur.
4. A bleeding diathesis may be associated with some forms and is due to thrombocytopenia and serum hyperviscosity.
5. Infections may result from immunodeficiency and/or neutropenia.
6. Renal dysfunction is associated with some tumors.

C. Laboratory features include the following.
1. Hyperglobulinemia is a consistent finding.
    a. A monoclonal, narrow-base, globulin spike is found in the beta or gamma region of the electrophoretogram (see Fig. 6.1).
        (1) This abnormal globulin is referred to as a paraprotein or M component.
        (2) It may be a complete immunoglobulin or light or heavy chain.
        (3) Monoclonal gammopathies may occur with lymphosarcoma.
    b. Depression of other immunoglobulins and normal immunoglobulins of the same class may lead to immunodeficiency; paraproteins are without immunoglobulin activity.
    c. Hypoalbuminemia may be evident.
2. Paraproteinuria occurs in approximately 20% of the cases.
    a. Light chains (Bence-Jones protein) are small enough to pass a normal glomerulus into the urine.
    b. Paraproteinuria is not detected by the usual reagent strip test for urine protein; urine electrophoresis is the most reliable test (see Fig. 6.1).
3. Abnormal bone marrow cytology is a usual diagnostic feature.
    a. Plasma cells in various stages of maturation are observed in marrow aspirates.
    b. The lesion may be missed unless an affected site is aspirated.
    c. Plasma cells may be observed in small numbers (usually less than 10%) in bone marrow aspirates from normal animals and from animals with a variety of other disease conditions.
4. Circulating plasma cells are uncommon.
5. Myelophthisis may result in nonregenerative anemia, thrombocytopenia, and leukopenia.
6. Hypercalcemia may result from osteolysis or pseudohyperparathyroidism.
7. Azotemia may accompany associated renal disease.
8. Hyperviscosity syndrome is a feature of some tumors.
    a. This syndrome is caused by high molecular weight IgM or polymerized IgA.
    b. Defective intrinsic clotting and platelet dysfunction together with thrombocytopenia and vascular lesions may lead to a bleeding diathesis.

D. Diagnosis
1. Two of the following are required for a diagnosis.
    a. Osteolytic lesion

        b. Neoplastic plasma cells
        c. Monoclonal gammopathy, excluding IgM types (IgM
           types are referred to as macroglobulinemia)
        d. Bence-Jones proteinuria
    2. Related disorders are:
        a. Macroglobulinemia, a neoplastic disorder associated
           with the excessive production of IgM
        b. Benign monoclonal gammopathy, a nonneoplastic
           disease

MYELOPROLIFERATIVE DISORDERS

This group of neoplastic diseases originates from cells normally produced by the bone marrow. Bone marrow hyperplasia, splenomegaly, hepatomegaly, and mild lymphadenopathy characterize these diseases. Sarcomatous masses are usually not observed; neoplastic cells infiltrate the organs of the monocyte-macrophage system (e.g., sinusoids of the lymph nodes, liver, spleen, and bone marrow). The diseases are most common in the cat, occasionally observed in the dog, and rare in other species.

  I. Granulocytic leukemia (Fig. 3.1)
    A. The blood picture may not be diagnostic on initial
       presentation; the disease should be followed with
       sequential hemograms.
    B. In the dog the leukocyte blood picture is variable. Two
       general blood pictures are observed.
      1. Neutrophilia with left shift (chronic granulocytic
         leukemia)
        a. The leukogram is similar to that of severe
           inflammation in which there is a leukemoid blood
           picture.
        b. This form of granulocytic leukemia is
           differentiated from a leukemoid blood picture by:
           (1) Following the course of the disease
           (2) Recognizing a source of inflammation that
               would cause a leukemoid blood picture
           (3) Observing some of the following cytologic
               abnormalities of neutrophils in blood and bone
               marrow smears
               (a) Immature forms
               (b) Uneven left shift
               (c) Variation in size and shape
               (d) Asynchronous maturation
               (e) Hypersegmentation
        c. The disease may terminate in a blast crisis.
      2. Neutrophilia with large numbers of blast forms (acute
         granulocytic leukemia)
        a. The blast cells must be differentiated from
           lymphoblasts and monoblasts.
        b. After using selective stains for cytoplasmic
           enzymes, blast neutrophils are positive for
           peroxidase and naphthol AS-D chloroacetate
           esterase, and negative for lipase and alpha
           naphthyl acetate esterase.

C. In the cat most cases are FeLV-positive.
    1. The leukogram usually exhibits sufficient dif-
        ferentiation to determine that the neutrophil is the
        neoplastic cell; it must be differentiated from a
        leukemoid blood picture (as described above for the
        dog).
    2. Granulocytic leukemia in the cat may be the terminal
        stage of a disease that has progressed from erythremic
        myelosis to erythroleukemia to granulocytic leukemia;
        it is similar to the Di Guglielmo syndrome of humans.
    3. A preleukemia or dysmyelopoietic form may occur in cats
        (Case 8).
        a. It is characterized by persistent neutropenia in
            the face of granulocytic hyperplasia in the bone
            marrow. Immature forms predominate in the marrow
            and may be found in small numbers in the blood. A
            nonregenerative anemia is often present.
        b. The disease may or may not progress to granulocytic
            leukemia; it has been called subleukemic granulo-
            cytic leukemia.
        c. These cats are usually FeLV-positive.
D. In both dogs and cats the following are found.
    1. Nonregenerative anemia, often very severe
    2. Thrombocytopenia with bizarre, large platelets
    3. Hypercellular bone marrow in which:
        a. Immature granulocytes predominate.
        b. Granulocytic immaturity may be more obvious than in
            peripheral blood.
        c. Erythroid cells and megakaryocytes are markedly
            reduced in number.

II. Eosinophilic leukemia. This rare myeloproliferative disorder is
     characterized by marked eosinophilia with variable maturation.
     Feline forms have not been shown to be caused by FeLV, and the
     disease has not been documented in the dog. Occasionally, an
     eosinophilic leukemoid blood picture may accompany alimentary
     lymphosarcoma in the cat.

III. Basophilic leukemia. Basophils predominate in the blood and
     bone marrow of this rare disease. The single feline case was
     FeLV-positive. Basophilic leukemia is differentiated from mast
     cell leukemia by the presence of segmented nuclei and more
     uniform granulation in neoplastic basophils.

IV. Monocytic leukemia. The disease is usually characterized by a
     marked monocytosis with immature forms. The bone marrow is
     hyperplastic as a result of immature monocytes, but the
     associated anemia is usually mild. Histochemically, monocytes
     are alpha naphthyl acetate esterase, lipase, and sometimes
     peroxidase positive and reveal bundles of cytoplasmic micro-
     filaments on electron microscopic examination. The disease may
     progress to the myelomonocytic form in the dog.

V.   Myelomonocytic leukemia
     A. This disorder is characterized by immature monocytes and
         neutrophils in the blood and bone marrow.

    B. Histochemical staining for neutrophil and monocyte markers are helpful and usually essential.
      1. Neutrophils are AS-D chloroacetate esterase positive.
      2. Monocytes are alpha naphthyl acetate esterase and lipase positive.
      3. Both cell types are Sudan black B, peroxidase, and PAS positive.
    C. Other laboratory findings may include:
      1. Macrocytic, normochromic, nonregenerative anemia
      2. Normal WBC count to marked leukocytosis
      3. Hypercellular bone marrow
      4. Thrombocytopenia
      5. Positive FeLV test in feline cases

VI. Erythremic myelosis (Fig. 3.1)
    A. This myeloproliferative disorder involves the erythroid series and occurs primarily in cats; it is caused by FeLV. A blast form of this disease was formerly called reticuloendotheliosis.
    B. Laboratory findings include:
      1. Severe nonregenerative anemia
      2. High nucleated RBC count in the absence of significant reticulocytosis or polychromasia
      3. Blast cells in the blood and bone marrow in varying numbers, from none to 95% of the nucleated cells
      4. Occasionally, megaloblastoid rubricytes and binucleated and mitotic cells in the blood and bone marrow
      5. Hyperplastic erythroid bone marrow with all stages of maturation present except in the blast form, where the primitive cell predominates.
    C. In the cat, the disease may progress to erythroleukemia and granulocytic leukemia.

VII. Erythroleukemia. This disease is a transition stage between erythremic myelosis and granulocytic leukemia. Characteristics of both diseases are present. It is described in FeLV-positive cats.

VIII. Megakaryocytic leukemia (megakaryocytic myelosis)
    A. The disease in the cat is FeLV-positive and is characterized by anemia, bizarre platelets in the blood, and an increase in megakaryocytes in the spleen and bone marrow. Undifferentiated cells may be observed in the blood.
    B. In the dog, anemia, thrombocytopenia, blast cells in the blood and bone marrow, and numerous megakaryocytes in various organs characterize the disease.

IX. Mast cell leukemia (systemic mastocytosis) (Fig. 3.1). Although not considered a strict hematopoietic cell neoplasm, mast cell neoplasms of cats often behave like myeloproliferative disorders. In the systemic form of the disease, a leukemic blood profile is commonly observed; neoplastic cells infiltrate the spleen, bone marrow, lymph nodes, and liver. The skin may be involved in some cases. These mast cells differ from basophils by their large size; round to oval nuclei; and large, prominently stained granules.

REFERENCES

Allan GS, Watson ADJ, Duff BC, et al: Disseminated mastocytoma and mastocytemia in a dog.
    J Am Vet Med Assoc 165:346, 1974.
Alroy J: Basophilic leukemia in a dog. Vet Pathol 9:90, 1972.
Andersen AC, Johnson RM: Erythroblastic malignancy in a beagle. J Am Vet Med Assoc
    141:944, 1962.
Barthel CH: Acute myelomonocytic leukemia in a dog. Vet Pathol 11:79, 1974.
Boudreaux MK, Blue JT, Durham SK, et al: Intravascular leukostasis in a horse with
    myelomonocytic leukemia. Vet Pathol 21:544, 1984.
Braund KG, Everett RM, Bartels JE, et al: Neurologic complications of IgA multiple myeloma
    associated with cryoglobulinemia in a dog. J Am Vet Med Assoc 174:1321, 1979.
Brumbough GW, Stitzel KA, Zinkl JG, et al: Myelomonocytic myeloproliferative disease in a
    horse. J Am Vet Med Assoc 180:313, 1982.
Burkhardt E, Saldern F, Huskamp B: Monocytic leukemia in a horse. Vet Pathol 21:394, 1984.
Cotter SM, Hardy WD, Essex M: Association of feline leukemia virus with lymphosarcoma and
    other disorders in the cat. J Am Vet Med Assoc 166:449, 1975.
Couto CG: Preleukemia syndrome in a dog. J Am Vet Med Assoc 184:1389, 1984.
Crow SE: Lymphosarcoma (malignant lymphoma) in the dog: Diagnosis and treatment. Compend
    Contin Educ Pract Vet 4:283, 1982.
Crow SE, Madewell BR, Henness AM: Feline reticuloendotheliosis: A report of four cases.
    J Am Vet Med Assoc 170:1239, 1977.
Dust A, Norris AM, Valli VED: Cutaneous lymphosarcoma with IgG monoclonal gammopathy,
    serum hyperviscosity and hypercalcemia in a cat. Can Vet J 23:235, 1982.
Ferrer JF: Bovine lymphosarcoma. Adv Vet Sci Comp Med 24:1, 1980.
Ferrer JF, Bhatt DM, Abt DA, et al: Serological diagnosis of infection with the putative
    bovine leukemia virus. Cornell Vet 65:527, 1975.
Ferrer JF, Marshak RR, Abt DA, et al: Relationship between lymphosarcoma and persistent
    lymphocytosis in cattle: A review. J Am Vet Med Assoc 175:705, 1979.
Fowler EH, Wilson GP, Roenigk WJ, et al: Mast cell leukemia in three dogs. J Am Vet Med
    Assoc 149:281, 1966.
Fraser CJ, Joiner GN, Jardine JH, et al: Acute granulocytic leukemia in cats. J Am Vet Med
    Assoc 165:355, 1974.
Garner FM, Lingeman CH: Mast-cell neoplasms of the domestic cat. Pathol Vet 7:517, 1970.
Gilmore CE, Gilmore VH, Jones TC: Reticuloendotheliosis, a myeloproliferative disorder of
    cats: A comparison with lymphocytic leukemia. Pathol Vet 1:161, 1964.
Green RA, Barton CL: Acute myelomonocytic leukemia in a dog. J Am Anim Hosp Assoc 13:708,
    1977.
Guerre R, Millet P, Groulade P: Systemic mastocytosis in a cat: Remission after
    splenectomy. J Small Anim Pract 20:769, 1979.
Hardy WD Jr: Hematopoietic tumors of cats. J Am Anim Hosp Assoc 17:921, 1981.
Hardy WD Jr: Feline leukemia virus non-neoplastic diseases. J Am Anim Hosp Assoc 17:941,
    1981.
Hardy WD Jr: The feline leukemia virus. J Am Anim Hosp Assoc 17:951, 1981.
Harvey JW: Myeloproliferative disorders in dogs and cats. Vet Clin North Am 11:349, 1984.
Harvey JW, Shields RP, Gaskin JM: Feline myeloproliferative disease: Changing
    manifestations in the peripheral blood. Vet Pathol 15:437, 1978.
Henness AM, Crow SE, Anderson BC: Monocytic leukemia in three cats. J Am Vet Med Assoc
    170:1325, 1977.
Hodgkins EM, Zinkl JG, Madewell BR: Chronic lymphocytic leukemia in the dog. J Am Vet Med
    Assoc 177:704, 1980.
Holscher MA, Collins RD, Cousar JB, et al: Megakaryocytic leukemia in a cat. Feline Pract
    13(4):8, 1983.
Holscher MA, Collins RD, Griffith BO: Megakaryocytic leukemia in a dog. Vet Pathol 15:562,
    1978.
Hoover EA, Kociba GJ: Bone lesions in cats with anemia induced by feline leukemia virus.
    J Natl Cancer Inst 53:1277, 1974.
Hribernik TN, Barta O, Gaunt SD, et al: Serum hyperviscosity syndrome associated with IgG
    myeloma in a cat. J Am Vet Med Assoc 181:169, 1982.
Jain NC, Madewell BR, Weller RE, et al: Clinical-pathological findings and cytochemical
    characterization of myelomonocytic leukaemia in five dogs. J Comp Pathol 91:17, 1981.
Jarrett WFH, Anderson LJ, Jarrett O, et al: Myeloid leukaemia in a cat produced
    experimentally by feline leukaemia virus. Res Vet Sci 12:385, 1971.
Latimer KS, Dykstra MJ: Acute monocytic leukemia in a dog. J Am Vet Med Assoc 184:852,
    1984.
Leifer LE, Matus RE, Patnaik AK, et al: Chronic myelogenous leukemia in the dog. J Am Vet
    Med Assoc 183:686, 1983.
Lester SJ, Searcy GP: Hematologic abnormalities preceding apparent recovery from feline
    leukemia virus infection. J Am Vet Med Assoc 178:471, 1981.
Linnabary RD, Holscher MA, Glick AD, et al: Acute myelomonocytic leukemia in a dog. J Am
    Anim Hosp Assoc 14:71, 1978.

Liska WD, MacEwen EG, Zaki FA, et al: Feline systemic mastocytosis: A review and results of splenectomy in seven cases. J Am Anim Hosp Assoc 15:589, 1979.

Liu S, Carb AV: Erythroblastic leukemia in a dog. J Am Vet Med Assoc 152:1511, 1968.

Loeb WF, Rininger B, Montgomery CA, et al: Myelomonocytic leukemia in a cat. Vet Pathol 12:464, 1975.

MacEwen EG, Drazner FH, McClelland AJ, et al: Treatment of basophilic leukemia in a dog. J Am Vet Med Assoc 166:376, 1975.

MacEwen EG, Hurvitz AI: Diagnosis and management of monoclonal gammopathies. Vet Clin North Am 7:119, 1977.

MacEwen EG, Hurvitz AI, Hayes A: Hyperviscosity syndrome associated with lymphocytic leukemia in three dogs. J Am Vet Med Assoc 170:1309, 1977.

MacEwen EG, Patnaik AK, Johnson GF, et al: Extramedullary plasmacytoma of the gastrointestinal tract in two dogs. J Am Vet Med Assoc 184:1396, 1984.

Mackey L: Feline leukaemia virus and its clinical effects in cats. Vet Rec 96:5, 1975.

Mackey LJ, Jarrett WFH, Lauder IM: Monocytic leukaemia in a dog. Vet Rec 96:27, 1975.

Madewell BR, Jain NC, Weller RE: Hematologic disorders preceding myeloid leukemia in three cats. Vet Pathol, 16:510, 1979.

Michel RL, O'Handley P, Dade AW: Megakaryocytic myelosis in a cat. J Am Vet Med Assoc 168:1021, 1976.

Miller C, Fish MB, Danelski TF: IgA multiple myeloma with multi-system manifestations in the dog: A case report. J Am Anim Hosp Assoc 18:53, 1982.

Miller JM: Bovine lymphosarcoma. Mod Vet Pract 61:588, 1980.

Mills JN, Eger CE, Robinson WE, et al: A case of multiple myeloma in a cat. J Am Anim Hosp Assoc 18:79, 1982.

Moulton JE: Tumors in domestic animals. Berkeley, University of California Press, 1978.

Onions DE: B- and T-cells in canine lymphosarcoma. Vet Rec 97:108, 1975.

Osborne CA, Perman V, Sautter JH, et al: Multiple myeloma in the dog. J Am Vet Med Assoc 153:1300, 1968.

Pollett L, Van Hove W, Mattheeuws D: Blastic crisis in chronic myelogenous leukaemia in a dog. J Small Anim Pract 19:469, 1978.

Ragan HA, Hackett PL, Dogle GE: Acute myelomonocytic leukemia manifested as myelophthisic anemia in a dog. J Am Vet Med Assoc 169:421, 1976.

Rebhun WC, Bertone A: Equine lymphosarcoma. J Am Vet Med Assoc 184:720, 1984.

Roberts MC: A case of primary lymphoid leukemia in a horse. Equine Vet J 9:216, 1977.

Schalm OW: Myeloproliferative disorder in a cat with a period of remission followed by a relapse two years later. Calif Vet 27(4):18, 1973.

Schalm OW: Manual of feline and canine hematology. Santa Barbara, Calif, Veterinary Practice Publishing Co, 1980.

Schalm OW, Theilen GH: Myeloproliferative disease in the cat, associated with C-type leukovirus particles in bone marrow. J Am Vet Med Assoc 157:1686, 1970.

Searcy GP, Orr JP: Chronic granulocytic leukemia in a horse. Can Vet J 22:148, 1981.

Shepard VJ, Dodds-Laffin WJ, Laffin RJ: Gamma A myeloma in a dog with defective hemostasis. J Am Vet Med Assoc 160:1121, 1972.

Shull RM, Osborne CA, Barrett RE, et al: Serum hyperviscosity syndrome associated with IgA multiple myeloma in two dogs. J Am Anim Hosp Assoc 14:58, 1978.

Silverman J: Eosinophilic leukemia in a cat. J Am Vet Med Assoc 158:, 1971.

Simon N, Holzworth J: Eosinophilic leukemia in a cat. Cornell Vet 57:579, 1967.

Sodikoff DH, Schalm OW: Primary bone marrow disease in the cat. III. Erythremic myelosis and myelofibrosis, a myeloproliferative disorder. Calif Vet 22(6):16, 1968.

Squire RA: A cytologic study of malignant lymphoma in cattle, dogs, and cats. Am J Vet Res 26:97, 1965.

Straub OC: Diagnosis of enzootic bovine leukosis: A comparison of haematological and immunodiffusion tests. Res Vet Sci 25:13, 1978.

Theilen GH, Fowler ME: Lymphosarcoma (lymphocytic leukemia) in the horse. J Am Vet Med Assoc 140:923, 1962.

Thrall MA: Lymphoproliferative disorders. Vet Clin North Am 11:321, 1981.

Valli VE, McSherry BJ, Dunham BM, et al: Histocytology of lymphoid tumors in the dog, cat, and cow. Vet Pathol 18:494, 1981.

Van Pelt RW, Conner GH: Clinicopathologic survey of malignant lymphoma in the dog. J Am Vet Med Assoc 152:976, 1968.

Ward JM, Sodikoff CH, Schalm OW: Myeloproliferative disease and abnormal erythrogenesis in the cat. J Am Vet Med Assoc 155:879, 1969.

Zawidzka ZZ, Jansen E, Grice HC: Erythremic myelosis in a cat. Pathol Vet 1:530, 1964.

4

Hemostasis

ESSENTIAL CONCEPTS

Hemostasis involves the interaction of blood vessels, platelets, and clotting factors to convert soluble fibrinogen to insoluble
fibrin and prevent hemorrhage. The fibrin clot is subsequently
removed by fibrinolysis.

I. Endothelial cell function
    A. Endothelium forms a nonthrombogenic surface, which is
        necessary for blood to flow freely.
    B. Secretory functions
        1. Endothelial cells synthesize von Willebrand's factor,
            which is absorbed by circulating platelets and
            necessary for their adherence to collagen.
        2. Endothelial cells secrete prostacyclin, a prostaglandin
            with a very short half-life.
            a. In health, small amounts of prostacyclin prevent
                platelet aggregation on the endothelial surface.
            b. During endothelial injury a synthetic burst of
                prostacyclin has local activity opposing
                hemostasis.
                (1) Platelet aggregation is inhibited.
                (2) Prostacyclin is a potent vasodilator.
                (3) Whereas the functions are counterproductive to
                    hemostasis, large areas of vascular endo-
                    thelial loss in disease favors unopposed
                    platelet activity and thrombosis.
        3. Injured cells release tissue thromboplastin (a
            lipoprotein) that initiates the extrinsic coagulation
            system and a protease that activates the intrinsic
            coagulation system.
        4. Venous endothelial cells release an activator of
            plasminogen that mediates fibrinolysis, another reason
            lack of endothelium favors thrombosis.
        5. Endothelial cells and fibroblasts secrete fibronectin,
            which is cross-linked to fibrin and is necessary for

fibrin attachment to cells or phagocytosis by
macrophages.
6. Endothelial cells secrete antithrombin III, which
combines with heparin and inhibits several factors of
coagulation.
C. Endothelial cells are dependent on circulating platelets to
maintain vascular integrity. Thrombocytopenia may allow
reversible endothelial cell attenuation and fenestration
culminating in petechiation.

II. Platelet function and production
A. Platelets adhere to exposed collagen within seconds after
injury, forming a hemostatic plug that is sufficient to
control bleeding from minute injuries of small vessels.
B. Adherent platelets release hemostatically active
substances.
1. Within milliseconds, adherent platelets undergo con-
formational change and release adenosine diphosphate
(ADP).
a. ADP is sticky and promotes a secondary wave of
platelet adherence.
b. ADP activates platelet phospholipase A2, initiating
synthesis of thromboxane A2, a prostaglandin with a
very short half-life. Secreted thromboxane A2
causes marked, irreversible platelet aggregation
and local, intense vasoconstriction.
2. Aggregated platelets undergo viscous metamorphosis, and
several substances associated with platelet membranes
(fibrinogen, factors V and VIII, and calcium) are
released within the gelatinous mass and localized at
the site of injury.
3. Platelet phospholipid released from the platelet
membrane accelerates intrinsic and common systems of
coagulation.
4. A variety of other substances are released by
aggregated platelets: a contractile protein, mitogens,
serotonin, a heparin antagonist, and others.
C. Platelets are produced by cytoplasmic demarcation of
megakaryocytes and released directly into the blood.
1. Maturation from megakaryoblast to platelet release
requires 4 to 5 days (in humans).
2. Platelet circulating life span is approximately 10
days.
3. Platelet production is regulated by the hormone thrombopoietin. Thrombopoietin concentration is controlled
by circulating platelet mass, not platelet number.
The hormone is adsorbed to the platelet surface; low
platelet mass has less adsorbed hormone, and more is
available for stimulating platelet production.
4. A splenic pool of platelets making up 20 to 30% of the
circulating platelet mass can affect platelet number.
Splenic contraction increases and splenic congestion
decreases the blood platelet number; such reactions do
not change platelet mass or platelet production.

III. Coagulation and fibrinolytic systems. Sequential clotting

factor activation yields thrombin, an enzyme that causes
fibrinogen polymerization to form fibrin (Fig. 4.1).
A. Components of the coagulation and fibrinolytic systems
    1. Enzymatic factors. Coagulation enzymes occur as
        zymogens in plasma and originate from liver. Factor VII
        may circulate in an active form.
        a. Clotting ability correlates with enzyme concen-
            tration. Partial deficiency causes partial loss of
            clotting potential and hemorrhage.
        b. Activated enzymatic factors are inhibited in
            vivo by the natural inhibitors, antithrombin III
            (complexed with heparin), and certain alpha-2-
            glycoproteins.
        c. Activated enzymatic factors are not consumed by the
            clotting reaction and are present in serum.
        d. The plasma half-life of these factors varies from
            hours to a few days. Factor VII has the shortest
            half-life, 4 to 6 hours.
        e. Enzymatic factors include:
            (1) Contact factors, XI and XII

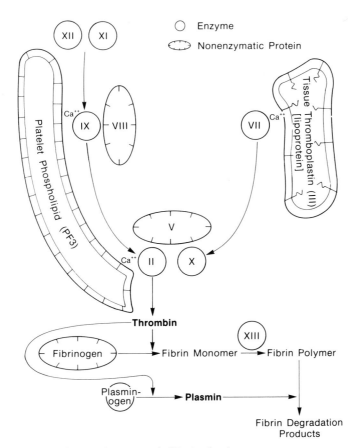

Fig. 4.1. Schema of coagulation and fibrinolysis.

(2) Vitamin K-dependent factors, II, VII, IX and X
(3) Plasminogen
(4) Clot stabilizing factor, XIII

    f. Intrinsic system clotting, involving factors XI,
XII, prekallikrein, and high molecular weight
kininogen, is activated when plasma interacts with
negatively charged substances: in vivo, collagen,
pyrophosphate from platelets, or endotoxin; in
vitro, glass, kaolin, or celite.

2. Nonenzymatic protein factors. These factors, origina-
ting from liver, associate with platelet membranes and
are localized during hemostasis by platelet aggregation, although each is present in plasma.

    a. Normal clotting can occur with partial deficiency.
Almost complete absence of a nonenzymatic factor is
necessary to cause hemorrhage or prolong clotting
time.

    b. Natural inhibitors of nonenzymatic proteins are not
described, but in vivo control is maintained by
localization within the platelet plug.

    c. Clotting consumes nonenzymatic factors; therefore,
they are absent in serum.

    d. Nonenzymatic protein factors include V, VIII, and
fibrinogen. These proteins also are said to be
"reactive proteins"; the plasma concentrations
increase during inflammatory or neoplastic
diseases. The plasma half-life is hours to days.

3. Platelet phospholipid. This substance, derived from
platelet membranes, provides a structural micelle upon
which coagulation factor activation is greatly
accelerated.

4. Tissue thromboplastin, factor III. This factor is
phospholipid complexed with a protein, thereby a
lipoprotein.

    a. The protein moiety gives the factor specificity to
react only with factor VII of the extrinsic system.

    b. Injured cells of any kind release factor III, and
extrinsic clotting proceeds instantly. Samples
obtained by clean venipuncture undergo intrinsic
clotting, with 5 to 15 minutes until clot formation. Samples contaminated by factor III during
difficult venipuncture may clot in 12 to 15
seconds.

5. Calcium. In hypocalcemia, life-threatening
neuromuscular diseases can occur, but sufficient
calcium is always available for hemostasis.
Anticoagulants such as EDTA, oxalates, or citrate
prevent clotting by binding calcium.

B. Thrombin

1. Thrombin, the essential reactant derived from the
intrinsic or extrinsic system, is activated factor II
(prothrombin).

2. Thrombin causes proteolytic cleavage of fibrinopeptides
from fibrinogen; the resultant fibrinogen molecules
polymerize, forming fibrin.

3. Thrombin has other activities, including activation of plasminogen and factors II, IX, and X. Therefore, thrombin accelerates both coagulation and fibrinolysis.
4. Thrombin is a potent platelet agonist.
C. Plasmin
1. Plasmin is activated plasminogen and hydrolyzes fibrin, forming fragments (fibrin–fibrinogen degradation products, FDP).
2. Plasmin is a nonspecific enzyme that can hydrolyze fibrinogen and factors V and VIII.
3. Fibrin degradation products are removed from a reactive site or circulation by macrophages. If FDP formation exceeds removal and the concentration increases, fibrin formation and platelet adherence are inhibited.

MEANS OF LABORATORY EVALUATION

I. Evaluation of platelets
A. Platelet count
1. Manual counting with a hemocytometer, using ammonium oxalate solution as blood diluent, is the most accurate method. Counting must be done within 4 to 5 hours after sample collection.
2. Automatic particle counters add little accuracy because of the lack of standards. Most systems require that erythrocytes be sedimented first; this is not possible with cattle, sheep, and goat blood.
3. The best of techniques may yield counts with up to 25% error.
4. Difficult venipuncture commonly causes contamination of the sample with tissue thromboplastin and platelet aggregation. Counts may be falsely low or contain larger error. Platelet aggregation is common in samples from cats and cattle.
5. Platelet number may be affected by splenic activity. Splenic congestion may cause a false low platelet count, and splenic contraction that accompanies excitement (epinephrine response) may cause a false high platelet count.
6. Whereas most species normally have 200,000 to 400,000 platelets/μl blood, counts less than 100,000/μl are considered clinically significant. Hemorrhage from thrombocytopenia alone will not occur in most species until counts are less than 25,000/μl.
B. Platelet evaluation on blood smear
1. Experienced technologists may report that platelets are normal, increased, or decreased based on their observation of the stained blood smear. Several techniques are used to estimate decreased numbers.
   a. Less than 3 or 4 platelets/oil immersion field is a significant thrombocytopenia.
   b. Six or 7 platelets/oil immersion field is approximately 100,000 platelets/μl.
   c. Less than 1 platelet/50 red blood cells denotes

thrombocytopenia, but the presence of anemia must be considered.
   d. The number of platelets per number of white blood cells (WBC) observed on the smear multiplied by the WBC/μl is an estimate of the platelet number/μl.
2. Platelet morphology (Fig. 1.4)
   a. Platelets are small flat disks with fine reddish granules. They uniformly average 2 to 4 μm in diameter in most species. Feline platelets vary more in size, and some are as large as erythrocytes. Equine platelets stain more faintly and may be difficult to see.
   b. Large platelets (megathrombocytes, shift platelets) may be found in thrombocytopenias caused by excessive platelet destruction or utilization and by infiltrative diseases of bone marrow regardless of platelet count. The large platelets may be round or elongated.
   c. Platelets with decreased granularity or vacuoles may be seen in feline leukemia virus infection and disseminated intravascular coagulation.
C. Examination of stained bone marrow smears for megakaryocytes
   1. Normal or increased numbers of megakaryocytes in a bone marrow smear from a thrombocytopenic patient usually indicate excessive platelet consumption or destruction as the primary mechanism.
   2. Too few or no megakaryocytes in a bone marrow smear from a thrombocytopenic patient usually indicate diminished production as the cause.
D. Bleeding time is an in vivo test that measures the functional ability of platelets to plug a minute wound.
   1. The test measures the duration of bleeding from a standardized incision of hairless skin or mucous membrane.
   2. Bleeding time is a simple clinical test to detect platelet function defects (e.g., von Willebrand's disease). The sensitivity of the test is low and a normal result may not eliminate platelet function defect from the differential diagnosis.
   3. If the animal is thrombocytopenic, bleeding time is prolonged and performing the test adds no new information about the patient.
   4. Coagulation factor deficiencies do not cause an abnormal bleeding time. If the standard procedure is altered by severing a larger vessel (e.g., canine toenail), prolonged bleeding caused by platelet function defect or coagulation factor deficiency cannot be differentiated.
   5. Blood vascular disease such as vitamin C deficiency (scurvy) causes prolonged bleeding time in humans and guinea pigs, but a similar disease has not been described in domestic animals.
E. Clot retraction measures the amount of clear serum appearing around the clot in a nonanticoagulated blood

          sample. Failure of serum separation denotes a platelet
          function defect and/or thrombocytopenia.

F. Other tests of platelet function are more sophisticated and
    not adapted to practice laboratories.

    1. Platelet adhesion measures the ability of platelets to
        adhere to surfaces.

    2. Platelet aggregation measures the ability of platelets
        to attach to one another.

G. Detection of antiplatelet antibody is available only in
    specialized laboratories.

    1. Fluorescent antibody tests can be done on blood or bone
        marrow smears.

    2. Several coagulation tests require generation of
        platelet phospholipid to shorten the clotting time.
        Modifications of these tests are used to detect
        antiplatelet antibody (e.g., platelet factor III test).

    3. ELISA tests are in the development stage.

H. Factor VIII antigen associated with von Willebrand's factor

    1. Canine-specific factor VIII antigen assay is available
        in laboratories specializing in disorders of hemostasis
        in animals.

    2. Factor VIII antigen activity is a measurement of von
        Willebrand's factor, which is required for platelet
        adherence to collagen.

    3. The assay is used to differentiate hemophilia A (factor
        VIII deficiency with normal factor VIII antigen
        activity) from von Willebrand's disease (factor VIII
        deficiency with deficiency of factor VIII antigen).

II. Evaluation of coagulation and fibrinolysis

  A. Activated clotting time (ACT)

    1. This test measures the time required for fibrin clot
        formation in fresh whole blood.

        a. ACT is very reproducible provided that careful
            attention is given to the technical requirements;
            i.e., the tube must be prewarmed and maintained at
            $37^{\circ}C$, and a good venipuncture is required. Failure
            to warm the tube may give false high values, and
            difficulty with the venipuncture contaminates the
            blood with tissue thromboplastin and falsely
            shortens the ACT.

        b. ACT tubes are commercially prepared and contain a
            substance that potentiates contact activation and
            makes the test more sensitive than Lee-White or
            capillary tube clotting times.

    2. Increased ACT indicates deficiency of coagulation
        factor(s) within the intrinsic or common system. The
        factor deficiency must be less than 5% of normal to
        prolong ACT.

    3. Slight prolongation of ACT occurs in thrombocytopenia
        if the platelet count is less than $10,000/\mu l$. This
        effect occurs as a result of lack of platelet
        phospholipid.

    4. The ACT tube can be used for subjective assessment of
        clot quality. The clot should be firm with clear serum

appearing by 1 to 2 hours after collection. A soft
friable clot that liquefies in 30 to 60 minutes
indicates excessive fibrinolysis or hypofibrinogenemia.

B. Citrated plasma clotting tests. Using plastic syringe and
test tubes, precisely 9 parts fresh whole blood is mixed
with 1 part 3.8% trisodium citrate. Plasma should be
separated from cells by centrifugation within 30 minutes
after bleeding. Unless the analysis is run immediately, the
plasma should be quickly frozen by immersion of the tube in
a mixture of dry ice and alcohol for transport to the
laboratory. Activity of factors VII and VIII is lost
quickly at room temperature, although species vary. Equine
factors may be more stable.

1. Activated partial thromboplastin time (APTT)

    a. APTT measures the time required for fibrin clot
        formation in citrated plasma after the addition of
        an activator of factor XII, a phospholipid that
        substitutes for platelet phospholipid, and
        recalcification.

    b. Reproducible results on bovine samples requires
        exact incubation time while conducting the assay.
        This specification is contrary to the variable
        incubation time allowed by reagent manufacturers
        that is satisfactory for most other species.

    c. Increased APTT indicates coagulation factor
        deficiency in the intrinsic or common system.

        (1) Factors must be less than 30% of normal to
             prolong APTT.

        (2) Fibrinogen must be less than 50 mg/dl to
             prolong APTT.

        (3) The sensitivity of the test can be increased
             by repeating the assay on saline-diluted
             citrated plasma. An already deficient factor
             may be reduced to less than 30% of normal by
             dilution.

    d. Therapeutic anticoagulation with heparin prolongs
        APTT and can be differentiated from factor defi-
        ciency by repeating the assay on a 1:1 mixture of
        patient's plasma and normal plasma; APTT will be
        normal if the disorder is a deficiency but will
        remain prolonged if the disorder is caused by
        heparin inhibition. Prolonged APTT caused by
        coumarin therapy cannot be differentiated from a
        true factor deficiency in this way.

    e. Fibrinogen, factor VIII, and factor V concentra-
        tions may increase in inflammatory disease, causing
        the APTT to be shorter than expected.

2. One-stage prothrombin time (OSPT)

    a. OSPT measures the time required for fibrin clot
        formation in citrated plasma after the addition of
        a tissue thromboplastin and recalcification.

    b. Reagents containing rabbit brain or synthetic
        tissue thromboplastin are preferred for animal

testing. Reagents that use human brain tissue thromboplastin give much longer OSPT values on animal samples. When in doubt about reference values, compare patient results with those of a clinically normal control animal.

    c. Increased OSPT indicates coagulation factor deficiency in the common system or factor VII deficiency.

        (1) Factors must be less than 30% of normal to prolong OSPT.

        (2) Fibrinogen must be less than 50 mg/dl to prolong OSPT.

        (3) The sensitivity of the test can be increased by repeating the assay on saline–diluted citrated plasma.

  3. Thrombin clotting time (TCT)

    a. TCT measures the time required for fibrin clot formation in recalcified, fresh citrated plasma after the addition of thrombin.

    b. Increased TCT occurs with hypofibrinogenemia (less than 100 mg/dl), dysfibrinogenemia, excessive FDP concentration, dysproteinemias, or heparinization.

  4. Other tests done on citrated plasma

    a. Correction studies on APTT and OSPT are based on a 1:1 mixture of patient's plasma and correcting reagents of known factor content. The procedure is used to identify specific factor deficiencies.

    b. Russell viper venom test (Stypven time) bypasses the extrinsic and intrinsic systems and measures the activity of factors X and V, prothrombin, and fibrinogen, the common system.

    c. Specific factor analysis, particularly for factors VIII (hemophilia A or von Willebrand's disease) and IX (hemophilia B) are available in specialized laboratories working on animal bleeding disorders.

C. Fibrinogen concentration (see Chapter 6)

  1. The TCT of diluted citrated plasma is inversely proportional to fibrinogen concentration. The TCT is compared with a standard fibrinogen preparation. This method is sensitive to detect marginally decreased fibrinogen concentration.

  2. Hypofibrinogenemia occurs in disseminated intravascular coagulation, severe hepatic insufficiency, and hereditary fibrinogen deficiency.

D. Fibrin-fibrinogen degradation products (FDP)

  1. Methods

    a. FDP are commonly detected by agglutination of latex particles coated with antihuman fibrinogen fragments. The reactivity across species makes the test useful on animal samples.

    b. Protamine paracoagulation and ethanol gel tests are qualitative indicators of FDP and are used by some laboratories.

        2. Increased FDP occurs in disseminated intravascular coagulation and following severe internal bleeding from any cause.

    E. Antithrombin III activity

        1. All available methods have not been tested on animal samples.

        2. Antithrombin III activity decreases in thrombotic diseases.

DIFFERENTIAL DIAGNOSIS OF BLEEDING OR THROMBOTIC DIATHESES BY LABORATORY FINDINGS

A routine hemostasis profile includes platelet count, APTT, OSPT, TCT, fibrinogen concentration, and FDP concentration. The common causes of abnormal hemostasis can usually be differentiated by the findings in this profile and attention to details of the clinical history. Definitive diagnosis of certain hereditary deficiencies may require application of specific tests outlined in the previous section of this chapter. Common findings in hemostasis profiles are outlined.

I. Thrombocytopenia; normal ACT, APTT, OSPT, and TCT; normal fibrinogen and FDP concentrations

    A. Disorders

        1. Destruction exceeding production of platelets occurs in immune-mediated thrombocytopenias (autoimmune, iso-immune, haptenic drug-induced), early ehrlichiosis and other rickettsial diseases, and hypersplenism (Case 2).

        2. Failure in platelet production occurs in aplastic anemia, myelophthisic disease, and cytotoxic chemotherapy.

    B. Variations in the profile in these diseases

        1. A slightly prolonged ACT can occur if platelets are less than 10,000/μl.

        2. Although platelet counts of less than 100,000/μl are significant, clinical signs of hemorrhage will not occur until the count is less than 25,000/μl in most species.

II. Thrombocytosis; normal ACT, APTT, OSPT, and TCT; normal fibrinogen and FDP concentrations

    A. Disorders

        1. Increased platelet production may accompany certain feline leukovirus-associated myeloproliferative syndromes.

        2. Thrombocytosis occurs during bleeding associated with trauma, blood-sucking parasites, or neoplasms (Case 1).

        3. Thrombocytosis usually accompanies iron-lack anemia.

    B. Variations in the profile in these diseases

        1. Thrombocytosis is commonly found during routine hematology and without conducting a hemostasis profile.

        2. Increased fibrinogen concentration is expected with several of the associated diseases.

III. Thrombocytopenia; prolonged ACT, APTT, OSPT, and TCT; decreased fibrinogen and increased FDP concentrations

  A. This profile indicates disseminated intravascular coagulation (DIC) (Case 10). Causes include neoplasia, endotoxemia, septicemia, massive necrosis, intravascular hemolysis, heat stroke, altered blood flow (shock, dehydration, dirofilariasis, bradycardia, polycythemia), and others.

  B. Variations in the profile in DIC

    1. If platelet count is low yet above 25,000/μl and hemorrhage is observed, coagulation factor deficiency also is indicated to account for the hemorrhage.

    2. Factors V and VIII and fibrinogen consumption exceeds production in DIC, and this accounts for the prolonged clotting times. However, the deficiency level may be above the level of sensitivity of the clotting tests, and ACT, APTT, OSPT, and TCT may be normal; or any combination of normal and prolonged values may be found. The key to diagnosis is concomitant thrombocytopenia and factor deficiency, a combination unique to DIC.

    3. In chronic DIC, all findings may be found within normal limits, except FDP concentration remains increased.

    4. DIC may be indicated by observing rapid clot lysis after conducting the ACT test.

IV. Normal platelet count; prolonged ACT, APTT, and OSPT; normal TCT; normal fibrinogen and FDP concentrations

  A. Disorders

    1. Vitamin K antagonism or deficiency is caused by ingestion of coumarin-type poisons and rarely by failure in intestinal absorption of fats (bile insufficiency) or coumarin anticoagulation therapy (Case 24).

    2. Other causes are therapeutic heparinization, hereditary factor X deficiency (Table 4.1), and hepatic insufficiency.

  B. Variations in the profile in these diseases

    1. Because of the relative insensitivity of the clotting tests, deficiency of prothrombin and factors VII, IX, or X may be mild and remain undetected, especially in hepatic insufficiency diseases. Saline dilution of the citrated plasma and repeating the APTT and OSPT may detect the deficiency.

    2. Early in the clinical course or after mild exposure to the coumarin-type poisons only OSPT may be prolonged with normal APTT and ACT. This occurs because factor VII has the shortest half-life among the vitamin K-dependent factors, and deficiency of factor VII develops earliest or alone in these circumstances.

    3. Increased FDP concentration may occur if internal bleeding is extensive.

V. Normal platelet count; prolonged ACT and APTT; normal OSPT and

TABLE 4.1. Hereditary Coagulation Disorders in Domestic Animals

Hemophilia A, factor VIII deficiency: sex-linked
  Canine: beagle, Chihuahua, collie, English bulldog, German
            shepherd, greyhound, Irish setter, Labrador retriever,
            miniature poodle, mongrel, samoyed, schnauzer, Shetland
            sheepdog, St. Bernard, vizsla, weimaraner
  Feline: domestic
  Equine: Arabian, standardbred, thoroughbred
Hemophilia B, factor IX deficiency: sex-linked
  Canine: Alaskan malamute, black-and-tan coonhound, cairn terrier,
            cocker spaniel, English sheepdog, French bulldog, Scottish
            terrier, Shetland sheepdog, St. Bernard
  Feline: British shorthair
Factor XI deficiency: autosomal
  Canine: English springer spaniel, great Pyrenees, Kerry blue
            terrier
  Bovine: Holstein
Factor X deficiency: autosomal
  Canine: cocker spaniel
Factor XII deficiency: autosomal
  Feline: domestic
Factor VII deficiency: autosomal incomplete dominance
  Canine: beagle, Alaskan malamute
Von Willebrand's disease, factor VIII and factor VIII-related antigen
  deficiencies: autosomal incomplete dominance
  Canine: Afghan hound, Airdale terrier, basset hound, boxer, cairn
            terrier, German shepherd, golden retriever, great Dane,
            Lakeland terrier, Irish setter, Labrador retriever, Lhasa
            apso, miniature schnauzer, papillon, Pembroke Welsh corgi,
            rottweiler, Scottish terrier, Shetland sheepdog, standard
            and miniature poodle, standard and toy Manchester terrier,
            Tibetan terrier, vizsla, Wheaten terrier
  Porcine: Poland China
Von Willebrand's disease, factor VIII and factor VIII-related antigen
  deficiencies: autosomal recessive
  Canine: Chesapeake Bay retriever, Scottish terrier
Prothrombin, factor II deficiency
  Canine: boxer, miniature pinscher
Afibrinogenemia: autosomal incomplete dominance
  Caprine: Saanen
Hypofibrinogenemia
  Canine: St. Bernard
Dysfibrinogenemia
  Canine: Russian wolfhound (borzoi)
  Equine: breed unknown
Platelet function defects
  Canine: basset hound, foxhound, otterhound, Scottish terrier
  Bovine: Simmental

    Note: Hemophilia A, von Willebrand's disease in dogs, and
hemophilia B are common; the others are rare.

TCT; normal fibrinogen and FDP concentrations
   A. Disorders include hereditary hemophilia A (factor VIII
       deficiency), hemophilia B (factor IX deficiency), von
       Willebrand's disease (factor VIII and factor VIII-related
       antigen deficiencies), factor XI deficiency, and factor XII
       deficiency (Table 4.1).
   B. Heterozygotes (carriers) of these deficiencies are not
       detected by the routine hemostasis profile.

VI. Normal platelet count; normal ACT, APTT, and TCT; prolonged
     OSPT; normal fibrinogen and FDP concentrations
   A. Disorders include the early stages or mild coumarin-type
       poisoning and hereditary factor VII deficiency (Table 4.1).
   B. For variations in the coumarin-type poisoning, see section
       IV.

REFERENCES

Badylak SF, Van Vleet JF: Alteration of prothrombin time and activated partial
   thromboplastin time in dogs with hepatic disease. Am J Vet Res 42:2053, 1981.
Bell TG, Smith WL, Oxender WD, et al: Biologic interaction of prostaglandins, thromboxane,
   and prostacyclin: Potential nonreproductive veterinary clinical applications. J Am Vet
   Med Assoc 176:1195, 1980.
Bowie EJW, Owen CA, Zollman PE, et al: Tests of hemostasis in swine: Normal values and
   values in pigs affected with von Willebrand's disease. Am J Vet Res 34:1405, 1973.
Byars TD, Green CE: Idiopathic thrombocytopenic purpura in the horse. J Am Vet Med Assoc
   180:1422, 1980.
Byars TD, Ling GV, Ferris NA, et al: Activated coagulation time (ACT) of whole blood in
   normal dogs. Am J Vet Res 37:1359, 1976.
Coffman J: Hemostasis and bleeding disorders: Equine practice. Vet Med Small Anim Clin
   75:1157, 1980.
Cotter SM, Brenner RM, Dodds WJ: Hemophilia A in three unrelated cats. J Am Vet Med Assoc
   172:166, 1978.
Dodds WJ: Bleeding disorders. In Ettinger SJ (ed): A textbook of veterinary internal
   medicine, Vol 2. Philadelphia, WB Saunders Co, 1975.
Dodds WJ: Coagulation and platelet function. 2. Normal coagulation in the horse. In
   Kitchen H, Krehbiel JD (eds): Proc 1st Int Symp Equine Hematol, East Lansing, Mich,
   1975.
Dodds WJ: Hemostasis and blood coagulation. In Kaneko JJ (ed): Clinical biochemistry of
   domestic animals, 3rd ed. New York, Academic Press, 1980.
Dodds WJ: Canine von Willebrand's disease. Vet Ref Lab, Inc, Newsletter 7(4):1, 1983.
Dodds WJ: Inherited coagulation disorders in the dog. In Practice 5:54, 1983.
Dodds WJ: Bleeding disease of small animals. Vet Ref Lab, Inc, Newsletter 7(4):1, 1984.
Dodds WJ: Bleeding disease of small animals. Vet Ref Lab, Inc, Newsletter 8(3):1, 1984.
Dodds WJ, White JG: Coagulation and platelet function. 1. The normal hemostatic mechanism.
   In Kitchen H, Krehbiel JD (eds): Proc 1st Int Symp Equine Hematol, East Lansing, Mich,
   1975.
Feldman BF: Coagulopathies in small animals. J Am Vet Med Assoc 179:559, 1981.
Feldman BF: Disseminated intravascular coagulation. Compend Contin Educ Pract Vet 3:46,
   1981.
Feldman BF, Madewell BR, O'Neill S: Disseminated intravascular coagulation: Antithrombin,
   plasminogen, and coagulation abnormalities in 41 dogs. J Am Vet Med Assoc 179:151,
   1981.
Gallop PM, Lian JB, Hauschka PV: Carboxylated calcium-binding proteins and vitamin K.
   N Engl J Med 302:1460, 1980.
Green RA: Bleeding disorders. In Ettinger SJ (ed): Textbook of veterinary internal
   medicine, Vol 2, 2nd ed. Philadelphia, WB Saunders Co, 1983.
Green RA: Clinical implications of antithrombin III deficiency in animal diseases. Compend
   Contin Educ Pract Vet 6:537, 1984.
Green RA, Kabel AL: Hypercoagulable state in three dogs with nephrotic syndrome: Role of
   acquired antithrombin III deficiency. J Am Vet Med Assoc 181:914, 1982.
Green RA, White F: Feline factor XII (Hageman) deficiency. Am J Vet Res 38:893, 1977.
Hall DE: Blood coagulation and its disorders in the dog. Baltimore, Williams and Wilkins
   Co, 1972.
Hoyer LW: The factor VIII complex: Structure and function. Blood 58:1, 1981.
Jackson CM: The biochemistry of prothrombin activation. Br J Haematol 39:1, 1978.

Jaffe EA: Endothelial cells and the biology of factor VIII. N Engl J Med 296:377, 1977.

Jain NC, Switzer JW: Autoimmune thrombocytopenia in dogs and cats. Vet Clin North Am 11:421, 1981.

Johnstone IB: Inherited defects of hemostasis. Compend Contin Educ Pract Vet 4:483, 1982.

Johnstone IB: The activated partial thromboplastin time of diluted plasma: Variability due to the method of fibrin detection. Can J Comp Med 48:198, 1984.

Kociba GJ: The diagnosis of hemostatic disorders. Vet Clin North Am 6:609, 1976.

Shattil SF, Bennett JS: Platelets and their membranes in hemostasis: Physiology and pathophysiology. Ann Intern Med 94:108, 1980.

Thomson GW, McSherry BJ, Valli VEO: Endotoxin induced disseminated intravascular coagulation in cattle. Can J Comp Med 38:457, 1974.

Wagner AE: Transport of plasma for prothrombin time testing in monitoring warfarin therapy in the horse. J Am Vet Med Assoc 178:306, 1981.

Wigton DH, Kociba GJ, Hoover EA: Infectious canine hepatitis: Animal model for viral-induced disseminated intravascular coagulation. Blood 47:287, 1976.

Wilkins RJ, Hurvitz AI, Dodds WJ: Immunologically mediated thrombocytopenia in the dog. J Am Vet Med Assoc 163:277, 1973.

Williams N, Levine RF: The origin, development and regulation of megokaryocytes. Br J Haematol 52:173, 1982.

5

Water, Electrolytes, and Acid Base

by **Jeanne Wright George,**
D.V.M., Ph.D.

TOTAL BODY WATER AND OSMOLALITY

I. Total body water. Total body water volume (hydration status) is controlled primarily by intake (thirst) and renal output. These control mechanisms respond to the effective circulation volume (i.e., the extracellular fluid that perfuses the tissues).
   A. Decreased total body water (Cases 4, 6, 11)
      1. Dehydration is expressed as decreased body weight (e.g., 10% dehydration is 10% decrease in body weight).
         a. Dehydration is best evaluated by accurate measurement of loss of body weight; this is rarely attained in clinical practice. Dehydration is most often inferred by evidence of hypovolemia.
         b. Careful clinical examination is essential for recognition of hypovolemia. Loss of skin elasticity, dryness of mucous membranes, retraction of eyes, and signs of shock are evidence of dehydration.
      2. Certain laboratory tests, especially increased blood urea nitrogen (BUN), plasma protein, packed cell volume (PCV), and urine specific gravity can help confirm the clinical finding of dehydration.
         a. Many other conditions alter these values (e.g., renal disease, anemia); therefore, they should be used only in conjunction with physical examination.
         b. Once baseline values are established for these analyses, day-to-day changes are fairly sensitive markers of change in hydration.
   B. Increased total body water (Cases 7, 12, 15, 18, 22)
      1. Increased body weight is the best measure of increased body water, but it is hard to evaluate in clinical practice. Increased total body water accumulates in

Jeanne Wright George is clinical assistant professor, Department of Clinical Pathology, College of Veterinary Medicine, University of California, Davis.

extracellular fluid (ECF) (e.g., edema, ascites, hydro-thorax). Clinical examination is used to identify sites of fluid accumulation.

2. Laboratory tests are helpful in confirming that the fluid accumulation is due to transudation rather than exudation (see Chapter 12).

C. Causes of change in total body water

1. The most common causes of dehydration, characterized by increased loss of body water and its solutes, are diarrhea, vomiting, and polyuria (Cases 4, 6).
    a. The exact composition of solute in the water lost determines electrolyte and pH abnormalities.
    b. Therapy must replace both water and solutes.

2. Pure or relative water loss is an uncommon cause of dehydration. Examples are decreased intake, which occurs when animals cannot drink or are deprived of water, and increased insensible water loss, which occurs with panting or sweating; dehydration follows the latter only if intake is prevented. Therapy is directed at replacing water.

3. Increased total body water, expansion of the ECF, is caused by retention of water and Na^+. Both are needed to increase the ECF compartment.
    a. Decreases in effective circulating volume produce increased secretion of aldosterone and increased thirst, leading to increased ECF. Causes include cardiac failure and hypoproteinemia (Cases 7, 18).
    b. Certain diseases that lead to body cavity fluid accumulation (liver disorders, serosal surface tumor metastasis) produce increased ECF by increase in aldosterone and other poorly defined mechanisms (Case 12).
    c. Therapy is directed at correcting the primary problem. Restriction of Na^+ intake and use of diuretics can aid in the reduction of ECF.

II. Extracellular osmolality. ECF osmolality is maintained around 300 milliosmoles (mOsm) (isotonicity) in health. Changes in ECF osmolality cause shifts between the ECF and intracellular fluid (ICF), as water moves passively to the compartment with the higher osmolality. Electrolytes and small molecules (glucose, urea) are the major contributors to osmolality. Large molecules such as proteins have little effect.

A. Serum osmolality

1. Serum osmolality is used as a measure of ECF osmolality, but it cannot be used as a measure of total body water.

2. Direct measurement, based on freezing point depression or vapor pressure, can be performed on an osmometer. Results are expressed as milliosmoles per kilogram.

3. Estimation of serum osmolality can be made from the concentrations of sodium and potassium if the BUN and glucose are normal: $mOsm/kg = 2[Na^+ + K^+(mEq/1)]$ (mEq = milliequivalents).

4. When BUN or glucose is high, another formula should be used: $mOsm/kg = 2[Na^+ + K^+(mEq/l)] + glucose\ (mg/dl)/18 + BUN\ (mg/dl)/2.8$.

B. Hyperosmolality
   1. All animals that are hypernatremic are hyperosmolal.
   2. Accumulation of other endogenous solutes can produce hyperosmolality (e.g., glucose, ketone bodies, BUN) (Cases 16, 17). Estimation of serum osmolality may not reveal an abnormality.
   3. Exogenous poisons that are small molecules can produce hyperosmolality (e.g., ethylene glycol). Estimation of serum osmolality may not reveal an abnormality.
   4. Accumulation of a solute that does not pass freely into the ICF produces water shifts from the ICF to the ECF (e.g., Na^+, glucose, ethylene glycol). Urea passes freely between the ECF and ICF and therefore does not produce water shifts.
      a. Shift of water to the ECF causes shrinkage of cells.
      b. Dehydration may be masked and hypovolemia may not be evident on physical examination because of these internal water shifts.
      c. Rapid return of hyperosmolal ECF to isotonicity causes cellular edema. Cerebral cellular edema can produce convulsions.

C. Hypo-osmolality
   1. Hypo-osmolality always is associated with hyponatremia (Case 6), but not all cases of hyponatremia are hypo-osmolal (e.g., when associated with hyperglycemia) (Case 16).
   2. Hypo-osmolality causes shifts of ECF water into the ICF and cellular swelling.
   3. Rapid development of hypo-osmolality can produce intravascular hemolysis.
   4. In dehydration, loss of ECF volume is amplified by movement of water into the ICF. Circulatory collapse and shock may occur.

DETERMINATION OF BLOOD GASES AND ELECTROLYTES

I. Blood gas analysis. Blood gas analysis measures the partial pressures of oxygen and carbon dioxide and hydrogen ion concentration.
   A. Sample management
      1. Heparinized whole blood must be measured immediately if it is kept at room temperature, or within 3 hours if kept on ice ($4^\circ C$).
      2. The sample should be collected from a large, free-flowing vessel and not exposed to air before measurement.
      3. Collect 2.5 ml blood in a plastic syringe containing 0.2 ml heparin, cap the needle with a rubber stopper, and deliver to the laboratory immediately.

4. Blood gas machines measure the sample at $37^{\circ}C$. Since actual in vivo concentrations are affected by body temperature, report the animal's body temperature when the sample is submitted to allow the laboratory to make the required corrections.
5. Only arterial blood samples are suitable for PO_2 determinations. Venous samples are adequate for pH and PCO_2 measurements.

B. Arterial partial pressure of oxygen (PO_2)
1. PO_2 can be used to determine the amount of O_2 dissolved in plasma: $O_2(mEq/l) = 0.01014 \times PO_2$.
2. PO_2 does not reflect the total O_2 carried in the blood. Most O_2 is combined with hemoglobin and does not contribute to PO_2.
3. The total O_2 concentration depends on total hemoglobin, O_2-carrying capability of hemoglobin, body temperature, blood pH, erythrocytic 2,3-diphosphoglycerate concentration, and PO_2. The percent saturation of hemoglobin is determined by PO_2.
4. High PO_2 can occur only when an animal is given gases with high O_2 content (e.g., via oxygen cage or anesthetic machine).
5. Low PO_2 (hypoxemia) can occur in respiratory disorders or with derangement of the respiratory control mechanisms (Case 25).

C. Partial pressure of carbon dioxide (PCO_2)
1. PCO_2 is proportional to the dissolved CO_2 in the plasma.
2. Dissolved CO_2 is in equilibrium with carbonic acid: $H_2CO_3(mEq/l) = 0.03 \times PCO_2$.
3. PCO_2 is a measure of alveolar ventilation. Decreased alveolar ventilation produces hypercapnia (high PCO_2) (Case 21); increased ventilation produces hypocapnia (low PCO_2) (Case 12).

D. Hydrogen ion concentration (pH)
1. Blood pH is maintained within narrow limits in health by proteinic, phosphate, and bicarbonate buffer systems. The bicarbonate buffer system is the only one measured for clinical evaluation.
2. Decrease in blood pH is acidemia. The condition producing this change is acidosis (Case 6).
3. Increase in blood pH is alkalemia. The condition producing this change is alkalosis (Cases 12, 25).

E. Bicarbonate (HCO_3^-)
1. HCO_3^- concentration is calculated from the pH and PCO_2 by the Henderson-Hasselbach equation: $pH = 6.1 + \log HCO_3^-/(0.03 \times PCO_2)$; 6.1 = pK of carbonic acid.
2. HCO_3^- concentration is maintained in health by conservation and production by the renal tubules.

II. Total CO_2 content (TCO_2). TCO_2 is another way of measuring plasma HCO_3^-. Its name comes from techniques used before the development of blood gas analysis. TCO_2 is the total CO_2 gas released when the sample is mixed with a strong acid.

A. Measurement
1. TCO_2 can be measured in serum or heparinized plasma.
    It is stable in samples handled for routine clinical
    chemistry.
2. Assays can be done by calculation from blood gas
    analyzer data, using UV spectrophotometry or ion-
    specific electrodes (see section IV).
3. A simple apparatus measuring TCO_2 is available for
    practice laboratories.
B. Components of TCO_2
1. HCO_3^- is the major contributor to TCO_2, and changes in
    TCO_2 concentration are interpreted as changes in HCO_3^-
    (Cases 4, 16, 21, 25).
2. Small amounts of TCO_2 come from dissolved H_2CO_3 and
    carbamino acids.

III. Acid base regulation
A. Ratio of HCO_3^-/H_2CO_3 ($HCO_3^-/(0.03 \times PCO_2)$)
1. The ratio is about 20:1 in most species (slightly less
    in the dog) in health.
    a. Decreases in the ratio produce acidemia, and
        increases produce alkalemia (Cases 6, 12, 25).
    b. The ratio, not the individual concentrations,
        determines pH.
2. If changes occur in either HCO_3^- or H_2CO_3, normal
    homeostatic mechanisms cause changes in the other to
    bring the ratio back to 20:1 (Case 14).
    a. Changes in HCO_3^- (called metabolic disorders)
        produce respiratory compensation (changes in PCO_2)
        within minutes.
    b. Changes in H_2CO_3 (called respiratory disorders)
        produce changes in HCO_3^- after a much longer
        period, often several days.
3. Compensation is an active physiologic process.
    Pathologic lesions in the respiratory or renal system
    interfere with normal compensation and potentiate the
    seriousness of the acid base disorder.
4. Serum electrolytes are needed to fully evaluate the
    cause of abnormal blood gases, pH, and HCO_3^-.
B. Patterns of acid base abnormalities
1. The common types of imbalance and laboratory differen-
    tiation are shown in Table 5.1. Note that compensation
    produces unidirectional change in the components of the
    buffer in order to restore the HCO_3^-/H_2CO_3 ratio (e.g.,
    if HCO_3^- is low, the compensatory change is a decrease
    in PCO_2).
2. Overcompensation does not occur. Shifts in HCO_3^- and
    PCO_2 in opposite directions indicate mixed respiratory
    and metabolic disorders (see Disorders of Respiratory
    Function).

IV. Electrolytes and anion gap. The electrolytes measured in most
     clinical situations are Na^+, K^+, Cl^-, and HCO_3^- as TCO_2.
A. Methods of measurement

TABLE 5.1. Laboratory Differentiation of Acid Base Imbalance

Condition	Blood pH	PCO$_2$	HCO$_3^-$*	HCO$_3^-$/H$_2$CO$_3$ Ratio†
Metabolic acidosis				
Uncompensated	▼	N	▼	▼
Partial compensation	▾	▾	▼	▾
Respiratory alkalosis‡				
Uncompensated	▲	▼	N	▲
Metabolic alkalosis				
Uncompensated	▲	N	▲	▲
Partial compensation	▴	▴	▲	▴
Respiratory acidosis				
Uncompensated	▼	▲	N	▼
Partial compensation	▾	▲	▴	▾

* Total CO$_2$ content is a value equivalent to HCO$_3^-$ concentration.
† H$_2$CO$_3$ concentration = PCO$_2$ × 0.03; HCO$_3^-$/H$_2$CO$_3$ = 20:1 in health.
‡ Partial compensation is unlikely.
▲ = marked changed.
▴ = mild change.
N = no change.

1. Sample management
   a. Serum is the best sample for electrolyte analysis. Heparinized plasma can be used.
   b. Serum should be separated from the clot as quickly as possible to prevent in vitro alteration.
2. Flame photometry
   a. Na$^+$ and K$^+$ can be measured by the intensity of light emitted when the sample is burned in a flame.
   b. Concentration is reported as mEq per liter of serum, although electrolytes are present only in the water phase of serum (about 96% of the volume in health).
   c. Factitious hyponatremia can occur in samples with increased nonaqueous phases (e.g., lipemia, increased protein concentration).
3. Coulombmetric titration
   a. Cl$^-$ can be measured by an electrical titration system (chloridimeter).
   b. Cl$^-$ is reported as mEq per liter of serum. The sample problems of false low values can occur with lipemia or increased protein concentration.
4. Ion-specific electrodes
   a. Many electrolytes can be measured, including Na$^+$, K$^+$, Cl$^-$, TCO$_2$, and ionized Ca^{++} (for sample handling of the latter, see Chapter 11).
   b. Measurement is based on electrical potential across a membrane designed to be selectively sensitive to a certain electrolyte.
   c. Machines are available to measure multiple electrolytes on one sample by a series of electrodes (e.g., Na$^+$, K$^+$, Cl$^-$, and TCO$_2$).
   d. Electrolytes are measured as mEq per liter of serum water. The increased nonaqueous phase (lipemia and hyperproteinemia) has no effect.
   e. Values in serum from healthy animals are about 1.04-fold greater than those of other techniques.

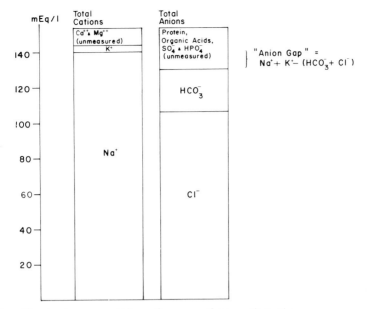

Fig. 5.1. The ionic composition of serum. Notice that the
anion gap equals unmeasured anions minus unmeasured cations and
that total anions equal total cations.

B. Anion gap calculation
    1. The anion gap (AG) is a calculated value ($Na^+ + K^+ - Cl^-$
       $- HCO_3^-$) that can aid in determining the cause of acid
       base abnormalities. Total serum cations equal those
       commonly measured ($Na^+ + K^+$) plus all remaining unmea-
       sured cations (UC). Total serum anions equal those
       commonly measured ($Cl^- + HCO_3^-$) plus all remaining
       unmeasured anions (UA) (Fig. 5.1).
    2. By the law of electrical neutrality:
       a. Total cations = total anions.
       b. $Na^+ + K^+ + UC = Cl^- + HCO_3^- + UA$.
    3. Rearrangement of the above equations gives:
       a. $Na^+ + K^+ - Cl^- - HCO_3^- = UA - UC$.
       b. $AG = UA - UC$.
    4. In health, the anion gap is around 10 to 20 mEq/1 in
       most species (15 to 25 mEq/1 in the dog and cat). The
       UC remain quite constant in health and disease. Most
       changes in AG occur because of changes in UA, such as
       small organic acids, albumin, and exogenous toxins.
    5. Increased anion gap occurs in many diseases, including
       lactic acidosis (lactate), diabetes mellitus and
       ketosis (ketones), renal insufficiency (salts of uremic
       acids), and certain toxicities (metabolites of ethylene
       glycol) (Cases 5, 16, 23). False high anion gap may
       occur with in vitro loss of HCO_3^- caused by improper
       sample handling.
    6. Decreased anion gap is rare. Causes include hemodilu-
       tion, hypoalbuminemia, and increase in certain cations
       (e.g., hypercalcemia). Any of these situations con-

comitant with diseases with increased anion gap may
temper the magnitude of anion gap change.

DISORDERS OF ELECTROLYTES AND METABOLIC ACID BASE IMBALANCE
      It is best to have complete electrolyte profiles (Na^+, K^+,
Cl^-), some measure of blood acid base status (blood gas analysis or
TCO_2), and determination of anion gap. Incomplete data may give false
information about the status of a patient and lead to inappropriate
treatment. Electrolyte and acid base profiles are used primarily for
assessment of severity of body fluid disorders rather than determination of a specific diagnosis. Sometimes they can be helpful in
substantiating a diagnosis. Rarely, an electrolyte pattern is
characteristic of a specific disease.

   I. Serum sodium
       A. Physiologic considerations
           1. Total ECF Na^+ = serum Na^+ × ECF volume.
           2. Na^+ maintains ECF osmolality and is essential for renal
               water retention, a control mechanism for hydration
               status.
           3. Serum Na^+ can be used as a measure of total body Na^+ if
               ECF volume (hydration status) is considered.
       B. Hyponatremia, normonatremia, and hypernatremia may occur

TABLE 5.2.   Mechanisms and Diseases Associated with Various Com-
             binations of Serum Na^+ Concentration and Hydration Status
Hyponatremia
   Decreased ECF H_2O (hypotonic dehydration): loss of Na^+-rich fluids;
      osmotic diuresis (diabetes mellitus), hypoaldosteronism, diarrhea
      (foals and horses), renal disease (cattle), salmonellosis (calves)
      (Cases 6, 23)
   Normal ECF H_2O (normal hydration): early hypoaldosteronism, early
      renal disease (cattle), rapidly occurring hyperglycemia, dietary
      salt deficiency (cattle), ruptured urinary bladder (foal), saliva
      loss (horse), treatment with low Na^+ fluids (5% dextrose) (Cases
      16, 19)
   Increased ECF H_2O (edema, ascites, hydrothorax): rare situation;
      treatment with excessive low Na^+ fluids during renal shutdown
      (Case 25)
Normonatremia
   Decreased ECF H_2O (isotonic dehydration): loss of isonatremic
      fluids; vomiting, diarrhea, renal disease, gut fluid sequestra-
      tion, exudation, hemorrhage (Cases 4, 11)
   Normal ECF H_2O (normal hydration): health
   Increase ECF H_2O (edema, ascites, hydrothorax): retention of water;
      liver disease (dog), hypoalbuminemia, cardiac failure (Cases 7,
      12, 15, 18, 22), treatment with isonatremic fluids during these
      diseases
Hypernatremia
   Decreased ECF H_2O (hypertonic dehydration): severe insensible H_2O
      loss; panting, sweating
   Normal ECF H_2O (normal hydration): salt poisoning; access to high
      salt diet with restricted water intake, force feeding properly
      formulated diet by pharyngostomy tube with inadequate water
      intake, consumption of seawater, osmoreceptor defect
   Increased ECF H_2O (edema, ascites, hydrothorax): rare situation;
      treatment with hypernatremic fluids during renal shutdown

with low, normal, or high ECF volume. The mechanisms and diseases responsible for each possibility are given in Table 5.2.

C. Hyponatremia with hyperkalemia and calculated Na^+/K^+ ratio less than 23:1 is very strong evidence for hypoaldosteronism (Addison's disease); some believe that a ratio less than 26:1 is suggestive.

II. Serum potassium
  A. Physiologic considerations
    1. Serum K^+ is maintained within narrow limits for normal neuromuscular and cardiac function.
    2. Serum K^+ is not a reliable indicator of total body K^+ because most is in the ICF. Serum K^+ can be altered by:
      a. Shifts of K^+ between the ICF and ECF (internal K^+ balance)
      b. Increases and decreases in total body K^+ (external K^+ balance)
      c. Mixed disorders of both internal and external types
    3. No clinical measure gives accurate evaluation of total body K^+ status.
    4. Since serum K^+ is affected by both internal and external K^+ balance or a combination of the two, both possibilities should be considered when determining proper K^+ therapy.
  B. Mechanisms and causes of hyperkalemia
    1. Hyperkalemia secondary to changes in internal K^+ balance may be due to:
      a. Acidemia
        (1) Hyperkalemia occurs in many acidotic patients because ICF K^+ exchanges with excess ECF H^+.
        (2) Hyperkalemia occurs most frequently in secretion (HCO_3^- loss) acidosis.
        (3) Hyperkalemia is less frequent in titration (organic acid excess) acidosis. It is thought that organic anions enter cells with the excess H^+ instead of cation exchange occurring.
        (4) Rapid alkalinization of the ECF of acidotic patients without K^+ supplementation may produce life-threatening hypokalemia.
        (5) External loss of K^+ may be greater than internal shifts in many disease states (e.g., diabetic ketoacidosis, severe diarrhea), producing normokalemia or hypokalemia in the face of acidemia (Case 6).
      b. Hyperosmolality. Hypertonicity can produce a shift of ICF K^+ to the ECF. This shift is independent of blood pH; the mechanisms are unknown.
      c. Tissue necrosis
        (1) Loss of cell membrane integrity produces efflux of ICF K^+ to the ECF.
        (2) Necrosis of a large mass of tissue, especially muscle, may release a large amount of K^+ and produce hyperkalemia (e.g., saddle thrombus in cats, white muscle disease in cattle).

    (3) Less severe cell damage may produce the same shifts; but restoration of normal cell function may cause rapid reversal of K^+ balance, leading to ECF K^+ depletion and hypokalemia.

   d. Insulin deficiency

    (1) Insulin facilitates the entry of K^+ into the ICF; therefore, deficiency of insulin may be accompanied by loss of ICF K^+ to the ECF and hyperkalemia. Usually, external K^+ loss in diabetes is so much greater than internal shift to ECF that hyperkalemia does not occur.

    (2) Administration of exogenous insulin causes rapid entry of K^+ into the ICF, and K^+ supplementation may be needed to prevent hypokalemia.

  2. Hyperkalemia secondary to changes in external K^+ balance may be due to:

   a. Anuria

    (1) Normally, most excess K^+ is lost in the urine.

    (2) Anuric renal disease or postrenal blockage (e.g., feline urologic syndrome) can produce hyperkalemia (Case 16).

   b. Hypoaldosteronism

    (1) Aldosterone is one of the mediators of renal K^+ excretion.

    (2) Hypoaldosteronism (Addison's disease) is characterized by hyperkalemia and hyponatremia (serum Na^+/K^+ ratio less than 23:1 is strong evidence, and less than 26:1 may be suggestive).

   c. Parenteral administration of K^+

    (1) Rapid administration of therapeutic K^+ may produce life-threatening hyperkalemia. In general, large animals are less susceptible to this problem than small animals.

    (2) Oral K^+ supplementation can be used in many conditions with less danger to the patient.

  3. Hyperkalemia can lead to life-threatening cardiac conduction abnormalities, bradycardia, and electrocardiogram changes.

 C. Mechanisms and causes of hypokalemia

  1. Hypokalemia secondary to changes in internal K^+ balance may occur in alkalosis.

   a. Low ECF H^+ concentrations may cause ICF H^+ to leave cells by exchanging with ECF K^+. This internal shift in K^+ is thought to be a minor cause of hypokalemia in alkalosis; certain diseases causing alkalosis also cause decreased ECF K^+ as a result of external shift in K^+ (Case 21).

   b. Shifts of K^+ to the ICF may occur with therapeutic alkalinization with parenteral fluids, producing hypokalemia in a patient that was normokalemic or hyperkalemic.

  2. Hypokalemia secondary to changes in external K^+ balance may be due to:

        a. Decreased oral intake. Anorectic animals
            (especially herbivores) may have negative K^+
            balance, especially during the 2 to 3 days needed
            for the kidneys to convert from K^+ excretion to K^+
            conservation (Cases 21, 23).
        b. Increased gastrointestinal losses. Loss of gastric
            and intestinal fluids, which are rich in K^+, can
            produce K^+ depletion (e.g., vomiting, abomasal
            disorders, and diarrhea) (especially severe in
            horses) (Case 19).
        c. Increased urinary loss (kaliuresis). Several
            conditions cause this, including polyuric states
            (e.g., osmotic diuresis, rapid rehydration),
            metabolic alkalosis and acidosis, increased
            mineralocorticoid secretion, and diuretics (Cases
            20, 23, 25).
     3. Loss of K^+ can potentiate the seriousness of a disease
        by producing life-threatening cardiac abnormalities,
        causing loss of renal concentrating ability, and
        perpetuating metabolic alkalosis (paradoxical
        aciduria).

III. Serum chloride
    A. Physiologic considerations
        1. Cl^- is the major anion of ECF.
        2. It is an important component of many secretions, such as
            NaCl, KCl, and HCl.
    B. Abnormalities
        1. Increase and decrease in serum Cl^- may parallel change
            in serum Na^+ concentration (Case 25).
        2. Loss of gastric or abomasal HCl leads to
            hypochloridemia with normonatremia (Cases 21, 23).
        3. Loss of HCO_3^- causes a relative increase in Cl^-,
            although a total body Cl^- deficit exists (see section
            IV B1) (Case 6).

IV. Metabolic acidosis
    A. Laboratory indication is a decreased plasma HCO_3^- or serum
       TCO_2 concentration.
        1. Moderate metabolic acidosis in most species is 15 to 20
            mEq/l, and 12 to 17 mEq/l in the dog and cat.
        2. Severe metabolic acidosis in most species is less than
            15 mEq/l, and less than 12 mEq/l in the dog and cat.
        3. Respiratory compensation is hyperventilation to exhale
            CO_2 and restore the HCO_3^-/H_2CO_3 ratio.
    B. Mechanisms and causes
        1. Secretion (HCO_3^- loss) acidosis
           a. HCO_3^- can decrease when fluids rich in $NaHCO_3$
              and/or $KHCO_3$ are lost from the body. Such fluids
              are:
              (1) Saliva in animals that cannot swallow,
                   especially ruminants (but not in the horse)
              (2) Intestinal and pancreatic secretions, either
                   trapped in the gut by obstruction or lost as
                   diarrhea (Cases 4, 6)

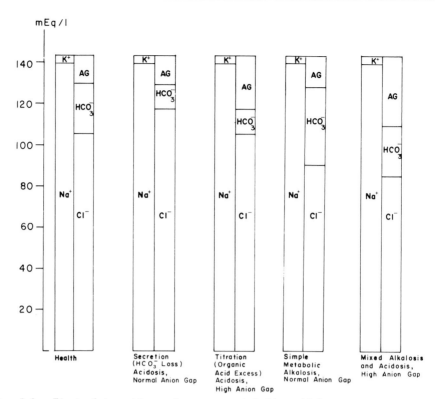

Fig. 5.2.   Electrolyte patterns in common metabolic acid base disorders.

          (3)   Urine rich in HCO_3^- in cases of renal tubular acidosis
     b.   The electrolyte pattern in secretion acidosis is (Fig. 5.2):
          (1)   Low plasma HCO_3^- or serum TCO_2
          (2)   High normal to high serum Cl^-
          (3)   Normal anion gap
          (4)   If hyponatremia exists, all the above values may be decreased.
  2.   Titration (organic acid excess) acidosis
     a.   Organic acid accumulation can lead to HCO_3^- loss by titration.
     b.   As HCO_3^- acts as a buffer, it is converted to the salt of the organic acid. For the acid HA: HA + $NaHCO_3 \rightarrow H_2CO_3$ + NaA; HCO_3^- concentration is decreased.
     c.   The presence of the salt of the acid (i.e., NaA in the above example) is recognized by an increased anion gap.
     d.   Clinically important organic acids include:
          (1)   Lactic acid in shock and grain overload
          (2)   Ketone bodies in diabetic ketoacidosis and ketosis of ruminants
          (3)   Uremic acids in renal failure (Case 16)

(4) Some organic poisons and their metabolites
(e.g., ethylene glycol and metaldehyde).
e. The electrolyte pattern in titration acidosis is
(Fig. 5.2):
(1) Low plasma HCO_3^- or serum TCO_2
(2) Normal serum Cl^-
(3) High anion gap
(4) If hyponatremia exists, all of the above
values may be decreased.

V. Metabolic alkalosis
A. Laboratory indication is an increase in plasma HCO_3^- or
serum TCO_2 (Fig. 5.2).
1. Moderate metabolic alkalosis in most species is 30 to
35 mEq/1 and 27 to 32 mEq/1 in the dog and cat.
2. Severe metabolic alkalosis in most species is greater
than 35 mEq/1 and greater than 32 mEq/1 in the dog and
cat.
3. Respiratory compensation by hypoventilation to retain
CO_2 and restore the HCO_3^-/H_2CO_3 ratio is restricted by
the need for O_2. Therefore, respiratory compensation is
often poor.
B. Loss of gastric or abomasal HCl is almost always the cause
of metabolic alkalosis (Case 21).
1. HCl is secreted by the following reaction: NaCl +
$H_2CO_3 \rightarrow$ HCl (secreted) + $NaHCO_3$ (retained in body
fluids). In health, the HCl is later reabsorbed in the
lower gastrointestinal tract, restoring the acid base
equilibrium.
2. Vomiting in monogastric animals leads to HCl loss.
3. In ruminants, abomasal or high gut obstruction leads to
reflux of abomasal contents into the rumen, sometimes
called "internal vomiting." Causes include physical
blockage (e.g., abomasal displacement or torsion) as
well as functional occlusion (e.g., vagal indigestion,
renal disease, and hypocalcemia).
4. Loss of HCl leads to a net gain in HCO_3^-; Cl^- is lost
as well as H^+, leading to alkalosis, hypochloridemia,
and normal to slightly increased anion gap.
C. Paradoxical aciduria in HCl loss, metabolic alkalosis
(Case 21)
1. Renal correction of metabolic alkalosis should be the
secretion of excess HCO_3^- and retention of H^+ ions to
restore the HCO_3^-/H_2CO_3 ratio. Often, the kidney cannot
correct the alkalosis. This condition is recognized by
an acid urine concomitant with metabolic alkalosis,
"paradoxical aciduria."
2. Paradoxical aciduria develops as the result of hypovolemia, hypochloridemia, and total body K^+ depletion.
a. Na^+ is retained by the kidney to restore body water
and ECF Na^+. Since Cl^- is deficient in the glomerular filtrate, HCO_3^- is reabsorbed as the anion with
Na^+.
b. Na^+ also can be reabsorbed by exchange and
secretion of H^+ or K^+. Since K^+ is deficient in the

plasma, H^+ is secreted into the urine.

    c. The loss of HCO_3^- from and the addition of H^+ to the renal filtrate leads to acid urine, and the retention of HCO_3^- perpetuates the state of metabolic alkalosis.

   3. Fluid therapy in cases of metabolic alkalosis with paradoxical aciduria should be directed at correcting the NaCl deficit. Such fluids include normal saline and Ringer's solution. When K^+ depletion is severe, treatment with parenteral or oral K^+ may be necessary to reverse paradoxical aciduria.

  D. Rare causes of metabolic alkalosis

   1. Hypokalemia associated with hypovolemia may lead to metabolic alkalosis. Possible clinical situations may include dehydration and concomitant diuretic use or mineralocorticoid excess, either exogenous or endogenous.

   2. Liver failure, especially in horses, may result in the presence of excess bases (NH_3 and amines) in circulation.

   3. Use of esophageal tubes for alimentation in the horse may lead to loss of saliva, which is rich in NaCl. The metabolic alkalosis with hyponatremia and hypochloridemia occurs after a few days of salivary loss.

VI. Mixed metabolic acidosis and alkalosis (Case 23)

  A. Laboratory findings are (Fig. 5.2):

   1. Plasma HCO_3^- or serum TCO_2 close to or within normal reference values

   2. Low serum Cl^-

   3. Very high anion gap. Measurement of blood gases or TCO_2 alone will never detect mixed metabolic alkalosis and acidosis; the high anion gap is an important indicator.

  B. Mechanisms and causes

   1. Vomiting may lead to hypovolemic shock. The increased HCO_3^- from the metabolic alkalosis is titrated by the lactic acid from shock. The HCO_3^- may drop close to or into the normal reference range, but the Cl^- remains low, and the anion gap is very high.

   2. Some conditions with titration acidosis may produce vomiting (e.g., diabetic ketoacidosis, renal failure). Vomiting increases HCO_3^- from the extremely low concentrations produced by the original condition. Serum Cl^- is low, and the anion gap is extremely high (often greater than 30 mEq/l).

   3. Restoration of ECF by low Cl^- fluids may cause correction of the acidosis but perpetuation of the alkalosis. Fluid therapy should include sufficient Cl^- and K^+ to correct both conditions.

DISORDERS OF RESPIRATORY FUNCTION

Although blood gas analysis is a relatively insensitive measure of pulmonary function and should be used as an adjunct to physical examination, radiology, and other diagnostic methods, arterial PO_2

and PCO_2 can be helpful in assessing severity of respiratory disorders. Differentiation of pathologic changes in PCO_2 from compensation for metabolic acid base disorders can be made only by evaluation
of a full blood gas and electrolyte profile.

I.   Arterial PO_2
     A. PO_2 is a measure of intrapulmonary gas exchange.
          1.   In health, regional distribution of air to areas of the
               lungs is balanced with regional blood flow.
          2. O_2 is almost 20 times less diffusible than CO_2 across
               the alveolar capillary barrier. Many intrapulmonary
               lesions can produce hypoxemia without altering CO_2
               exchange.
     B.   Conditions that cause hypoxemia accompanied by normal PCO_2
          (Case 25) or by low PCO_2 caused by hyperventilation are:
          1.   Perfusion/diffusion abnormalities, which include many
               cases of pneumonia, pulmonary edema, and pulmonary
               thrombosis.
          2.   Decreased intrapulmonary gas diffusion, which is caused
               by thickened alveolar septae, pulmonary fibrosis, and
               pulmonary edema.
     C.   Conditions that cause hypoxemia accompanied by increased
          PCO_2 (hypoxemia and respiratory acidosis) all are caused by
          decreased alveolar ventilation. Diseases and circumstances
          are listed in Table 5.3.

II. Arterial PCO_2
     A.   Arterial PCO_2 is a measure of alveolar ventilation.
          1.   Minute-to-minute neurologic control of PCO_2 occurs in
               health.
          2.   In chronic hypoxemia the aortic and carotid bodies,
               responding to total O_2 content, can become the major
               controllers of respiration.
          3.   Well-ventilated areas of the lungs can compensate for
               regions with poor gas exchange, causing hypoxemia with
               normal PCO_2 as described above.
     B.   Respiratory acidosis
          1.   Hypercapnia (high $PaCO_2$) indicates hypoventilation.
          2.   Hypoventilation can occur with deranged central
               control, failure of the mechanical apparatus of

TABLE 5.3.   Hypoventilatory Diseases and Circumstances Associated with
             Hypoxemia and Respiratory Acidosis (Low PaO_2, High $PaCO_2$)

Abnormalities of neurogenic control
  Anesthesia, sedation, head trauma
Muscular or mechanical failure in breathing
  Pneumothorax, pleural effusion, muscular weakness associated with
  coonhound paralysis, myasthenia gravis, neurotoxins (botulism,
  tetanus), paralytic drugs (succinylcholine)
Pulmonary abnormalities
  Pneumonia (severe*), pulmonary edema (severe*), chronic obstructive
  lung disease, airway obstruction (calf diphtheria, tracheal
  collapse)

  *Less severe pneumonia and pulmonary edema may lead to hypoxemia
without respiratory acidosis.

TABLE 5.4. Causes of Hyperventilation and Respiratory Alkalosis
Altered respiratory control
  Fear or anxiety (panting), fever, hepatic encephalopathy,
  convulsions, heat exposure
Hypoxemia
  Hypotension, pulmonary vascular shunts, pulmonary fibrosis,
  pneumonia, pulmonary edema
Iatrogenic causes
  Mechanical ventilation, rapid correction of metabolic acidosis

breathing, and severe pulmonary abnormalities. The diseases and circumstances associated with these mechanisms are listed in Table 5.3.

3. Hypoxemia exists in all causes of respiratory acidosis because O_2 exchange is always less efficient than CO_2 exchange.

C. Respiratory alkalosis
  1. Hypocapnia (low $PaCO_2$) indicates hyperventilation and is always associated with altered respiratory control. Specific conditions are listed in Table 5.4.
  2. The respiratory centers may be influenced by physiologic (e.g., heat control) or pathologic (e.g., hepatic encephalopathy) stimuli (Case 12).
  3. Hypoxemia produces hypocapnia unless diffuse, severe lung damage prevents alveolar ventilation (see above discussion on arterial PO_2).

D. Mixed respiratory and metabolic acid base disorders
  1. The laboratory findings that indicate this mixed disorder are:
     a. Lack of expected compensation (e.g., normal PCO_2 and abnormal HCO_3^- or abnormal PCO_2 and normal HCO_3^-) (Case 25).
     b. PCO_2 and HCO_3^- changes both producing alkalosis or acidosis (e.g., low PCO_2 and high HCO_3^- or high PCO_2 and low HCO_3^-).
  2. Respiratory compensation occurs within minutes after the onset of a blood pH abnormality. It should be expected in short-term as well as long-term metabolic disorders.
  3. Metabolic compensation may lag several days after the onset of a respiratory disorder. Acute respiratory conditions may need to be reevaluated after 3 to 4 days to determine if compensation has occurred.
  4. Mixed disorders may lead to severe blood pH abnormalities; therapy should be directed to return blood pH to normal limits.

REFERENCES

Behr MF, Hackett RP, Bentinck-Smith J, et al: Metabolic abnormalities associated with rupture of the urinary bladder in neonatal foals. J Am Vet Med Assoc 178:263, 1981.
Bia M, Thier SO: Mixed acid base disturbances: A clinical approach. Med Clin North Am 62:347, 1981.
Brobst D: Pathophysiologic and adaptive changes in acid-base disorders. J Am Vet Med Assoc 183:773, 1983.
Clark WT, Jones BR, Clark J: Blood oxygen and carbon dioxide tensions in normal dogs and dogs with respiratory failure. J Small Anim Pract 18:535, 1977.

Cornelius LM, Rawlings CA: Arterial blood gas and acid-base values in dogs with various diseases and signs of disease. J Am Vet Med Assoc 178:992, 1981.

Cox M: Potassium homeostasis. Med Clin North Am 65:363, 1981.

Crawford MA, Kittleson MD, Fink GD: Hypernatremia and adipsia in a dog. J Am Vet Med Assoc 184:818, 1984.

Cronin RE, Knochel JP: The consequences of potassium deficiency. Contemp Issues Nephrol 2:205, 1978.

DuBose TD: Metabolic alkalosis. Semin Nephrol 1:281, 1981.

Edwards DF, Richardson DE, Russell RG: Hypernatremic, hypertonic dehydration in a dog with diabetes insipidus and gastric dilation-volvulus. J Am Vet Med Assoc 182:973, 1983.

Eiler H, Lyke WA, Johnson R: Internal vomiting in the ruminant: Effect of apomorphine on ruminal pH in sheep. Am J Vet Res 42:202, 1981.

Feig PU, McCurdy DK: The hypertonic state. N Engl J Med 297:1444, 1977.

Gabow PA, Kaehny WD, et al: Diagnostic importance of an increased serum anion gap. N Engl J Med 303:854, 1980.

Gabuzda GJ: Sodium in clinical medicine. In Moses C (ed): Sodium in medicine and health: A monograph. Baltimore, Reese Press Pub, 1980.

Gilbert R: Spirometry and blood gases. Henry JB (ed): Clinical diagnosis and management by laboratory methods, 16th ed. Philadelphia, WB Saunders Co, 1979.

Gingerich DA, Murdick PW: Experimentally induced intestinal obstruction in sheep: Paradoxical aciduria in metabolic alkalosis. Am J Vet Res 36:663, 1975.

Gingerich DA, Murdick PW: Paradoxic aciduria in bovine metabolic alkalosis. J Am Vet Med Assoc 166:227, 1975.

Green RA: Perspectives in clinical osmometry. Vet Clin North Am 8:287-300, 1978.

Groer: Physiology and pathophysiology of the body fluids. St. Louis, CB Mosby Co, 1981.

Haskins SC: Sampling and storage of blood for pH and blood gas analysis. J Am Vet Med Assoc 174:429, 1977.

Hughes DE, Sokolowski JH: Sodium chloride poisoning in the dog. Canine Pract 5:28, 1978.

Kaehny WD: Respiratory acid-base disorders. Med Clin North Am 67:915, 1983.

Karselis KC: Electrolyte instrumentation: Then and now. Am J Med Tech 48:329, 1982.

Narins RG, Emmitt M: Simple and mixed acid-base disorders: A practical approach. Medicine 59:161, 1980.

Narins RG, Gardner B: Simple acid-base disturbances. Med Clin North Am 65:321, 1981.

Oh MS, Carroll HJ: Current concepts: The anion gap. N Engl J Med 297:814, 1977.

Polzin DJ, Stevens JB, Osborne CA: Clinical application of the anion gap in evaluation of acid-base disorders in dogs. Compend Contin Educ Pract Vet 4:1021, 1982.

Sebastian A, Hulter HN, Rector FC: Metabolic alkalosis. Contemp Issues Nephrol 2:101, 1978.

Shull RM: The gaps game. Vet Clin Pathol 7(2):19, 1978.

Shull RM: The value of anion gap and osmolal gap in veterinary medicine. Vet Clin Pathol 7(3):12, 1978.

Stick JA, Robinson E, Krehbiel JD: Acid-base and electrolyte alterations associated with salivary loss in the pony. Am J Vet Res 42:733, 1981.

Tasker JB: Fluids, electrolytes and acid-base balance. In Kaneko JJ (ed): Clinical biochemistry of domestic animals, 3rd ed. New York, Academic Press, 1980.

Thrall MA, Grauer GF, Mero KN: Clinicopathologic findings in dogs and cats with ethylene glycol intoxication. J Am Vet Med Assoc 184:37, 1984.

Westenfelder C, Nascimento L: Respiratory acidosis and alkalosis. Semin Nephrol 1:220, 1981.

Whitlock RH, Kessler MJ, Tasker JB: Salt (sodium) deficiency in dairy cattle: Polyuria and polydipsia as prominent clinical features. Cornell Vet 65:512, 1975.

6

Proteins, Lipids, and Carbohydrates

PLASMA PROTEINS

I. Functions and origins
   A. Plasma contains certain proteins that are incorporated into the clot and are not found in serum (i.e., fibrinogen and factors V and VIII).
   B. Collectively these proteins perform a nutritive function, exert a colloidal osmotic pressure, and aid in the mainte- nance of acid base balance. Individual proteins serve as enzymes, antibodies, coagulation factors, and transport substances.
   C. Albumin and most of the alpha and beta globulins are synthesized by the liver, but immunoglobulins are secreted by B lymphocytes and plasma cells in the lymphoid organs.

II. Means of measurement
   A. Total protein
      1. It is usually measured as serum protein.
      2. The colorimetric biuret method is used by most laboratories. It is very accurate in the ranges usually found in serum but is not precise at very low levels (less than 1 g/dl).
      3. Precipitation (trichloroacetic acid) and dye-binding (Coomassie blue) methods have been used to quantitate small amounts of protein found in fluids such as urine and cerebrospinal fluid.
      4. Refractometry can be used to measure plasma, serum, or body fluid protein, since proteins in solution cause a change in refractive index that is proportional to their concentration.
         a. Modern refractometers are calibrated to read protein directly as grams per deciliter.
         b. The assumption is made that other solutes in plasma and serum remain constant from sample to sample. Abnormally high concentrations of glucose, urea,

sodium, chloride, or lipid will result in false
high readings.
    c. The serum, plasma, or body fluid must be clear.
Hemolysis causes mild elevations, and lipemia
interferes; but icterus does not alter the reading.
B. Albumin
   1. The clinical procedure in common use is bromcresol
green dye binding.
    a. It may give false high results with low albumin
levels as a result of attachment of dye to other
proteins.
    b. Bilirubin, anticonvulsants, and certain antibiotics
compete with albumin for the dye and cause a color
shift different from that caused by albumin; a
false low reading may result.
   2. Electrophoretic separation of albumin and other
proteins allows for more accurate determination (Fig.
6.1).
C. Fibrinogen
   1. It may be determined indirectly by refractometry by
measuring the plasma protein concentration before and
after precipitating the fibrinogen by heating to 56°C
for 10 minutes. The difference in the two readings is
assumed to be fibrinogen. This method is too
insensitive to detect hypofibrinogenemia.
   2. Fibrinogen may be determined from a measurement of the
thrombin time with use of a standard curve.
D. Globulins
   1. Most globulin concentrations listed on chemistry
profiles are calculated by subtracting albumin
concentration from total protein concentration.
   2. Globulins and albumin can be separated and quantitated
by electrophoresis (Fig. 6.1). Because of overlap of
the various globulin fractions, it may be difficult to
precisely identify the division between fractions. A
helpful landmark is the midpoint of the electrophoreto-
gram, which should lie between the alpha-2 and beta-1
peaks.
   3. Immunochemical methods, immunoelectrophoresis, and
radial immunodiffusion allow for specific identification and quantitation.
   4. The zinc sulfate turbidity test has been used as a
screening test to determine absorption of colostral
immunoglobulins in foals and calves. Visual turbidity
after mixing 6 ml zinc sulfate solution (205 mg/1
boiled distilled water) with 0.1 ml serum indicates
greater than 400 to 500 mg IgG/dl and colostral
absorption. Dam's serum can be used as a positive
control. Other types of turbidity tests for the same
purpose as this test are also described (e.g., sodium
sulfite precipitation test).
   5. Refractometric total serum protein values greater than
5 g/dl in neonates has been used to indicate colostral
immunoglobulin absorption. False-negative findings
limit the usefulness of this method.

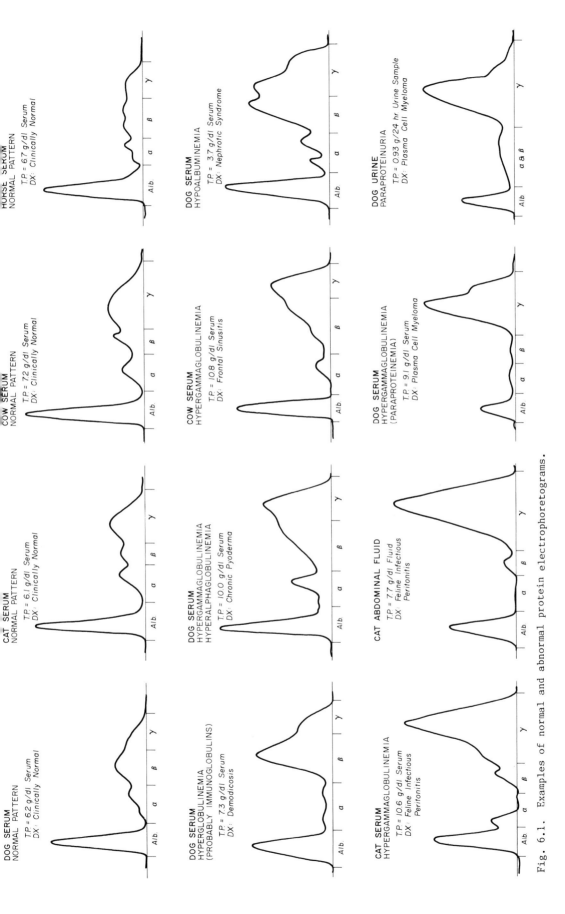

Fig. 6.1. Examples of normal and abnormal protein electrophoretograms.

E. Albumin/globulin (A/G) ratio. This arithmetic value has
    been used to aid in interpretation of total protein values.
    The ratio will remain normal if both fractions are uni-
    formly altered and be abnormal if an alteration in one
    fraction predominates.

III. Protein abnormalities (dysproteinemias)
    A. Hyperproteinemia
        1. Spurious (dehydration) (Case 4)
            a. The packed cell volume (PCV) is also increased. A
                rise in protein concentration is a better index of
                dehydration than the PCV, but neither is reliable
                if the magnitude of the fluid loss is not great
                (see discussion on dehydration in Chapter 5).
            b. The A/G ratio is normal.
        2. Hyperalbuminemia. An increase in this protein fraction
            does not occur except spuriously during dehydration.
        3. Hyperfibrinogenemia commonly occurs in inflammatory
            (Cases 5, 6, 23) or neoplastic disease.
            a. This change is most consistent in the bovine
                species.
            b. Dehydration causes moderate increase and can be
                differentiated from true hyperfibrinogenemia by
                calculating the plasma protein/fibrinogen ratio
                (PP/F) (e.g., PP = 8.4 g/dl, F = 600 mg/dl,
                PP/F = 8.4/0.6 = 14).
                (1) PP/F greater than 15 is consistent with
                     dehydration or normal fibrinogen
                     concentration.
                (2) PP/F less than 10 is consistent with true
                     fibrinogen increase.
        4. Hyperglobulinemia (Cases 10, 22)
            a. Alpha globulins. Acute phase reactants (e.g.,
                haptoglobin, alpha-2 macroglobulin, alpha-1 anti-
                trypsin), which migrate in this zone, are often
                increased after tissue injury or inflammation (Fig.
                6.1).
            b. Beta globulins. Transferrin, beta lipoprotein,
                complement-3, and some immunoglobulins migrate in
                this zone. Increases have been associated with
                active liver disease and strongylosis; this
                fraction is often increased in association with
                increases in gamma globulin when an intense immune
                response is in effect (Fig. 6.1).
            c. Gamma globulins
                (1) Polyclonal gammopathies are characterized by
                     an increased globulin fraction with a broad-
                     based electrophoretic peak composed of a
                     heterogeneous mixture of immunoglobulins. They
                     are associated with chronic inflammatory
                     diseases, immune-mediated diseases, and some
                     lymphoid neoplasms (Fig. 6.1).
                (2) Monoclonal gammopathies are characterized by
                     an increased globulin fraction with a narrow-
                     based electrophoretic peak, no wider than the

albumin peak, caused by a single immunoglobulin class produced by a single clone of
cells (Fig. 6.1) (see Chapter 3, II. Plasma
cell myeloma).

B. Hypoproteinemia
1. Hypoalbuminemia (Fig. 6.1)
    a. Diminished production is associated with intestinal
       malabsorption, malnutrition, exocrine pancreatic
       insufficiency (Case 17), and chronic liver disease
       (Case 12).
    b. Accelerated loss occurs with hemorrhage (Case 1),
       renal disease (proteinuria) (Case 15), protein-
       losing enteropathies (Case 18), severe exudative
       skin diseases, burns, and high-protein effusions.
    c. If albumin is selectively lost (e.g., glomerular
       disease, hepatic insufficiency), the A/G ratio will
       be low; but if there is a concomitant loss of
       globulins, panhypoproteinemia and a normal A/G
       ratio occur.
    d. Compensatory increases in globulins may occur in
       hypoalbuminemic states.
2. Hypoglobulinemia
    a. Failure of passive colostral transfer or colostrum
       deprivation leads to a very low gamma globulin
       level.
    b. Combined immunodeficiency disease of foals is the
       result of a failure to synthesize immunoglobulins
       and defective cell-mediated immunity. Low levels of
       immunoglobulin are evident after catabolism of
       maternal antibody, and a lymphopenia is present.
    c. Other diseases characterized by deficiency of
       immunoglobulin include agammaglobulinemia,
       selective IgM deficiency, and transient
       hypogammaglobulinemia.
    d. Globulins may be lost with albumin during
       hemorrhage (Case 1), exudation, and protein-losing
       enteropathies (Case 18).
3. Hypofibrinogenemia. Disseminated intravascular
   coagulation is characterized by decreased plasma
   fibrinogen, but the total amount of this protein that
   is lost is not sufficient to be manifested as a
   hypoproteinemia (Case 10).

PLASMA LIPIDS
    The four major components of plasma lipids are cholesterol,
cholesterol esters, triglycerides, and phospholipids. They traverse
in plasma attached to peptides; the lipid-peptide complexes are
called lipoproteins. A variety of conditions alter plasma lipid
concentrations and may cause overt lipemia.

I. Basic concepts
   A. Exogenous lipids
      1. Dietary lipids are digested to monoglyceride and free
         fatty acids, which are absorbed by mucosal epithelium.

      2. Mucosal cells synthesize triglycerides and combine them
with lesser amounts of phospholipids, cholesterol
esters, and a protein to form chylomicra, which are
secreted into intestinal lymph.

      3. Chylomicra enter plasma from the thoracic duct;
following action of plasma lipoprotein lipase, they are
removed by liver, adipose, or other tissues.

      4. In large amounts, chylomicra can be grossly visible in
blood, causing a "cream of tomato soup" quality, or in
plasma, causing it to be whitish and opaque.

B. Endogenous lipids

      1. Plasma lipoproteins synthesized by the liver and
secreted into plasma are of several types.

         a. Very low-density lipoproteins (VLDL) are composed
of triglycerides and cholesterol in the approximate
ratio of 5:1.

         b. Low-density lipoproteins (LDL) are composed
principally of cholesterol with small amounts of
triglycerides.

         c. High-density lipoproteins (HDL) are rich in protein
with small amounts of cholesterol and
triglycerides.

      2. The fate of endogenous lipids is poorly understood, but
plasma lipoprotein lipase is required for clearance
from blood.

      3. Hyperlipidemias involving one or more of the endogenous
lipids may occur; when triglyceride-rich lipoproteins
are involved, grossly visible lipemia may occur.

C. Effects of lipemia on other laboratory tests and management
of the problem

      1. Major effects of lipemia in vitro

         a. Lipemia enhances hemolysis, and hemolyzed serum may
alter test results (e.g., lipase is markedly
inhibited by hemoglobin).

         b. Turbidity of the serum may impair spectrophoto-
metric determinations (e.g., glucose values are
falsely high).

         c. Serum Na^+ and K^+ measured by flame photometry on
lipemic samples are falsely low.

         d. Plasma protein measured by refractometry is falsely
high in lipemic samples.

      2. Management of lipemia for purposes of acquiring better
laboratory specimens

         a. Fasting for 24 hours should eliminate lipemia.

         b. In cases where lipemia persists after fasting, in
vivo clearing of plasma may be enhanced by giving
intravenous heparin-sodium (dose in dogs, 100
IU/kg) and collecting a sample 15 minutes later.

         c. Refrigeration of lipemic serum and collection below
the lipid layer may be sufficient.

II. Methods of determination and clinical significance

A. Lipemia-refrigeration test

      1. Turbidity of plasma or serum indicates the presence of
triglyceride-rich lipoproteins and/or chylomicra; the

specimen is refrigerated for 4 to 8 hours.
a. A flocculent layer on top and clearing of the sample indicate chylomicra.
b. Persistent turbidity of the sample indicates triglyceride-rich lipoproteins.
c. Certain lipemias have both types of lipids.
2. Lipemia may occur postprandially, secondary to endocrine, hepatic, pancreatic, or renal diseases, or rarely as a primary disorder of lipid metabolism.

B. Cholesterol
1. High serum cholesterol concentration reflects a high level of the cholesterol-rich lipoproteins LDL and VLDL. These lipoproteins may increase secondary to endocrine, hepatic, or renal diseases or rarely as a primary disorder of lipid metabolism (Cases 15, 20).
2. Serum cholesterol concentration tends to be inversely related to thyroid hormone activity.

C. Triglyceride
1. Fasting samples should be analyzed because postprandial hypertriglyceridemia occurs 4 to 6 hours after eating regardless of diet type; high-fat diets may cause postprandial lipemia composed of triglyceride-rich chylomicra.
2. Hypertriglyceridemia primarily indicates chylomicranemia and/or increased VLDL; these changes occur postprandially and secondary to endocrine, hepatic, pancreatic (Case 19), and renal diseases.
3. In vivo lipoprotein lipase clears plasma of triglyceride-rich lipoproteins. Activity of this enzyme is enhanced by insulin, thyroid hormone, glucagon, and heparin.

D. Lipoprotein electrophoresis
1. Serum lipoproteins can be identified by their position relative to serum protein positions and quantitated.
2. The lipoprotein types identified by electrophoretic position are VLDL, prebeta globulin zone; LDL, beta globulin zone; HDL, alpha globulin zone; and chylomicra, remain at origin.

III. Disorders causing secondary hyperlipidemias
A. Hypothyroidism. Cholesterol utilization decreases, and lipoprotein lipase activity is reduced. Hyperlipidemia varies from mild increase in cholesterol and HDL concentrations to marked lipemia with hypercholesterolemia; hypertriglyceridemia; and increased chylomicra, VLDL, LDL, and HDL.
B. Diabetes mellitus. Lipoprotein lipase activity is decreased. Hypertriglyceridemia is marked, but cholesterol is mildly increased.
C. Equine hepatic lipidosis syndrome. Hyperlipidemia varies from mild hypertriglyceridemia and clear plasma to marked lipemia with severe hypertriglyceridemia and increased VLDL.
D. Other causes of secondary hyperlipidemia in which the mechanism and characteristics remain unclear are:

1. Canine acute pancreatitis
2. Canine hepatic disease, especially associated with
    cholestasis (feline hepatic lipidosis syndrome is not
    associated with lipemia)
3. Nephrotic syndrome
4. Exogenous corticosteroids (canine hyperadrenocorticism
    is not associated with lipemia)

IV. Primary hyperlipidemia. Idiopathic hyperlipemia with
     hypertriglyceridemia occurs in miniature schnauzers. A fasting
     hyperchylomicranemia also has been described in dogs.

PLASMA CARBOHYDRATES

       Glucose metabolism and blood glucose concentration are abnormal
in many diseases, and hyperglycemia or hypoglycemia are common
laboratory findings. Disorders of glucose caused by diseases of the
endocrine pancreas are described in greater detail in Chapter 11.
Ketones and lactate are organic anions that may be produced in excess
during abnormal carbohydrate metabolism, and laboratory assessment of
them is described in this section.

I. Glucose
    A. Hormonal control and maintenance of blood glucose
        1. Factors that increase blood glucose concentration are
            as follows.
            a. Digestion and intestinal absorption:
                (1) Cause an increased concentration for 2 to 4
                     hours postprandially in simple-stomached
                     animals
                (2) Cause minimal or no increase in ruminants
                     because most of the dietary carbohydrates are
                     fermented to volatile fatty acids. The primary
                     source of ruminant blood glucose is hepatic
                     gluconeogenesis from the fatty acids.
            b. Hepatic glycogenolysis and gluconeogenesis,
                stimulated by glucagon secreted in response to
                hypoglycemia, increase blood glucose concentration.
                In addition to glucagon:
                (1) Catecholamines stimulate glycogenolysis.
                (2) Glucocorticoids stimulate gluconeogenesis.
            c. Interference with insulin-mediated uptake of
                glucose by liver, skeletal muscle, and fat
                increases blood glucose concentration.
                (1) This antiinsulin effect is caused by
                     catecholamines, glucocorticoids, and growth
                     hormone.
                (2) The hyperglycemic effect can be induced by
                     progesterone-mediated secretion of growth
                     hormone.
        2. Insulin is the only metabolic factor that decreases
            blood glucose concentration (for more details, see
            Chapter 11, Endocrine Pancreas).

B. Means of evaluating glucose metabolism
    1. Blood glucose
        a. Proper sample management is imperative to correct
            interpretation of blood glucose values.
            (1) Sampling a frightened animal should be avoided
                 to prevent the hyperglycemic effect of
                 catecholamines.
            (2) If the history precludes the likelihood of
                 hypoglycemia, the simple-stomached animal
                 should be fasted at least 12 hours to avoid
                 postprandial hyperglycemia.
            (3) If the history indicates the possibility of
                 hypoglycemia (neurologic signs or clinical
                 circumstances often associated with
                 hypoglycemia), fasting is avoided and the
                 baseline glucose concentration is determined.
                 (a) If the baseline value is normal, begin
                      the fast and sample every 2 hours.
                 (b) Hypoglycemia is confirmed if blood
                      glucose concentration falls below 40
                      mg/dl, whereas greater than 50 mg/dl
                      after a 24-hour fast excludes
                      hypoglycemia from further consideration.
            (4) Serum or plasma should be separated from blood
                 cells if more than 30 minutes occur between
                 sample collection and assay.
                 (a) In vitro glycolysis by blood cells
                      decreases blood glucose concentration by
                      about 10% per hour at room temperature.
                 (b) An alternative to serum or plasma
                      separation is use of the anticoagulant
                      sodium fluoride, which inhibits
                      glycolysis.
            (5) Lipemia markedly interferes with the accuracy
                 of glucose measurement. Management of lipemia
                 is described earlier in this chapter (see
                 Plasma Lipids).
        b. Assay techniques are primarily colorimetric, but
            reagent sticks read visually or with a reflectance
            meter for estimating glucose in fresh whole blood
            are available. The sticks may reliably detect
            hyperglycemia, but hypoglycemia may be missed in
            canine blood.
    2. Urine glucose (see Chapter 9)
        a. The resorptive capacity of the proximal renal
            tubule is exceeded when blood glucose concentration
            exceeds 180 mg/dl in most species. The bovine renal
            threshold is 100 mg/dl.
        b. If hyperglycemia is transient and since urine
            collects over time in the urinary bladder, positive
            urinary glucose tests may be encountered in animals
            in which simultaneously measured blood glucose
            concentration is below the renal threshold.
    3. Serum insulin and amended insulin/glucose ratio (see

Chapter 11, Endocrine Pancreas). These measurements are used to detect hyperinsulinism and have largely replaced glucose tolerance tests for that purpose.

4. Glucose tolerance tests
   a. Indications
      (1) Intravenous or oral glucose tolerance tests may be used to detect hyperinsulinism. The tests have been largely replaced by the amended insulin/glucose ratio because failure of tumor cells to release insulin in response to hyperglycemia is a common feature that renders the tolerance test nondiagnostic.
      (2) Intravenous or oral glucose tolerance tests may be used to detect glucose intolerance in animals with persistent hyperglycemia below the renal threshold. Once persistent hyperglycemia exceeds the renal threshold, glucose tolerance testing adds no further diagnostic information.
      (3) In dogs in which diabetes mellitus has been confirmed, the intravenous glucose tolerance test combined with the measurement of serum insulin after the glucose injection may be used to identify the type of diabetes mellitus (see Chapter 11, Endocrine Pancreas). The type is identified by the insulin response pattern.
      (4) The most common use of the oral glucose tolerance test is to assess intestinal absorption.
   b. Dosages and interpretive guidelines. Blood glucose concentration is measured after a 12-hour fast (if the animal is not hypoglycemic) and at appropriate intervals after administration.
      (1) Oral glucose tolerance test (Fig. 6.2)
         (a) In the dog, give 1 g glucose/lb body weight per os. In the horse, give 1 g glucose/kg as a 20% solution via stomach tube.
         (b) Samples for blood glucose measurement are collected at 30-minute intervals.
         (c) Blood glucose concentration should reach about 160 mg/dl by 30 to 60 minutes and return to baseline values by 120 to 180 minutes in normal dogs. In the horse, blood glucose concentrations should reach about 175 mg/dl by 120 minutes and return to baseline values by 360 minutes.
         (d) Failure to reach the maximal levels may be interpreted to indicate intestinal malabsorption. Vomiting or delayed gastric emptying are additional causes. Increased glucose tolerance and lower than normal peak values may be seen in hypothyroidism, adrenal insufficiency, hypopituitarism, and hyperinsulinism.
         (e) Failure to return to baseline values

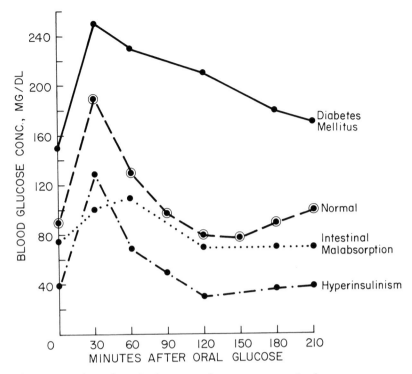

Fig. 6.2. Examples of oral glucose tolerance curves in dogs.

within the expected time may be interpreted to indicate glucose intolerance (a
feature of diabetes mellitus, hyperadre-
nalism, hyperthyroidism, and hepatic
insufficiency).
(2) Intravenous glucose tolerance test
    (a) After a 12-hour fast, the dog is given
         0.5 g glucose/kg intravenously over a
         30-second period; blood samples are
         collected at 5, 15, 25, 35, 45, and 60
         minutes after administration.
    (b) The results of the glucose measurements
         are plotted on log scale versus time on
         arithmetic scale, and the time required
         for the glucose value to decrease by one-
         half is calculated (normally 45 minutes
         or less in the dog).
    (c) Prolonged glucose disappearance indicates
         intolerance (the same diseases as
         described for the oral test above).
    (d) Serum insulin can be measured on the
         samples. The normal canine insulin
         response is a 5- to 10-fold increase at
         5 minutes and return to baseline at 60
         minutes after glucose administration.
         (To classify diabetes mellitus by type,
         see Chapter 11, Endocrine Pancreas).

TABLE 6.1. Causes of Hyperglycemia and Glucosuria
Persistent hyperglycemia
  Acromegaly (glucosuria)
  Diabetes mellitus (glucosuria)*
  Hyperadrenocorticism
  Hyperglucagonemia
  Hyperpituitarism (glucosuria in the horse)
Transient hyperglycemia
  Ammonia toxicosis (ruminants)
  Bovine milk fever (glucosuria)
  Bovine neutrologic diseases (glucosuria)*
  Drugs (ACTH, glucocorticoids, fluids, ketamine, morphine,
    phenothiazine, xylazine) (glucosuria, especially in cattle)
  Excessive insulin dosage in diabetic dogs (wide glucose fluctuation
    with posthypoglycemic hyperglycemia) (glucosuria)
  Fear or exertional catecholamine release (glucosuria in cattle)
  Hyperthyroidism
  Moribund animals (glucosuria, especially in cattle)
  Pain-induced catecholamine and glucocorticoid release
  Postprandial
  Ovine enterotoxemia (glucosuria)
  Ovine listeriosis
  Ovine transport tetany
  Pancreatitis
        *Ketosis may occur in animals with these diseases.

   C. Hyperglycemia disorders (Cases 5, 16, 17, 20, 21, 23).
       Diseases and circumstances associated with persistent or
       transient hyperglycemia and glucosuria are listed in Table
       6.1.
   D. Hypoglycemia disorders. Diseases and circumstances
       associated with hypoglycemia are listed in Table 6.2.

II. Ketones
   A. Basic concepts
       1. The ketone bodies (anions of buffered ketoacids) are
           acetoacetate, beta hydroxybutyrate, and acetone. The
           former two are intermediary metabolites of lipid
           metabolism, and the latter is a waste product.
       2. Ketone production always increases when carbohydrate

TABLE 6.2. Causes of Hypoglycemia
Adrenocortical insufficiency
Aflatoxicosis in horses
Exertional extreme (hunting dog, endurance-ride horse)
Glycogen storage diseases
Gram-negative septicemia
Hepatic insufficiency (paradoxically, prolonged postprandial
  hyperglycemia and glucose intolerance)
Hyperinsulinism (islet cell neoplasm, insulin therapy overdose)
Hypopituitarism
Juvenile hypoglycemia in toy and miniature breed dogs
Ketosis in cattle
Malabsorption
Neonatal hypoglycemia
Neoplasms
Pregnancy toxemia in sheep
Starvation

depletion and increased gluconeogenesis occur. In this circumstance, oxaloacetate depletion in Krebs cycle and suppressed lipogenesis lead to acetacetyl coenzyme A production, the precursor to ketogenesis.

3. The renal threshold for ketones is low, and ketonuria usually precedes detectable ketonemia.

B. Measurement of ketone bodies

1. Qualitative tests employ the nitroprusside reaction, which is specific for acetoacetate and to a lesser extent acetone; beta hydroxybutyrate does not react. The degree of reaction does not correlate with severity of ketosis.

2. Specimens of milk, urine, or serum should be fresh to avoid false-negative reaction from degradation of acetoacetate.

a. Milk may be tested directly.

b. Urine should be diluted 1:10 with water to avoid false-positive reactions.

c. Serum should be diluted to 1:1 with water to avoid false-positive reactions.

3. Ketonemia may be suspected indirectly when the calculated anion gap (see Chapter 5) is high. Diabetic ketonemia is primarily beta hydroxybutyrate, which does not react with the nitroprusside reagents; a negative serum ketone test would not exclude ketonemia as the cause of a high anion gap.

C. Causes of ketonemia and ketonuria include starvation, diabetes mellitus (Case 17), bovine ketosis, ovine pregnancy toxemia, high fat diet, and bovine hepatic lipidosis syndrome.

III. Lactate

A. Basic concepts

1. Lactate is the organic anion of buffered lactic acid.

2. Endogenous lactic acid production increases as tissue perfusion and oxygenation decrease. It diffuses immediately into extracellular fluid and dissociates into hydrogen ion and lactate.

3. Enteric organisms produce an increased exogenous source of lactic acid in conditions of carbohydrate overload. Absorbed lactic acid dissociates also.

B. Measurement of lactate

1. Blood samples for quantitative lactate analysis must be collected into sodium fluoride anticoagulant, which prevents in vitro glycolysis and increased lactate production.

2. Hyperlactatemia may be suspected indirectly when the calculated anion gap (see Chapter 5) is high and clinical circumstances are consistent with lactic acid production.

C. Causes of hyperlactatemia include shock, grain overload, sustained heavy exercise, and abdominal crisis in horses that is characterized by torsion, strangulation, or rupture. Prognosis is poor with very high blood lactate levels.

REFERENCES

Angsubhakorn S, Poomvises P, Romruen K, et al: Aflatoxicosis in horses. J Am Vet Med Assoc
    178:274, 1981.
Atkins CE: Disorders of glucose homeostasis in neonatal and juvenile dogs: Hyperglycemia.
    Compend Contin Educ Pract Vet 5:851, 1983.
Atkins CE: Disorders of glucose homeostasis in neonatal and juvenile dogs: Hypoglycemia,
    Part I. Compend Contin Educ Pract Vet 6:197, 1984.
Atkins CE: Disorders of glucose homeostasis in neonatal and juvenile dogs: Hypoglycemia,
    Part II. Compend Contin Educ Pract Vet 6:353, 1984.
Barsanti JA, Duncan JR: Determination of the concentration of protein in the cerebrospinal
    fluid with a new dye-binding method. Vet Clin Pathol 7(3):6, 1978.
Bartley JC: Lipid metabolism and its disorders. In Kaneko JJ (ed): Clinical biochemistry
    of domestic animals, 3rd ed. New York, Academic Press, 1980.
Bauer JE: Plasma lipids and lipoproteins of fasted ponies. Am J Vet Res 44:379, 1983.
Bentinck-Smith J, Tasker JB: Special topics in clinical pathology. Cornell Vet 68:307,
    1978.
Bergman EN: Glucose metabolism in ruminants as related to hypoglycemia and ketosis.
    Cornell Vet 63:341, 1973.
Blaisdell FS, Dodds WJ: Evaluation of two microhematocrit methods for quantitating plasma
    fibrinogen. J Am Vet Med Assoc 171:340, 1977.
Breitschwerdt EB, Barta O, Waltman C, et al: Serum proteins in healthy basenjis and
    basenjis with chronic diarrhea. Am J Vet Res 44:326, 1983.
Breitschwerdt EB, Loar AS, Hribernik TN, et al: Hypoglycemia in four dogs with sepsis.
    J Am Vet Med Assoc 178:1072, 1981.
Campbell MD: Determination of plasma fibrinogen concentration in the horse. Am J Vet Res
    42:100, 1981.
Case GL, Phillips RW, Cleek JL: Lactic acid and glucose metabolism in healthy, lactic-acid
    infused, and diarrheic calves. Am J Vet Res 41:1035, 1980.
Chastain CB: Intensive care of dogs and cats with diabetic ketoacidosis. J Am Vet Med
    Assoc 179:972, 1981.
Church DB, Watson ADJ: Whole blood glucose determination in dogs using dextrostix and the
    eyetone reflectance colorimeter. J Small Anim Pract 20:163, 1979.
Coffman JR: Clinical application of serum protein electrophoresis in the horse.
    Proc Am Assoc Equine Pract, Philadelphia, 1968.
Coffman JR: Blood glucose. 1. Factors affecting blood levels and test results. Vet Med
    Small Anim Clin 74:719, 1979.
Coffman JR: Blood glucose. 2. Clinical application of blood glucose determination. Vet Med
    Small Anim Clin 74:855, 1979.
Coffman JR: Plasma lactate determinations. Vet Med Small Anim Clin 74:997, 1979.
Coffman JR: The plasma proteins. Vet Med Small Anim Clin 74:1168, 1979.
Coffman JR: Plasma protein electrophoresis. Vet Med Small Anim Clin 74:1251, 1979.
Deem DA, Traver DS, Thacker HL, et al: Agammaglobulinemia in a horse. J Am Vet Med Assoc
    175:469, 1979.
Dewhirst MW, Stamp GL, Hurvitz AI: Idiopathic monoclonal (IgA) gammopathy in a dog. J Am
    Vet Med Assoc 170:1313, 1977.
DiBartola SP, Reynolds HA: Hypoglycemia and polyclonal gammopathy in a dog with plasma
    cell dyscrasia. J Am Vet Med Assoc 180:1345, 1982.
Feldman EC, Nelson RW: Insulin-induced hyperglycemia in diabetic dogs. J Am Vet Med Assoc
    180:1432, 1982.
Finco DR, Duncan JR, Schall WD, et al: Chronic enteric disease and hypoproteinemia in 9
    dogs. J Am Vet Med Assoc 163:262, 1973.
Frantz ID, Medina G, Faeusch HW: Correlation of dextrostix values with true glucose in the
    range less than 50 mg/dl. J Pediatr 87:417, 1975.
Gay CC, Sullivan ND, Wilkinson JS: Hyperlipemia in ponies. Aust Vet J 54:459, 1978.
Hardie EM, Barsanti JA: Treatment of canine actinomycosis. J Am Vet Med Assoc 180:537,
    1982.
Havel RJ: Caloric homeostasis and disorders of fuel transport. N Engl J Med 287:1186,
    1972.
Herdt TH, Liesman JS, Gerloff BJ, et al: Reduction of serum triacylglycerol-rich
    lipoprotein concentrations in cows with hepatic lipidosis. Am J Vet Res 44:293, 1983.
Herdt TH, Stevens JB, Linn J, et al: Influence of ration composition and energy balance on
    blood beta-hydroxybutyrate (ketone) and plasma glucose concentrations of dairy cows in
    early lactation. Am J Vet Res 42:1177, 1981.
Herdt TH, Stevens JB, Olson WG, et al: Blood concentrations of beta-hydroxybutyrate in
    clinically normal Holstein-Friesian herds and in those with a high prevalence of
    clinical ketosis. Am J Vet Res 42:503, 1981.
Hill FWG, Kidder DE: The oral glucose tolerance test in canine pancreatic malabsorption.
    Br Vet J 128:207, 1972.
Hopkins FM, Dean DF, Green W: Failure of passive transfer in calves: Comparison of field
    diagnostic methods. Mod Vet Pract 65:625, 1984.

Hsu WH, Hembrough FB: Intravenous glucose tolerance test in cats: Influenced by
   acetylpromazine, ketamine, morphine, thiopental and xylazine. Am J Vet Res 43:2060,
   1982.
Hurvitz AI, Kehoe JM, Capra JD, et al: Bence Jones proteinemia and proteinuria in a dog.
   J Am Vet Med Assoc 159:1112, 1971.
Hurvitz AI, MacEwen EG, Middaugh CR, et al: Monoclonalcryoglobulinemia with
   macroglobulinemia in a dog. J Am Vet Med Assoc 170:511, 1977.
Jackson RF, Bruss ML, Growney PJ, et al: Hypoglycemia-ketonemia in a pregnant bitch. J Am
   Vet Med Assoc 177:1123, 1980.
Jacobs KA, Bolton JR: Effect of diet on the oral glucose tolerance test in the horse. J Am
   Vet Med Assoc 180:884, 1982.
James RC, Chase GR: Evaluation of some commonly used semiquantitative methods for urinary
   glucose and ketone determinations. Diabetes 23:474, 1974.
Jasper DE, Jain NC: Postprandial lipemia in dogs. Calif Vet 18(3):27, 1964.
Jones BR, Wallace A, Harding DRK, et al: Occurrence of idiopathic, familial
   hyperchylomicronaemia in a cat. Vet Rec 112:543, 1983.
Kaneko JJ: Carbohydrate metabolism. In Kaneko JJ (ed): Clinical biochemistry of domestic
   animals, 3rd ed. New York, Academic Press, 1980.
Kaneko JJ: Serum proteins and the dysproteinemias. In Kaneko JJ (ed): Clinical
   biochemistry of domestic animals, 3rd ed. New York, Academic Press, 1980.
Koterba A, Carlson GP: Acid-base and electrolyte alterations in horses with exertional
   rhabdomyolysis. J Am Vet Med Assoc 180:303, 1982.
Kreisberg RA: Lactate homeostasis and lactic acidosis. Ann Intern Med 92:227, 1980.
Kurtz H, Quast J: Effects of continuous intravenous infusion of Escherichia coli endotoxin
   into swine. Am J Vet Res 43:262, 1982.
Lewis LD, Phillips RW, Elliott CD: Changes in plasma glucose and lactate concentrations
   and enzyme activities in the neonatal calf with diarrhea. Am J Vet Res 36:413, 1975.
Manning PJ: Thyroid gland and arterial lesions of beagles with familial hypothyroidism
   and hyperlipoproteinemia. Am J Vet Res 40:820, 1979.
Marsh CL, Mebus CA, Underdahl NR: Loss of serum proteins via the intestinal tract in
   calves with infectious diarrhea. Am J Vet Res 30:163, 1969.
McEwan AD, Fisher EW, Selman IE, et al: A turbidity test for the estimation of immune
   globulin levels in neonatal calf serum. Clin Chim Acta 27:155, 1970.
McGuire TC, Crawford TB, Hallowell AL, et al: Failure of colostral immunoglobulin transfer
   as an explanation for most infections and deaths of neonatal foals. J Am Vet Med Assoc
   170:1302, 1977.
McGuire TC, Pfeiffer NE, Weikel JM, et al: Failure of colostral immunoglobulin transfer in
   calves dying from infectious disease. J Am Vet Med Assoc 169:713, 1976.
McGuire TC, Poppie MJ, Banks KL: Hypogammaglobulinemia predisposing to infection in foals.
   J Am Vet Med Assoc 166:71, 1975.
Molla A: Estimation of bovine colostral immunoglobulins by refractometry. Vet Rec 107:35,
   1980.
Moore JN, Johnson JH, Traver DS, et al: A review of lactic acidosis with particular
   reference to the horse. J Equine Med Surg 1(3):96, 1977.
Naylor JM: Diseases of lipid metabolism in large animals. Proc Annu Meeting Am Coll Vet
   Intern Med, 1982.
Naylor JM, Kronfeld DS, Ackland H: Hyperlipemia in horses: Effects of undernutrition and
   disease. Am J Vet Res 41:899, 1980.
Osbaldiston GW: Serum protein fractions in domestic animals. Br Vet J 128:386, 1972.
Perryman LE, McGuire TC: Evaluation of immune system failures in horses and ponies. J Am
   Vet Med Assoc 176:1374, 1980.
Perryman LE, McGuire TC, Poppie MJ, et al: Primary immunodeficiency disorders in foals.
   Pathogenesis and differential diagnosis. Proc 4th Int Conf Equine Infect Dis, Paris,
   France, 1976.
Pfeiffer NE, McGuire TL: A sodium sulfite-precipitation test for assessment of colostral
   immunoglobulin transfer to calves. J Am Vet Med Assoc 170:809, 1977.
Poppie MJ, McGuire TC: Combined immunodeficiency in foals of Arabian breeding: Evaluation
   of mode of inheritance and estimation of prevalence of affected foals and carrier mares
   and stallions. J Am Vet Med Assoc 170:31, 1977.
Roberts MC, Hill FWG: The oral glucose tolerance test in the horse. Equine Vet J
   5:171, 1973.
Rogers WA: Lipemia in the dog. Vet Clin North Am 7:637, 1977.
Rogers WA, Donovan EF, Kociba GJ: Idiopathic hyperlipoproteinemia in dogs. J Am Vet Med
   Assoc 166:1087, 1975.
Rogers WA, Donovan EF, Kociba GJ: Lipids and lipoproteins in normal dogs and in dogs with
   secondary hyperlipoproteinemia. J Am Vet Med Assoc 166:1092, 1975.
Rumbaugh GE, Ardans AA, Ginno D, et al: Measurement of neonatal equine immunoglobulins for
   assessment of colostral immunoglobulin transfer: Comparison of single radial
   immunodiffusion with the zinc sulfate turbidity test, serum electrophoresis,
   refractometry for total serum protein, and the sodium sulfite precipitation test. J Am
   Vet Med Assoc 172:321, 1978.

Rumbaugh GE, Ardans AA, Ginno D, et al: Identification and treatment of colostrum-deficient foals. J Am Vet Med Assoc 174:273, 1979.

Schalm OW: Hypoproteinemia in the dog. Calif Vet 28(8):6, 1974.

Scherston B, Kuhl C, Hollender A, et al: Blood glucose measurements with dextrostix and new reflectance meter. Br Med J 3:384, 1974.

Schotman AJH, Kroneman J: Hyperlipemia in ponies. Neth J Vet Sci 2:60, 1969.

Strombeck DR, Krum S, Meyer D, et al: Hypoglycemia and hypoinsulinemia associated with hepatoma in a dog. J Am Vet Med Assoc 169:811, 1976.

Strombeck DR, Rogers Q, Freedland R, et al: Fasting hypoglycemia in a pup. J Am Vet Med Assoc 173:299, 1978.

Tennant B, Baldwin BH, Braun RK, et al: Use of the glutaraldehyde coagulation test for detection of hypogammaglobulinemia in neonatal calves. J Am Vet Med Assoc 174:848, 1979.

Turnwald GH: Hypoglycemia. Part I. Carbohydrate metabolism and laboratory examination. Compend Contin Educ Pract Vet 5:932, 1983.

Turnwald GH: Hypoglycemia. Part II. Clinical aspects. Compend Contin Educ Pract Vet 6:115, 1984.

Whitlock RH, Tasker JB: Hyperglycemia in ruminants. Bull Am Soc Vet Clin Pathol 1(2):5, 1972.

Wilkins RJ: A micro-spectrophotometric method for the determination of protein with CSF. Bull Am Soc Vet Clin Pathol 3(4):3, 1974.

Wilson DE: The clinical laboratory and hyperlipidemia: A clinician's view. Med Technol 47:551, 1981.

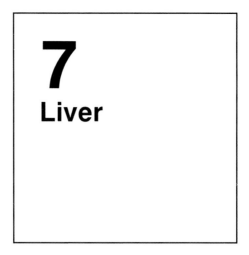

7
Liver

HEPATIC ABNORMALITIES DETECTED BY LABORATORY TESTS

I. Hepatocellular injury
    A. Change in cell permeability allows leakage of intracellular
        substances into extracellular fluid.
        1. Leakage may occur with sublethal cell injury or with
            necrosis.
        2. Enzymes soluble in hepatic cytosol are the usual
            diagnostic indicators of change in permeability.
        3. In general, the magnitude of increase in enzyme
            activity in extracellular fluid (serum) correlates with
            the number of affected hepatocytes.
    B. Increased intracellular to extracellular concentration
        gradient occurs with enzyme induction, and the activity of
        the induced enzyme increases in extracellular fluid.
        1. Induction may occur by increased enzyme synthesis,
            decreased enzyme degradation (intracellular), or
            stimulated activity without an increase in number of
            molecules.
        2. Most known inducible enzymes are of the mixed function
            oxidase system; although not of this type, certain
            diagnostic enzymes also may be induced.
        3. Distinction between induction and leakage as the cause
            of increased activity in extracellular fluid is often
            impossible.
    C. Certain types of injury may affect a single hepatocyte
        function without associated hepatic lesions or interference
        with other functions. The best example is failure in
        carboxylation of coagulation factors II, VII, IX, and X in
        coumarin poisoning (see Chapter 4).
    D. Decreased functional mass of hepatocytes is acquired in a
        variety of chronic progressive liver diseases.
        1. Most hepatic functions do not become insufficient until
            70 to 80% of the hepatocellular mass is lost.
        2. Diminished mass is reflected in several tests.

       a.   Severe hepatic insufficiency leads to hypo-
albuminemia and hypoproteinemia (see Chapter 6).
       b.   Diminished glycogen storage capacity causes
prolonged postprandial hyperglycemia or anorexia-
related hypoglycemia (see Chapter 6).
       c.   Reduced availability of hepatocyte receptors causes
decreased clearance of certain exogenous dyes from
blood; these may detect 50 to 60% decrease in
functional mass.

II.   Cholestasis. Cholestasis implies that products of bile occur in
abnormal concentrations in blood; it may develop by physical
obstruction of biliary flow or by metabolic abnormality of
hepatocytes.
   A.   Obstruction of bile flow may occur with lesions affecting
bile canaliculi, bile ductules or ducts, the common bile
duct or gallbladder, and interference with drainage into
the intestine.
       1.   Obstruction of bile flow causes leakage of bile into
interstitial tissue, drainage by lymphatics, and
ultimately increased concentration of bile components
in blood (e.g., bilirubin and bile acid).
       2.   Certain components in some species have a low renal
threshold and appear in urine.
   B.   Metabolic causes of cholestasis may be hereditary (e.g.,
Dubin-Johnson syndrome in Corredale sheep) or acquired with
certain drugs or toxicants; distinction between an
obstructive or a metabolic mechanism for cholestasis may be
difficult.
   C.   Cholestasis is detected by several types of tests.
       1.   Bile products such as bile acid and bilirubin can be
measured in blood and urine.
       2.   Exogenous dyes given intravenously and cleared from
blood by hepatocytes are excreted in bile; blood
concentration remains abnormally high during
cholestasis.
       3.   Bile stasis may cause induction of certain diagnostic
enzymes.

III.   Altered hepatic blood flow
   A.   Chronic passive congestion is one form of altered hepatic
blood flow, and centrilobular hypoxemia is a principal
consequence.
       1.   Hepatocellular injury characterized by change in
permeability and, in severe cases, decreased functional
mass may be detected by laboratory tests.
       2.   Removal of certain exogenous dyes from blood by hepato-
cytes may be diminished by reduced hepatic blood flow.
   B.   Portal venous-systemic venous shunting of blood impairs
delivery of portal substances to the liver.
       1.   Certain substances (e.g., ammonia) are normally
absorbed by the intestine and removed efficiently by
hepatocytes after delivery from portal blood.
       2.   The decreased availability of normal hepatotrophic
factors in portal blood leads to hepatic atrophy, and

once decreased functional hepatic mass reaches a critical level, it may be detected by laboratory tests (see above).

3. Exogenous dyes may be abnormally cleared in portosystemic shunts as a result of some combination of inadequate portal blood flow and hepatic atrophy.

IV. Altered Kupffer cell activity. Kupffer cells may be involved in the pathogenesis of many hepatic diseases, but diminished Kupffer cell mass in chronic fibrosing disorders is probably the only alteration detectable by laboratory test. Diminished Kupffer cell mass allows delivery of enteric substances (normally phagocytized by these cells) to the systemic lymphoid tissues; hyperimmunoglobulinemia results.

HEPATIC LABORATORY TESTS

I. Serum enzyme tests
   A. Alanine aminotransferase (ALT). Synonym is glutamic pyruvic transaminase (GPT).
      1. ALT is a cytosol enzyme that catalyzes the reaction: alanine + alpha ketoglutarate $\rightleftharpoons$ pyruvate + glutamate. The reaction involves alanine biosynthesis from carbohydrate intermediate metabolites or the reverse.
      2. The enzyme is considered to be nearly specific for liver in diagnostic use in dogs and cats. The plasma half-life of ALT in the dog is estimated to be about 60 hours and is shorter in the cat.
      3. The enzyme is stable in serum or plasma for several days at zero to 4°C. Hemolysis should be avoided. Although activity is expressed in international units, laboratories may run the assay at different temperatures or with other variables, and reference values should be established at each laboratory (see Appendix I).
      4. Serum ALT activity increases with change in hepatocellular permeability (sublethal injury and necrosis) (Case 11). Guidelines for interpretation are as follows.
         a. The magnitude of increase roughly parallels the number of cells affected in acute disease.
         b. Several days after the occurrence of massive necrosis, activity may be misleadingly low as a result of exhausted enzyme supply from necrotic cells.
         c. Correlation between serum activity and clinical manifestation of hepatic insufficiency is poor. In chronic progressive liver diseases typically fewer hepatocytes are undergoing necrosis at any one time, and serum ALT activity may be unimpressive compared to the degree of hepatic insufficiency. In acute hepatic sublethal injury or necrosis with very high serum ALT activity, signs of hepatic insufficiency may be minimal.

        d.   In acute liver diseases, a 50% or more decrease in serum ALT over the time of one half-life would be a favorable finding; however, in chronic progressive liver diseases, declining serum activity may be due to decreasing functional mass of hepatocytes as the liver undergoes fibrosis.

    5.   Serum ALT activity may increase as a result of enzyme induction in hepatocytes. Glucocorticoids induce hepatic ALT as a consequence of gluconeogenic activity (Case 20).

    6.   Species differences for ALT are as follows.

        a.   The enzyme may be considered liver-specific in dogs and cats.

        b.   Hepatic ALT in horses, cattle, sheep, goats, and pigs is very low, which precludes its use for detecting liver disease in these species. Serum ALT increases moderately in cattle, sheep, and swine with muscular diseases.

B. Aspartate aminotransferase (AST). Synonym is glutamic oxaloacetic transaminase (GOT).

    1.   Two or more AST isoenzymes, located in cytosol and mitochondria respectively, catalyze the reaction: asparate + alpha ketoglutarate $\rightleftharpoons$ glutamate + oxaloacetate. The reaction involves aspartate biosynthesis from carbohydrate intermediates or the reverse.

    2.   The enzyme occurs in almost all cells, but it is considered a diagnostic enzyme for liver and muscle disease because of its high activity in these tissues (see Chapter 10). The plasma half-life of AST is approximately 12 hours in the dog, shorter in cats, 18 hours in swine, and probably longer in horses and cattle.

    3.   Considerations regarding AST assay are similar to those mentioned above for ALT.

    4.   Serum AST activity increases with change in hepatocellular permeability (sublethal injury and necrosis), and the guidelines for interpretation are the same as given for ALT above (Case 5).

    5.   Serum AST activity also increases with change in muscular permeability (sublethal injury and necrosis). Guidelines for interpretation are given in Chapter 10 (Case 13).

    6.   Species differences for AST are as follows.

        a.   In the dog and cat, ALT is used more frequently because of its liver specificity. ALT activity is usually greater than AST activity in animals with liver disease when both assays are done. Comparatively, the sensitivity to detect liver disease may not be greatly different (e.g., in canine neoplasia metastatic to the liver, 87% of the cases had increased AST activity and 62% had increased ALT activity).

        b.   Because of its common availability in veterinary and medical laboratories and in spite of its liver and muscle specificity, AST is widely used in large animals to detect liver disease.

C. Alkaline phosphatase (ALP)

1. ALP applies to a group of enzymes with broad substrate specificity that catalyze the hydrolysis of monophosphate esters at an alkaline pH.

   a. Little is known about intracellular functions, but the enzymes are bound to intracellular microsomal membranes and do not leak out of the cell during conditions of increased permeability. .

   b. Some believe that only newly synthesized (induced) ALP escapes from cells having normal cell membrane permeability.

   c. ALP isoenzymes are in every tissue; high activities occur in liver, bone, intestine, kidney, placenta, and leukocytes.

   d. The various ALP isoenzymes can be isolated from tissues and identified by their electrophoretic characteristics; isoenzyme identification of serum ALP can be used to identify the tissue of origin. This identification is available in a limited number of veterinary laboratories.

2. Serum ALP activity in healthy animals is primarily of hepatic origin in dogs, cats, and horses. Placental ALP isoenzyme may be found in the serum of healthy pregnant mares and queens, and bone ALP isoenzyme may be found in very young, healthy growing animals.

   a. The serum half-life of ALP isoenzymes in dogs and cats has been experimentally studied.

      (1) Hepatic ALP isoenzyme half-life in plasma is estimated to be 3 days in the dog and 5.8 hours in the cat.

      (2) Intestinal, renal, and placental ALP isoenzymes have less than 6-minute half-life in canine plasma.

      (3) Intestinal ALP isoenzyme has about a 2-minute half-life in feline plasma.

   b. ALP isoenzymes with plasma half-life in minutes can be excluded from consideration when interpreting abnormally high total serum ALP activity.

3. Causes for increased serum ALP activity are as follows. Differentiation requires consideration of other clinical and laboratory findings on the case in question.

   a. Cholestasis causes hepatic ALP induction and increased serum activity; the enzyme is induced in affected and unaffected hepatic lobes during localized cholestatic lesions (Case 11).

      (1) Intrahepatic cholestasis tends to cause a progressive increase.

      (2) Extrahepatic obstructions of individual bile ducts cause a progressive increase, but serum activity may plateau or even decline if recanalization occurs.

      (3) The potential magnitude of serum ALP increase

in cholestatic diseases is marked.

    (4) Serum ALP increase may be considered a sensitive indicator of cholestasis; in early stages or mild circumstances, it precedes development of hyperbilirubinemia or other indicators of cholestasis.

b. Drugs induce hepatic ALP and increase serum activity.

    (1) These include primidone, phenobarbital, deildrin, glucocorticoids, and certain other compounds.

    (2) Both endogenous and exogenous glucocorticoids induce hepatic ALP (Case 20).

    (3) In serum ALP isoenzyme profiles of dogs with glucocortoid-induced, high serum ALP activity, a specific steroidal isoenzyme that moves slightly more anodal than the normal hepatic isoenzyme may be found.

    (4) The potential magnitude of serum ALP increase is marked in drug-induced circumstances.

c. Conditions characterized by increased osteoblastic activity may increase serum ALP activity.

    (1) These conditions include primary and secondary hyperparathyroidism, bone healing, and osteosarcoma (Case 14).

    (2) In the dog, in contrast to cholestasis and drug induction, the potential magnitude of serum ALP increase in these diseases is very mild.

d. Frequently, high serum ALP activity is found on routine biochemical testing, and the mechanism cannot be determined (i.e, other clinical or laboratory findings may not indicate either hepatic disease, hepatic ALP induction, or bone disease) (Case 19).

e. In acute toxic liver injury with very high serum ALT or AST activity, ALP is usually normal or only mildly increased; during recovery stages serum ALP may continue to increase for several days while the activities of the other enzymes decrease.

f. In certain old dogs, occasionally malignant neoplasms of a variety of types (e.g., mammary gland adenocarcinoma, squamous cell carcinoma, hemoangiosarcoma) are associated with extremely high serum ALP activity.

5. Species differences for interpretation of serum ALP activity

a. Differences in half-life of isoenzymes in serum have been noted above.

b. Canine liver normally contains about three times more ALP activity than feline liver. This fact plus the more rapid disappearance of hepatic ALP from plasma in cats reflect the much less dramatic values in this species compared with those in the dog.

        c. Certain feline hepatic hyperbilirubinemic disorders are accompanied by normal serum ALP activity (e.g., some cases of feline infectious peritonitis). In view of the concept described above, this observation remains unexplained.

        d. Reference values for serum ALP in cattle and sheep are wide, which reduces the sensitivity for detecting cholestatic liver disease.

D. Gamma glutamyltransferase (GGT) (synonym, gamma glutamyl transpeptidase)

    1. GGT is a carboxypeptidase that cleaves C-terminal glutamyl groups and transfers them to peptides or other acceptors such as glycylglycine. The enzyme is involved in glutathione metabolism, and it is associated with microsomal membranes (95% of cellular GGT activity) and cytosol (5%).

    2. Most cells contain GGT, but renal convoluted tubular cells and canalicular surfaces of hepatocytes and bile duct epithelium contain the greatest activity. Serum GGT activity is primarily of hepatic origin in health and disease; renal GGT is delivered to urine in nephrosis (routine serum assay for GGT will not work on urine).

    3. Serum GGT activity increases with cholestasis.

    4. Species differences for GGT are as follows.

        a. GGT offers no advantages over ALP for detecting cholestasis in dogs and cats, except it can be considered liver-specific.

        b. Serum GGT activity increases in cholestatic diseases of horses, cattle, sheep, and swine; it is more useful than ALP in these species because of the narrow reference values.

        c. Some reports indicate that serum GGT activity may increase in horses, cattle, and sheep with acute hepatic necrosis.

E. Other serum enzymes used to detect liver injury

    1. Sorbitol dehydrogenase (SDH) (synonym, iditol dehydrogenase)

        a. Hepatocytic cytosol contains high SDH activity in all animals, and increased serum SDH indicates acute change in hepatocellular permeability (Case 5).

        b. The plasma SDH half-life is extremely short; in acute hepatotoxicities, serum activity may return to normal limits in 4 or 5 days after the insult, which is often before the animal is evaluated by clinical or laboratory means.

    2. Other enzymes that increase in serum with hepatic necrosis include arginase, glutamate dehydrogenase, ornithine carbamyltransferase, isocitric dehydrogenase (tissue specificity similar to AST), and lactate dehydrogenase (see Chapter 10).

    3. Leucine aminopeptidase (LAP) and 5'nucleotidase behave similarly to ALP. In cats LAP does not increase in obstructive biliary disease.

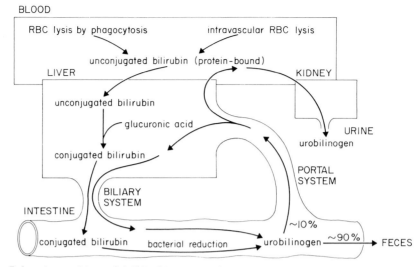

Fig. 7.1. An outline of bilirubin excretion.

II. Tests of hepatic uptake, conjugation, and secretion
    A. Bilirubin
        1. Bilirubin originates from senescent erythrocytes (about
            80%) in the macrophages of spleen, liver, and bone mar-
            row and from nonheme porphyrins (about 20%) (Fig. 7.1).
            a. Bilirubin is transported in plasma bound to
                albumin, globulin, and other proteins.
            b. Hepatic uptake of bilirubin, dissociated from the
                plasma protein at the cell membrane, is followed by
                conjugation principally to glucuronic acid; minimal
                extrahepatic conjugation by some tissues such as
                renal tubular epithelium may occur. Conjugation
                renders the bilirubin water soluble.
            c. Conjugated bilirubin is secreted into bile
                canaliculi and delivered to the intestine where
                most is converted to urobilinogen by intestinal
                flora and excreted.
            d. Small amounts of urobilinogen are reabsorbed into
                portal blood and removed by hepatocytes or excreted
                into urine. Small amounts of intestinal conjugated
                bilirubin are hydrolyzed to the unconjugated form
                and reabsorbed into blood.
        2. Methods of bilirubin assay are based on the diazo
            reaction. With the addition of reagent, color develops
            rapidly (direct reaction); after addition of alcohol,
            further color development allows measurement of total
            bilirubin.
            a. The direct reaction measures conjugated bilirubin
                (although a small percentage of serum unconjugated
                bilirubin may react directly). The concentration of
                prehepatic or unconjugated bilirubin (free or
                protein-bound bilirubin) is determined by the
                numerical difference between total and direct-
                reacting measurements.

       b. Most methods yield reproducible total bilirubin
values, but values for direct-reacting bilirubin
are quite variable. No significance should be
placed on the direct-reacting value when total
bilirubin is within the normal range.

       c. Sample management is important to evaluation of
hyperbilirubinemia. Serum total bilirubin may drop
by as much as 50%/hour in direct exposure to
sunlight or artificial fluorescent lighting (400 to
600 nm wavelength).

3. Measurement of urine bilirubin is done by qualitative
methods; bilirubin, if present in urine, will usually
be conjugated, water soluble bilirubin (see Chapter 9).

4. Measurement of urobilinogen in urine is done by
semiquantitative methods. Urinary urobilinogen is
unstable, and results are poorly reproducible. Many
healthy animals have urine with no detectable
urobilinogen in their urine, which makes the test of
little clinical value in veterinary medicine.

5. Causes of hyperbilirubinemia and bilirubinuria may be
classified as follows.

       a. "Retention" or hemolytic hyperbilirubinemia is
characterized by unconjugated bilirubin as the
predominant form in serum. Bilirubinuria may or may
not accompany the hyperbilirubinemia.

          (1) Hemolytic disorders with overproduction of
pigment are the primary causes (see Chapter 1)
(Case 3).

          (2) Inadequate hepatic uptake or defective
conjugation may occur in certain hepatic
diseases, leading to "retention."

          (3) Massive internal hemorrhage may be followed by
a transient retention hyperbilirubinemia.

       b. "Regurgitation" or cholestatic hyperbilirubinemia
is characterized by conjugated bilirubin as the
predominant form in serum. Bilirubinuria
accompanies the hyperbilirubinemia and may precede
it in animals with a low renal threshold such as
the dog.

          (1) Intrahepatic or extrahepatic obstruction of
bile flow causes leakage of bilirubin into the
interstitium, the lymphatic system, and hence
to blood (see discussion on cholestasis
earlier in this chapter). Serum ALP increase
is a far more sensitive indicator of this
phenomenon and precedes the development of
hyperbilirubinemia.

          (2) Defective secretion of conjugated bilirubin
also may be a cause.

       c. "Combined" hyperbilirubinemia is characterized by
increased unconjugated and conjugated bilirubin in
serum, without one form predominating markedly over
the other, and usually bilirubinuria. It develops
by both the retention and regurgitation mechanisms
defined above (Case 11).

          (1) Acute or chronic hepatic diseases, usually

with necrosis or decreased functional mass and diffuse fibrosis, are the causes. From a practical standpoint, this form of hyperbilirubinemia cannot be readily differentiated from regurgitation hyperbilirubinemia with intrahepatic obstruction or from retention hyperbilirubinemia with reduced hepatic uptake.

(2) In general, the more complete the physical obstruction to bile flow, the greater the conjugated bilirubin proportion of serum total bilirubin.

6. Species differences and guidelines for interpretation of bilirubin tests follow (Table 7.1).

a. Hyperbilirubinemia in dogs and cats usually can be classified using the above categories (retention, regurgitation, or combined).

(1) Hemolytic hyperbilirubinemias have conjugated bilirubin (direct-reacting) less than 50% of serum total bilirubin.

(2) Extrahepatic biliary obstructions have greater than 50% direct-reacting bilirubin.

(3) Intrahepatic causes of hyperbilirubinemia are variable. From 20 to 60% of total bilirubin may be direct-reacting; that is, a few cases (more in cats than in dogs) cannot be differentiated from hemolytic hyperbilirubinemia without using other laboratory findings.

b. Dogs have a low renal threshold for conjugated bilirubin.

(1) Bilirubinuria commonly precedes developing hyperbilirubinemia.

(2) Healthy dogs with urine specific gravity in excess of 1.040 often have trace bilirubinuria; this finding is more common in males than females.

c. In most species, regurgitation and combined hyperbilirubinemias are preceded by increased serum ALP or GGT activity; certain cases in cats are an exception (e.g., some cases of feline infectious peritonitis).

d. The hyperbilirubinemia associated with canine

TABLE 7.1.   Comparative Findings in Cholestatic and Hemolytic Hyperbilirubinemias

Finding	Normal	Hemolytic Disease	Cholestatic Disease Partial	Complete
Total bilirubin	Normal	+++	+	++
Conjugated bilirubin		▲	▲	▲
Unconjugated bilirubin		▲	▲	▲
Urine bilirubin	- or trace	+	++	+++
Urine urobilinogen	+ or -	++	+ or -	-
Color of feces	Normal	Orange	Normal	Acholic

Note: See text for species differences; size of arrow corresponds to relative magnitude of change; + = positive, - = negative.

leptospirosis is of the regurgitation type, whereas
leptospirosis in cattle, sheep, and swine causes a
retention hyperbilirubinemia.

    e. Equine hyperbilirubinemia is predominantly unconjugated, and the magnitude may be quite marked.

       (1) Hyperbilirubinemia associated with hemolysis typically has less than 25% of total bilirubin that is direct-reacting.

       (2) Direct-reacting bilirubin usually ranges from 15 to 40% of total bilirubin in hyperbilirubinemias caused by intrahepatic or extrahepatic obstruction.

       (3) Anorexia commonly is associated with hyperbilirubinemia in horses; total bilirubin is usually less than 10 mg/dl and less than 25% is direct reacting. The mechanism is diminished hepatic uptake of bilirubin.

    f. Hyperbilirubinemia in cattle, sheep, goats, and swine is almost always retention in type.

       (1) Hemolytic diseases are more common than hepatic diseases as causes of hyperbilirubinemia in these species.

       (2) Hyperbilirubinemia occurs in a variety of bovine diseases, usually accompanied by anorexia and rumen stasis, and is characterized as retention-type (hemolytic) rather than regurgitation-type. Overt hepatic disease and anemia may not be features of these diseases, and the mechanism is obscure.

       (3) Extrahepatic biliary obstruction will cause some increase in direct-reacting bilirubin in cattle; otherwise, measurable conjugated bilirubin is rarely found in hyperbilirubinemic cattle.

       (4) The magnitude of hyperbilirubinemia in cattle is usually minimal compared to similar diseases in dogs or horses.

       (5) Inadequate hepatic uptake and defective conjugation cause unconjugated hyperbilirubinemia in certain mutant Southdown sheep (similar to human Gilbert's syndrome).

       (6) Conjugated hyperbilirubinemia from decreased hepatic secretion occurs in certain mutant Corredale sheep (similar to human Dubin-Johnson syndrome).

B. Sulfobromophthalein (BSP) excretion test

    1. BSP dye is rapidly removed from blood, conjugated by hepatocytes, and excreted in bile. The rate of removal from blood is a function of:

      a. Volume of distribution of the dye

      b. Rate of hepatic blood flow

      c. Availability of carrier protein

      d. Functional hepatic mass

      e. Hepatocellular conjugation and secretion

       f. Patency of the biliary system

2. Two procedures are used.

       a. In the dog and cat the amount of BSP retention in blood is determined 30 minutes after a single intravenous injection of 5 mg BSP/kg body weight.

       b. In large animals the rate of clearance (i.e., the amount of dye cleared from blood per unit of time) is determined and reported as half-time for disappearance (T 1/2). Plasma samples are collected after a single intravenous injection of 1.0 gram BSP (body weight need not be determined).

3. Interpretation of BSP retention or clearance values

       a. Anasarca, ascites, and obesity may cause an expanded volume of distribution of dye; the effect on retention or clearance should be minimal unless the expanded extracellular fluid is high in protein content, in which case faster clearance or lower retention values might underestimate hepatic dysfunction (Case 7).

       b. Diminished hepatic blood flow caused by postsinusoidal obstruction or cardiac insufficiency decreases effective delivery of dye to hepatocytes and causes retention or reduced clearance (Case 7).

       c. Portal venous–systemic venous shunting of blood may cause retention or reduced clearance of BSP if hepatic mass also is reduced; dye removal in animals with shunts is normal if hepatic mass and hepatic arterial supply are normal (Case 12).

       d. In hypoalbuminemia a higher proportion of albumin molecules are bound to BSP, and albumin interaction with hepatocyte receptors (a normal dynamic event) would favor enhanced BSP uptake; in severe hypoalbuminemia, the BSP value may underestimate hepatic dysfunction (Case 7).

       e. BSP retention or reduced clearance occurs with about 55% loss of functional hepatic mass (other factors being normal).

       f. BSP retention or reduced clearance is always found in hyperbilirubinemic conditions.

          (1) In regurgitation–type hyperbilirubinemia, BSP in bile escapes back to blood via interstitial fluid and lymph drainage.

          (2) In retention–type (hemolytic) hyperbilirubinemia, uptake of free bilirubin and BSP by hepatocytes is competitive, and the system is saturable; therefore, BSP retention or reduced clearance is expected during hemolytic disease.

       g. Drugs that bind to plasma albumin may compete with BSP for carrier binding and decrease hepatocellular uptake, causing BSP retention or reduced clearance.

       h. A dog with a histologically normal liver and defective intracellular hepatic carrier system with marked BSP retention has been described.

     C. Indocyanine green (ICG) clearance
         1. The principles affecting removal of ICG from blood by liver and the considerations for interpretation of ICG values are essentially the same as those for the BSP excretion test.
         2. The procedure for measurement is more complicated for the veterinary practitioner than that for BSP.
             a. A preinjection plasma sample is required for preparation of a blank and standard in the laboratory.
             b. Reconstituted dye is administered intravenously at a dose of 0.5 mg ICG/kg body weight; but a portion of the same dye lot, stable for only 24 hours, must accompany the plasma samples to the laboratory for preparation of a standard solution.
             c. Measurement of the dye in the laboratory requires a spectrophotometer capable of producing an 805-nm wavelength of light, relatively uncommon among laboratory instruments.
     D. Bile acids
         1. Two bile acids, cholic acid and chenodeoxycholic acid, are synthesized by hepatocytes, conjugated primarily with glycine or taurine, and secreted into bile.
             a. The bile acids, secreted as anions, may be stored in the gallbladder and delivered to the intestine after the ingestion of food.
             b. Bile acids are required for dietary fat emulsification, a prerequisite for fat digestion and absorption and for absorption of fat-soluble vitamins A, D, E, and K.
             c. About 95% of bile acids are reabsorbed into portal blood, taken up by the liver, and resecreted into bile (enterohepatic circulation).
         2. Serum bile acids are assayed by radioimmune assay or enzyme-linked, spectrophotometric systems; most assays measure the principal bile acid of man and dog, cholylglycine.
         3. Increased serum bile acid concentration occurs with cholestasis; the abnormality tends to parallel change in ALP activity in experimentally obstructed dogs.
         4. Acute toxic hepatic necrosis increases serum bile acid concentration of dogs, ponies, sheep, and calves.

III. Tests for portal blood clearance
     A. Plasma ammonia and ammonia tolerance test
         1. Most plasma ammonia is produced by microbial deamination of urea and exogenous dietary amines in the intestinal tract. Ammonia absorbed from the intestine is carried in portal venous blood to the liver where it is efficiently removed.
         2. Several reliable methods for laboratory measurement of plasma ammonia are available in most veterinary laboratories.

a. Careful sample management is critical for accurate
    results.
    (1) Ammonia-free heparin is recommended for sample
         collection; other anticoagulants may cause
         false high values.
    (2) Simple-stomached animals should be fasted at
         least 8 hours before sample collection.
    (3) Blood should be placed in an ice bath
         immediately after collection and the plasma
         separated within 30 minutes; hemolysis will
         cause false high values.
    (4) Separated plasma must be assayed within 60
         minutes if held at refrigerator temperature;
         delay causes false high values.
    (5) Quick-freezing plasma by immersion and
         swirling the tube in a mixture of dry ice and
         ethanol and maintaining at $-20^{\circ}C$ will preserve
         ammonia levels at least 2 days.
b. If the baseline fasting plasma ammonia level is not
    abnormally high, additional information may be
    obtained with the ammonia tolerance test.
    (1) Ammonium chloride solution (20% w/v) is
         administered at the dosage of 0.5 ml/kg body
         weight via stomach tube or by forced drinking
         as a mixture with chocolate milk.
    (2) A 30-minute postfeeding plasma sample is
         collected for ammonia assay.
    (3) Interpretation of the absolute value and the
         magnitude of increase over the baseline value
         are useful. In healthy dogs the postfeeding,
         plasma ammonia value is about two to two and
         one-half times the baseline value.
c. Whereas in vivo acid base status affects the plasma
    balance between ammonia and ammonium ion, the
    laboratory assay is conducted by conversion
    entirely to ammonia, and acid base status does not
    require consideration for interpretation of
    results.
3. Guidelines for interpretation of plasma ammonia
    concentration
    a. Baseline fasting ammonia is increased with portal
        venous-systemic venous shunting of blood (Case 12).
        (1) Congenital shunts and hyperammonemia are
             described in dogs, calves, cats, and horses.
        (2) Acquired shunts may develop in chronic
             fibrosing liver diseases.
        (3) If an ammonia tolerance test is done when
             baseline plasma ammonia is high, consideration
             for possible physiopathologic consequences of
             hyperammonemia should be given.
        (4) If an ammonia tolerance test is done in a dog
             with shunts in spite of a high baseline value,
             the postfeeding plasma ammonia value will be
             about two to two and one-half times the

baseline value. If the value is greater than two and one-half times the baseline, it may indicate reduced functional hepatic mass secondary to shunting of blood.

    (5) Shunts are unlikely if baseline plasma ammonia is within normal limits.

  b. In dogs with up to 60% loss of functional hepatic mass and no portal venous-systemic venous shunting of blood, baseline plasma ammonia remains within normal limits.

    (1) If the ammonia tolerance test is done in dogs with 60% or more loss of hepatic mass and no shunts, postfeeding plasma ammonia value may be about five times the baseline value.

    (2) Apparently with this degree of reduced functional mass, hepatocellular receptors for ammonia can be saturated using the ammonia tolerance test as defined above.

  c. Hyperammonemia can be found in ammonia toxicosis in ruminants.

  d. Congenital deficiency of certain urea cycle enzymes and hyperammonemia are described in the dog.

B. Plasma branched chain/aromatic amino acid ratio

  1. The plasma concentration and precise distribution of amino acids varies with diet and rate of intestinal absorption; uptake following absorption is by all cells, but particularly by hepatocytes.

  2. Amino acid analysis is available in a limited number of academic or commercial laboratories and is conducted by automated analyzers or chromatography.

  3. The ratio of branched chain to aromatic amino acid concentrations in serum decreases from greater than three in healthy dogs to less than one in dogs with portal venous-systemic venous shunting of blood or chronic active hepatitis.

    a. Branched chain amino acid concentration is thought to be low because of enhanced utilization by muscle and adipose tissues induced by insulin.

    b. In diseases such as portal venous-systemic venous shunting or chronic active hepatitis, higher fasting insulin level occurs, and insulin stimulates incorporation of branched chain amino acids into protein by muscle.

C. Plasma globulin concentration

  1. Plasma proteins are discussed in detail in Chapter 6.

  2. In chronic liver disease, reduced mass of Kupffer cells allows wider dissemination of enteric-derived foreign protein into the monocyte-macrophage population. Unlike Kupffer cells, splenic and lymphoid macrophages process antigen for lymphocytic antibody production, and hyperimmunoglobulinemia or polyclonal gammapathy occurs.

D. Dye excretion tests. BSP and ICG tests were included in the previous section because unless hepatic mass is significantly reduced by concomitant atrophy or other lesions portal venous-systemic venous shunting alone will not cause dye retention or reduced clearance.

IV. Tests related to hepatic synthesis
     A. Glucose
         1. Glucose is discussed in detail in Chapter 6.
         2. In chronic liver disease, prolonged postprandial hyperglycemia from decreased functional hepatic mass and/or anorexia-associated hypoglycemia from reduced glycogen storage capability may be observed.
     B. Albumin and albumin/globulin (A/G) ratio
         1. Plasma proteins are discussed in detail in Chapter 6.
         2. In chronic liver disease, reduced functional hepatic mass leads to decreased synthesis of albumin and certain nonimmunogenic globulins causing hypoalbuminemia and decreased A/G ratio.
             a. This change occurs very late in the course of disease; from 60 to 80% loss of functional mass may have occurred before hypoalbuminemia is observed.
             b. In affected dogs, serum albumin is typically 1.5 to 2.5 g/dl.
     C. Citrated plasma clotting tests: one-stage prothrombin time and activated partial thromboplastin time
         1. These tests are discussed in detail in Chapter 4.
         2. The liver synthesizes the vitamin K-dependent factors II, VII, IX, and X as well as certain other coagulation factors.
             a. Coagulation factors have short plasma half-life, and diminished synthesis as a result of reduced functional hepatic mass may cause decreased plasma concentrations.
             b. The citrated plasma clotting tests become abnormal if any coagulation factor is reduced to less than 30% of normal; some increased sensitivity can be achieved by sample dilution (see Chapter 4).
         3. The sensitivity of the citrated plasma clotting tests, using diluted plasma, is comparable to the diagnostic enzymes for detecting hepatic disease in dogs; such animals seldom have a bleeding dyscrasia.
         4. If clinical hemorrhage accompanies otherwise confirmed hepatic disease in animals, the usual laboratory assessment of hemostasis should be conducted (see Chapter 4).
     D. Bile acids. Bile acids are synthesized and secreted by liver but were included in the section on uptake, conjugation, and secretion of organic anions above.

CATEGORIES OF HEPATIC LESIONS AND LABORATORY TEST PATTERNS

The liver is affected in a wide variety of diseases. Many have hepatic lesions and laboratory abnormalities without clinical manifestations of liver involvement. This section is an attempt to place hepatic lesions into a perspective consistent with general patterns of hepatic laboratory test abnormalities. Causes of each lesion category are summarized in Table 7.2.

TABLE 7.2. Categories of Hepatic Lesions and Causes
_____
Multiple focal (microscopic) hepatic necrosis
  Any bacterial septicemia, salmonellosis, tularemia, pseudo-
  tuberculosis, listeriosis, tuberculosis, toxoplasmosis, nocardiosis,
  Tyzzer's disease, equine viral rhinopneumonitis and shigellosis,
  canine herpes, ovine pasteurellosis, porcine pseudorabies,
  infectious bovine rhinotracheitis
Centrilobular lesions associated with local hypoxia
  Cardiac insufficiency diseases, space-occupying mediastinal lesions,
  severe anemias, shock, equine and bovine monensin toxicity
Acute submassive or massive necrosis, toxic hepatopathy
  Blue-green algae, halothane, gossypol, alsike clover (sheep),
  cocklebur (pig), birdsfoot trefoil (sheep), clay pigeon (pig),
  selenium (sheep), moldy hay (horse), phosphorus, aflatoxin, carbon
  tetrachloride, chloroform, ferrous salt, and drug toxicities;
  infectious canine hepatitis; Rift Valley fever; Theiler's disease
  (horse); hepatosis dietetica (pig)
Large focal (gross) hepatic lesions (localized in one or more lobes)
  Hepatic abscess, bovine bacillary hemoglobinuria, infarction, feline
  infectious peritonitis (dry form), bovine necrobacillosis
Diffuse hepatic lipidosis
  Diabetes mellitus, feline hepatic lipidosis syndrome, equine lipemia
  and hepatic lipidosis syndrome, bovine hepatic lipidosis (fat cow
  syndrome), ovine pregnancy toxemia
Steroid hepatopathy
  Exogenous corticosteroids and hyperadrenocorticism (dog)
Cholangiohepatitis, cholangitis, extrahepatic biliary obstruction
  Cholangitis and cholangiohepatitis (dog, cat); feline lymphocytic
  cholangitis; gallstones, abscesses, neoplasms, or other obstructive
  lesions in region of bile duct; feline Platynosomum sp. infection;
  ruminant thysanosomiasis
Chronic, progressive, primary liver diseases
  Aflatoxin, pyrrolyzidine alkaloid, alsike clover (horse, cattle),
  Lantana sp., and copper (sheep) toxicities; ovine facial eczema;
  Bedlington terrier hepatopathy; Doberman pinscher hepatopathy;
  chronic active hepatitis (dog, horse); porcine stephanuriasis;
  distomiasis; echinococcosis; hepatic cirrhosis
Portal venous-systemic venous shunts
  Acquired with chronic, progressive, primary liver diseases;
  congenital shunts (dog, cat, horse, cattle)
Primary and metastatic hepatic neoplasms
  Hepatoma, hepatic carcinoma, carcinoid, bile duct carcinomas,
  myeloproliferative diseases (dog, cat), lymphosarcoma, metastatic
  adenocarcinomas and sarcomas
_____

I. Multiple focal hepatic necrosis
    A. Clinical features and characteristics
        1. The lesion is usually an incidental finding at necropsy
            and often of diagnostic importance for infectious
            diseases. No clinical signs of liver disease occur, and
            the cause of death is usually extrahepatic.
        2. The microscopic foci of necrosis are randomly dispersed
            within hepatic lobules throughout the liver.
    B. Laboratory findings (assuming antemortem evaluation)
        1. Diagnostic enzyme activity denoting hepatocellular
            cytosol leakage is abnormal.
        2. Tests detecting cholestasis or altered hepatic blood
            flow are normal.

II. Centrilobular lesions associated with local hypoxia
    A. Clinical features and characteristics

        1. Animals usually are under veterinary care for cardiac diseases or diseases with anemia. Clinical signs of liver disease are not observed in most cases. In cardiac insufficiency disease, especially in dogs, a high-protein ascites may occur (see Chapter 12).

        2. Hypoxic injury of centrilobular cells, farthest from hepatic arterial supply, causes progressive hepatocellular necrosis and eventually replacement, centrilobular fibrosis.

   B. Laboratory findings

        1. Diagnostic enzyme activity denoting hepatocellular cytosol leakage is mildly increased in serum.

        2. Tests of cholestasis are seldom abnormal because biliary drainage toward the periphery of hepatic lobules is unaffected.

        3. Retention or decreased clearance of BSP or ICG reflects diminished hepatic blood flow.

        4. Tests related to specific hepatic synthetic or metabolic functions and those dependent on portal blood delivery to the liver are usually normal.

III. Acute submassive or massive hepatic necrosis (toxic hepatopathy)

   A. Clinical features and characteristics

        1. Clinical signs may reflect acute hepatic involvement (e.g., anorexia, vomiting, icterus, signs of hepato-encephalopathy in large animals); in some cases no signs occur in spite of massive necrosis. Disseminated intravascular coagulation syndrome may occur in some cases.

        2. The diffuse hepatic necrosis is usually arranged in various patterns (e.g., centrilobular, midzonal, periportal, confluent) within each hepatic lobule, depending on the cause. The occurrence of inflammation and fibrosis also depends on the cause and longevity.

   B. Laboratory findings

        1. Diagnostic enzyme activity denoting hepatocellular leakage or induction increases dramatically in serum. After the toxic insult, the activity of the enzymes with short serum half-lives may fall rapidly (e.g., ALT, SDH), whereas those more often associated with induction slowly increase (e.g., ALP, GGT).

        2. Hyperbilirubinemia of the regurgitation type and cholestasis may or may not occur.

        3. BSP or ICG retention or reduced clearance occurs if the amount of hepatic loss by necrosis is at least 60% or if cholestasis occurs.

        4. Serum albumin and glucose concentrations usually are not abnormal, but the citrated plasma clotting tests may be abnormal.

        5. Tests dependent on portal blood delivery to liver are usually normal.

IV. Large focal hepatic lesions

   A. Clinical features and characteristics

        1.   Clinical signs referable to hepatic involvement are usually absent.

        2.   The lesions (abscesses or infarcts) affect one or more hepatic lobes but usually involve a small proportion of the total hepatic mass.

B.   Laboratory findings

        1.   In ruminant hepatic abscessation, quite often the only laboratory abnormality is polyclonal gammopathy secondary to chronic bacterial disease.

        2.   In more acute conditions activity of hepatocellular, cytosol-leakage enzymes may be increased in serum.

        3.   Other laboratory tests are usually normal.

        4.   In some cases of the dry form of feline infectious peritonitis involving liver, hyperbilirubinemia occurs that cannot be explained on the basis of the localized hepatic lesions.

V.   Hepatic lipidosis

   A.   Clinical features and characteristics

        1.   The clinical signs are related to the general disease condition involved (e.g., diabetes mellitus), or as in the cat, sudden complete anorexia and sometimes icterus may relate directly to hepatic involvement; large animals may show signs of hepatoencephalopathy.

        2.   The liver is enlarged and diffusely affected by fatty change.

   B.   Laboratory findings

        1.   Activity of hepatocellular, cytosol-leakage enzymes is increased in serum as a result of permeability change.

        2.   BSP or ICG retention or reduced clearance usually occurs, but the mechanism is not clear unless evidence for cholestasis is found.

        3.   If hepatocellular swelling from fat accumulation is severe, physical obstruction of bile canaliculi occurs and tests of cholestasis are abnormal.

        4.   Hyperammonemia may occur (cats and horses).

        5.   Serum albumin concentration and citrated plasma clotting tests are usually normal.

VI.   Steroid hepatopathy

   A.   Clinical features and characteristics

        1.   Clinical signs relative to liver lesions are usually absent in this canine problem, but history of corticosteroid therapy or signs of hyperadrenocorticism should be present.

        2.   The reversible lesion consists of large, irregular foci of hepatocellular vacuolar change, randomly dispersed within hepatic lobules; hepatic glycogen and lipid content are increased.

   B.   Laboratory findings

        1.   Activity of hepatocellular, cytosol-leakage enzymes is mildly increased in serum as a result of permeability change.

        2.   ALP is markedly increased as a result of corticosteroid-stimulated induction.

       3.   BSP retention and mild hyperbilirubinemia are sometimes found.

       4.   Plasma ammonia, serum albumin, and other tests are usually normal.

VII.   Cholangitis/cholangiohepatitis/extrahepatic biliary obstruction

    A.   Clinical features and characteristics

       1.   Clinical signs in affected animals, especially cats, are intermittent or episodic and often referable to hepatic disease (anorexia, lethargy, pyrexia, vomiting, weight loss, hepatomegaly, icterus). In animals with complete biliary obstructions, acholic feces and hemorrhage may occur.

       2.   The lesions vary from extensive cellular infiltration, necrosis, and fibrosis centered on the biliary tract in the inflammatory conditions to mild periductal fibrosis and little or nor parenchymal change in the extrahepatic biliary obstructions.

    B.   Laboratory findings

       1.   Activity of hepatocellular, cytosol-leakage enzymes in serum is mildly increased.

       2.   ALP or GGT activities are markedly and progressively increased in serum as a result of the inductive effect of cholestasis.

       3.   Other tests of cholestasis are abnormal. In extrahepatic biliary obstructions, serum direct-reacting bilirubin predominates in dogs and cats and is usually greater than 25% of the total in horses; in affected cattle a small amount of total bilirubin may be direct-reacting.

       4.   Serum albumin and plasma ammonia are usually normal.

       5.   Citrated plasma clotting tests may be abnormal, particularly in nearly complete biliary obstructions, as a result of decreased intestinal absorption of fat-soluble vitamin K.

VIII.   Chronic, progressive, primary liver diseases

    A.   Clinical features and characteristics

       1.   Clinical signs of hepatic disease and insufficiency are common (e.g., anorexia, weight loss, vomiting, polyuria, polydipsia, low-protein ascites, icterus, hepatomegaly or small liver, signs of hepatoencephalopathy, and photodynamic dermatitis in herbivores). Some diseases are associated with specific clinical signs.

       2.   The lesions vary with the etiology; in some types, specific histologic features may be diagnostic. In general, zonal, diffuse, or piecemeal necrosis; fibrosis; variable inflammatory cell infiltration; bile duct hyperplasia; and micro- or macronodular hyperplasia occur in varying combinations and severity.

    B.   Laboratory findings

       1.   Activity of hepatocellular, cytosol-leakage enzymes in serum is increased but may steadily decline as the disease progresses and fewer cells remain.

2. All tests affected by cholestasis are typically abnormal.
3. Baseline plasma ammonia may be increased if portal venous-systemic venous shunts are acquired.
4. Normal baseline ammonia with ammonia intolerance to oral challenge with an ammonium salt may occur if the functional hepatic mass is reduced by at least 60%.
5. Serum albumin and A/G ratio decrease.
6. In monogastric animals, postprandial hyperglycemia or anorexia-associated hypoglycemia may occur.
7. Citrated plasma clotting tests may be abnormal.
8. Polyclonal gammopathy is common.

IX. Portal venous-systemic venous shunting of blood. The acquired shunts occur with chronic, progressive, primary liver diseases described above.
   A. Clinical features and characteristics
      1. Clinical signs of hepatic insufficiency and hepatic encephalopathy develop in young animals affected with congenital shunts.
      2. The early hepatic lesion is atrophy, although other changes occur as the disease progresses.
   B. Laboratory findings
      1. If only hepatic atrophy occurs, activity of hepatocellular, cytosol-leakage enzymes is normal.
      2. Tests of cholestasis are normal.
      3. BSP or ICG retention or reduced clearance occurs if some degree of reduced functional mass (atrophy) accompanies the shunt but will remain normal when atrophy is minimal.
      4. Baseline plasma ammonia is abnormal.
      5. Serum albumin and other tests are usually normal unless atrophy or other lesions greatly reduce the functional mass of liver.

X. Primary or metastatic hepatic neoplasia. The clinical and laboratory features in affected dogs and cats may be difficult to distinguish from chronic, progressive, primary hepatic diseases described above. No significant correlation between the extent of neoplastic involvement and the biochemical changes have been noted. Some indicate that AST may be abnormal in a higher percentage of canine cases than is ALT.

REFERENCES

Anderson PH, Berrett S, Brush PJ, et al: Biochemical indicators of liver injury in calves with experimental fascioliasis. Vet Rec 100:43, 1977.
Anderson PH, Matthews JG, Berrett S, et al: Changes in plasma enzyme activities and other blood components in response to acute and chronic liver damage in cattle. Res Vet Sci 31:1, 1981.
Asquith RL, Edds GT, Aller WW, et al: Plasma concentrations of iditol dehydrogenase (sorbitol dehydrogenase) in ponies treated with aflatoxin B1. Am J Vet Res 41:925, 1980.
Atwell RB, Farmer TS: Clinical pathology of the "caval syndrome" in canine dirofilariasis in northern Australia. J Small Anim Pract 23:675, 1982.
Badylak SF, Van Vleet JF: Alterations of prothrombin time and activated partial thromboplastin time in dogs with hepatic disease. Am J Vet Res 42:2053, 1981.

Badylak SF, Van Vleet JF: Tissue gammaglutamyl transpeptidase activity and hepatic ultrastructural alterations in dogs with experimentally induced glucocorticoid hepatopathy. Am J Vet Res 43:649, 1982.

Bennett AM, Davies JD, Gaskell CJ, et al: Lobular dissecting hepatitis in the dog. Vet Pathol 20:179, 1983.

Bishop L, Strandberg JD, Adams RJ, et al: Chronic active hepatitis in dogs associated with leptospires. Am J Vet Res 40:839, 1979.

Bissell DM: Formation and elimination of bilirubin. Gastroenterology 69:519, 1975.

Boyd JW: The comparative activity of some enzymes in sheep, cattle and rats: Normal serum and tissue levels and changes during experimental liver necrosis. Res Vet Sci 3:256, 1962.

Boyd JW: The mechanisms relating to increases in plasma enzymes and isoenzymes in diseases of animals. Vet Clin Pathol 12(2):9, 1983.

Braun JP, Rico AG, Benard P: Tissue and blood distribution of gamma-glutamyl transferase in the lamb and in the ewe. Res Vet Sci 25:37, 1978.

Brobst DF, Schall WD: Needle biopsy of the canine liver and correlation of laboratory data with histopathologic observations. J Am Vet Med Assoc 161:382, 1972.

Brown CM, Ainsworth DM, Personett LA, et al: Serum biochemical and haematological findings in two foals with focal bacterial hepatitis (Tyzzer's disease). Equine Vet J 15:375, 1983.

Bunch SE, Castleman WL, Hornbuckle WE, et al: Hepatic cirrhosis associated with long-term anticonvulsant drug therapy in dogs. J Am Vet Med Assoc 181:357, 1982.

Burrows CF, Chiapella AM, Jezyk P: Idiopathic feline hepatic lipidosis: The syndrome and speculations on its pathogenesis. Fla Vet J (winter):18, 1981.

Calhoun MC, Veckert DN, Livingston CW, et al: Effects of bitterweed (Hymenoxys odorata) on voluntary feed intake and serum constituents of sheep. Am J Vet Res 42:1713, 1981.

Center SA, Baldwin BH, King JM, et al: Hematologic and biochemical abnormalities associated with induced extrahepatic bile duct obstruction in the cat. Am J Vet Res 44:1822, 1983.

Center SA, Bunch SE, Baldwin BH, et al: Comparison of sulfobromophthalein and indocyanine green clearances in the dog. Am J Vet Res 44:722, 1983.

Center SA, Bunch SE, Baldwin BH, et al: Comparison of sulfobromophthalein and indocyanine green clearances in the cat. Am J Vet Res 44:727, 1983.

Coffman J: Clinical chemistry and pathophysiology of horses. Enzymology, part 2. Vet Med Small Anim Clin 74:1791, 1979.

Cornelius CE: Biochemical evaluation of hepatic function in dogs. J Am Anim Hosp Assoc 15:259, 1979.

Cornelius CE: Liver function. In Kaneko JJ (ed): Clinical biochemistry of domestic animals, 3rd ed. New York, Academic Press, 1980.

Cornelius CE, Himes JA: New concepts in canine hepatic function. J Am Anim Hosp Assoc 9:147, 1973.

Cornelius LM, DeNovo RC: Icterus in cats. In Kirk RW (ed): Current veterinary therapy VIII. Philadelphia, WB Saunders Co, 1983.

Cornelius LM, Thrall DE, Halliwell WH, et al: Anomalous portosystemic anastomoses associated with chronic hepatic insufficiency in six young dogs. J Am Vet Med Assoc 167:220, 1975.

DeNovo RC, Prasse KW: Comparison of serum biochemical and hepatic functional alterations in dogs treated with corticosteroids and hepatic duct ligation. Am J Vet Res 44:1703, 1983.

Divers TJ, Warner A, Vaale WE, et al: Toxic hepatic failure in newborn foals. J Am Vet Med Assoc 183:1407, 1983.

Doige CE, Lester S: Chronic active hepatitis in dogs: A review of fourteen cases. J Am Anim Hosp Assoc 17:725, 1981.

Dorner JL, Hoffmann, WE, Long GB: Corticosteroid induction of an isoenzyme of alkaline phosphatase in the dog. Am J Vet Res 35:1457, 1974.

Dumas MB, Spano JS: Characterization of equine alkaline phosphatase isoenzymes based on their electrophoretic mobility by polyacrylamide gel disc electrophoresis. Am J Vet Res 41:2076, 1980.

Dunavant ML, Rich LJ: Clinical applications of serum enzyme determinations. Bull Am Soc Vet Clin Pathol 3(1):3, 1974.

Easley JC, Carpenter JL: Hepatic arteriovenous fistula in two Saint Bernard pups. J Am Vet Med Assoc 166:167, 1975.

Eckersall PD, Nash AS: Isoenzymes of canine alkaline phosphatase: An investigation using isoelectric focusing and related to diagnosis. Res Vet Sci 34:310, 1983.

Edwards DE, McCracken MD, Richardson DC: Sclerosing cholangitis in a cat. J Am Vet Med Assoc 182:710, 1982.

Engelking LR, Gronwall R: Bile acid clearance in sheep with hereditary hyperbilirubinemia. Am J Vet Res 40:1277, 1979.

Everett RM, Duncan JR, Prasse KW: Alkaline phosphatase, leucine aminopeptidase, and alanine aminotransferase activities with obstructive and toxic hepatic disease in cats. Am J Vet Res 38:963, 1977.

Everett RM, Duncan JR, Prasse KW: Alkaline phosphatases in tissues and sera of cats. Am J Vet Res 38:1533, 1977.

Ford EJH: Activity of gamma-glutamyl transpeptidase and other enzymes in the serum of
  sheep with liver or kidney damage. J Comp Pathol 84:231, 1974.
Freedland RA, Kramer JW: Use of serum enzymes as aids to diagnosis. Adv Vet Sci Comp Med
  14:61, 1970.
Froscher BG, Nagode LA: Isoenzymes of equine alkaline phosphatase. Am J Vet Res 40:1514,
  1979.
Gartner RJW, Ryley JW, Beattie AW: Values and variations of blood constituents in grazing
  Hereford cattle. Res Vet Sci 7:424, 1966.
Gelehrter TD: Enzyme induction, Part 1. N Engl J Med 244:522, 1976.
Gelehrter TD: Enzyme induction, Part 2. N Engl J Med 244:589, 1976.
Gelehrter TD: Enzyme induction, Part 3. N Engl J Med 244:646, 1976.
Gerber H: Serum enzyme determination in equine medicine. Equine Vet J 1:129, 1969.
Griffiths GL, Lumsden JH, Valli VEO: Hematologic and biochemical changes in dogs with
  portosystemic shunts. J Am Anim Hosp Assoc 17:705, 1981.
Gronwall R: Effects of fasting on hepatic function in ponies. Am J Vet Res 36:145, 1975.
Gronwall R, Engelking LR, Anwer MS, et al: Bile secretion in ponies with biliary fistulas.
  Am J Vet Res 36:653, 1975.
Gronwall R, Engelking LR, Noonan N: Direct measurement of biliary bilirubin excretion in
  ponies during fasting. Am J Vet Res 41:125, 1980.
Guelfi JF, Braun JP, Benard P, et al: Value of so-called cholestasis markers in the dog.
  Res Vet Sci 33:309, 1982.
Hamilton JM, Knight D: Alkaline phosphatase levels in canine mammary neoplasia. Vet Rec
  93:121, 1973.
Harrison FA, Saunders RC, Brikas P: Plasma clearance of bromosulphthalein in surgically
  prepared sheep. Br Vet J 138:127, 1982.
Himes JA, Cornelius CE: Hepatic excretion and storage of sulfobromophthalein sodium in
  experimental hepatic necrosis in the dog. Cornell Vet 63:424, 1973.
Hirsch VM, Doige CE: Suppurative cholangitis in cats. J Am Vet Med Assoc 182:1223, 1983.
Hoffman WE: Diagnostic value of canine serum alkaline phosphatase and alkaline phosphatase
  isoenzymes. J Am Anim Hosp Assoc 13:237, 1977.
Hoffman WE, Dorner JL: Alkaline phosphatase and alkaline phosphatase isoenzymes in the
  cat. Vet Clin Pathol 6(3):21, 1977.
Hoffman WE, Dorner JL: Disappearance rates of intravenously injected canine alkaline
  phosphatase isoenzymes. Am J Vet Res 38:1553, 1977.
Hoffman WE, Dorner JL: Serum half-life of intravenously injected intestinal and hepatic
  alkaline phosphatase isoenzymes in the cat. Am J Vet Res 38:1637, 1977.
Javitt NB: Hepatic bile formation, Part 1. N Engl J Med 295:1464, 1976.
Javitt NB: Hepatic bile formation, Part 2. N Engl J Med 295:1511, 1976.
Johnson GF, Zawie DA, Gilbertson SR, et al: Chronic active hepatitis in Doberman
  pinschers. J Am Vet Med Assoc 180:1438, 1982.
Jones S, Blackmore DJ: Observations on the isoenzymes of aspartate aminotransferase in
  equine tissues and serum. Equine Vet J 14:311, 1982.
Kantek Navarro CE, Kociba GJ, Kowalski JJ: Serum biochemical changes in dogs with
  experimental Leptospira interrogans serovar icterohaemorrhagica infection. Am J Vet Res
  42:1125, 1981.
Kaplan MM: Current concepts: Alkaline phosphatase. N Engl J Med 286:200, 1972.
Klei TR, Tolbert BJ, Ochoa R, et al: Morphologic and clinicopathologic changes following
  Strongylus vulgaris infections of immune and nonimmune ponies. Am J Vet Res 43:1300,
  1982.
Kramer JW: Clinical enzymology. In Kaneko JJ (ed): Clinical biochemistry of domestic
  animals, 3rd ed. New York, Academic Press, 1980.
Levesque DC, Oliver JE, Cornelius LM, et al: Congenital portacaval shunts in two cats:
  Diagnosis and surgical correction. J Am Vet Med Assoc 181:143, 1982.
Maddison JE: Portosystemic encephalopathy in two young dogs: Some additional diagnostic
  and therapeutic considerations. J Small Anim Pract 22:731, 1981.
McConnell MF, Lunsden JH: Biochemical evaluation of metastatic liver disease in the dog.
  J Am Anim Hosp Assoc 19:173, 1983.
McSherry BJ, Lumsden JH, Valli VE, et al: Hyperbilirubinemia in sick cattle. Can J Comp
  Med 48:237, 1984.
Meyer DJ: Serum gamma-glutamyl transferase as a liver test in cats with toxic and
  obstructive hepatic disease. J Am Anim Hosp Assoc 19:1023, 1983.
Meyer DJ, Noonan NE: Liver tests in dogs receiving anticonvulsant drugs (diphenylhydantoin
  and primidone). J Am Anim Hosp Assoc 17:261, 1981.
Meyer DJ, Strombeck DR, Stone EA, et al: Ammonia tolerance test in clinically normal dogs
  and in dogs with portosystemic shunts. J Am Vet Med Assoc 173:377, 1978.
Mia AS, Koger HD: Comparative studies on arginase and transaminases in hepatic necrosis in
  various species of domestic animals. Vet Clin Pathol 8:9, 1979.
Miller DM, Crowell WA, Stuart BP: Acute aflatoxicosis in swine: Clinical pathology,
  histopathology, and electron microscopy. Am J Vet Res 43:273, 1982.
Moore WE, Feldman BF: The use of isoenzymes in small animal medicine. J Am Anim Hosp Assoc
  10:420, 1974.
Morrow DA, Hillman D, Dade AW, et al: Clinical investigation of a dairy herd with the fat
  cow syndrome. J Am Vet Med Assoc 174:161, 1979.

Moss DW, Butterworth PJ: Enzymology and medicine. London, Pitman Medical, 1974.

Muchiri DJ, Bridges CH, Ueckert DN, et al: Photosensitization of sheep on kleingrass pasture. J Am Vet Med Assoc 177:353, 1980.

Mullowney PC, Tennant BC: Choledocholithiasis in the dog: A review and a report of a case with rupture of the common bile duct. J Small Anim Pract 23:631, 1982.

Noonan NE: Variations of plasma enzymes in the pony and the dog after carbon tetrachloride administration. Am J Vet Res 42:674, 1981.

Patnaik AK, Hurvitz AI, Lieberman PH, et al: Canine hepatocellular carcinoma. Vet Pathol 18:427, 1981.

Polzin DJ, Stowe CM, O'Leary TP, et al: Acute hepatic necrosis associated with the administration of mebendazole to dogs. J Am Vet Med Assoc 179:1013, 1981.

Prasse KW, Bjorling DE, Holmes RA, et al: Indocyanine green clearance and ammonia tolerance in partially hepatectomized and hepatic devascularized, anesthetized dogs. Am J Vet Res 44:2320, 1983.

Prasse KW, Mahaffey EA, DeNovo R, et al: Chronic lymphocytic cholangitis in three cats. Vet Pathol 19:99, 1982.

Reid IM, Harrison RD, Collins RA: Fasting and refeeding in the lactating dairy cow. J Comp Pathol 87:253, 1977.

Rich LJ, Dunavant ML: Serum enzymes in bovine practice. Bovine Pract 5:8, 1972.

Rich LJ, Spano JS: Biochemical profiles in small animals: Diseases of pancreas, kidney, and liver. J Am Anim Hosp Assoc 10:349, 1974.

Rico AG, Braun JP, Benard P, et al: Tissue distribution and blood levels of gamma-glutamyl transferase in the horse. Equine Vet J 9:100, 1977.

Rogers WA: Source of serum alkaline phosphatase in clinically normal and diseased dog: A clinical study. J Am Vet Med Assoc 168:934, 1976.

Saini PK, Saini SK: Immunochemical study of canine intestinal, hepatic, and osseous alkaline phosphatase. Am J Vet Res 39:1510, 1978.

Schall WD: Laboratory diagnosis of hepatic disease. Vet Clin North Am 6:679, 1976.

Schall WD, Chapman WL, Finco DR, et al: Cholelithiasis in dogs. J Am Vet Med Assoc 163:469, 1973.

Schmid R: Bilirubin metabolism in man. N Engl J Med 287:703, 1972.

Scott DW, Hoffer RE, Amand WB, et al: Cholelithiasis in a dog. J Am Vet Med Assoc 163:254, 1973.

Sherding RG: Hepatic encephalopathy in the dog. Compend Contin Educ Pract Vet 1:55, 1979.

Strombeck DR: Clinicopathologic features of primary and metastatic neoplastic disease of the liver in dogs. J Am Vet Med Assoc 173:267, 1978.

Strombeck DR, Gribble D: Chronic active hepatitis in the dog. J Am Vet Med Assoc 173:380, 1978.

Strombeck DR, Quallo C: Hepatic sulfobromophthalein uptake and storage defect in a dog. J Am Vet Med Assoc 172:1423, 1978.

Strombeck DR, Meyer DJ, Freedland RA: Hyperammonemia due to urea cycle enzyme deficiency in two dogs. J Am Vet Med Assoc 166:1109, 1975.

Strombeck DR, Rogers Q: Plasma amino acid concentrations in dogs with hepatic disease. J Am Vet Med Assoc 173:93, 1978.

Strombeck DR, Rogers W, Gribble D: Chronic active hepatic disease in a dog. J Am Vet Med Assoc 169:802, 1976.

Strombeck DR, Weiser MG, Kaneko JJ: Hyperammonemia and hepatic encephalopathy in the dog. J Am Vet Med Assoc 166:1105, 1975.

Tennant B, Baldwin B, Evans CD, et al: Diseases of the equine liver. Proc 21st Am Assoc Equine Pract, 1975.

Thornburg LP, Rottinghaus GB, Glassberg R: Drug induced hepatic necrosis in a dog. J Am Vet Med Assoc 183:327, 1983.

Thornburg LP, Simpson S, Digilio K: Fatty liver syndrome in cats. J Am Anim Hosp Assoc 18:397, 1982.

Traub JL, Rantanen N, Reed S, et al: Cholelithiasis in four horses. J Am Vet Med Assoc 181:59, 1982.

Treacher RJ, Collis KA: The effect of protein intake on the activities of liver specific enzymes in the plasma of dairy cows. Res Vet Sci 22:101, 1977.

Twedt DC, Sternlieb I, Gilbertson SR: Clinical, morphologic, and chemical studies on copper toxicosis of Bedlington terriers. J Am Vet Med Assoc 175:269, 1979.

Van Vleet JF, Alberts JO: Evaluation of liver function tests and liver biopsy in experimental carbon tetrachloride intoxication and extrahepatic bile duct obstruction in the dog. Am J Vet Res 29:2119, 1968.

Watson TG, Croll NA: Clinical changes caused by the liver fluke Metorchis conjunctis in cats. Vet Pathol 18:778, 1981.

Weisiger R, Gollan J, Ockner R: An albumin receptor on the liver cell may mediate hepatic uptake of sulfobromophthalein and bilirubin (abstract). Gastroenterology 79:1065, 1980.

Young JT: Source, fate, and possible significance of elevated serum alkaline phosphatase in nonicteric animals with partial biliary obstruction. J Am Anim Hosp Assoc 10:415, 1974.

Zimmerman HJ: Intrahepatic cholestasis. Arch Intern Med 139:1038, 1979.

8
Digestive System

Laboratory evaluation of the exocrine pancreas is directed toward two categories of disease: (1) inflammation and necrosis, and (2) exocrine insufficiency. Exocrine insufficiency results in maldigestion and also malabsorption, which must be differentiated from that caused by intestinal disease.

LABORATORY DETECTION OF PANCREATIC INFLAMMATION AND NECROSIS
This disease occurs primarily in the dog and is uncommon in other species. Most of the information available relates to the dog.

I. Serum enzymes
    A. Amylase
        1. Characteristics
            a. Only alpha amylase is present in animals; it is secreted in the active form, which hydrolyzes 1,4 glycoside linkages forming disaccharides and mono-saccharides. Several isoenzymes exist.
            b. The pancreas, liver, and small intestine are sources of serum amylase. Salivary amylase is not present in domestic animals except the pig.
            c. Serum amylase activity in health is derived primarily from extrapancreatic sources; canine values are 5 to 10 times that of humans.
            d. Serum amylase is inactivated by the kidney.
            e. Older methods (saccharogenic), which measure reducing substances generated by amylase on a starch substrate, should not be used because maltase found in normal canine serum will have an additive effect on the number of reducing units.
        2. Interpretation of hyperamylasemia
            a. Increased serum amylase activity may occur with pancreatitis (Case 19).
                (1) Increased serum amylase activity is caused by enzyme leakage from degenerating pancreatic acinar cells or obstructed ducts directly into

145

venules or into the blood via lymphatics.

(2) The higher the serum activity (a three- to fourfold increase), the more likely the cause is pancreatic disease.

(3) Because pancreatitis is not the only cause of hyperamylasemia, serum amylase should be used in conjunction with serum lipase in the diagnosis of acute pancreatic disease.

(4) Normal serum amylase values occasionally may be found with acute pancreatic disease.

  b. High serum amylase activity may occur in nonpancreatic disease.

(1) Renal disease

(2) Intestinal obstruction

(3) Both increases and decreases in serum amylase activity have been reported following corticosteroid administration.

B. Lipase

  1. Characteristics

    a. Pancreatic lipase, phospholipase A and B, and cholesterol ester hydrolase are secreted in the active form.

    b. Lipase activity is optimum at an alkaline pH and is enhanced by bile.

    c. The procedures used require more time than those for amylase; therefore, lipase is not as useful as a "stat." procedure.

    d. Hemolysis inhibits enzyme activity.

    e. The kidney is involved in lipase degradation.

  2. Interpretation of hyperlipasemia

    a. A two-fold or more increase in serum activity usually indicates acute pancreatic disease (Case 19).

    b. Normal values seldom occur in the presence of acute pancreatic disease.

    c. Increased activity can occur in renal and hepatic disease and following corticosteroid administration.

II. Other laboratory findings in pancreatic inflammation and necrosis

  A. Routine test findings include the following.

    1. Neutrophilic leukocytosis with a left shift, lymphopenia, eosinopenia, and occasionally monocytosis

    2. Fasting hyperlipemia

      a. Lipoprotein lipase, a plasma lipemia-clearing enzyme produced by the pancreas, may be inactivated in pancreatic necrosis, resulting in a transient lipemia.

      b. Diabetes mellitus may be a sequela to severe pancreatic necrosis and cause hyperlipemia.

    3. High packed cell volume and plasma protein concentration resulting from fluid shifts and vomiting (relative polycythemia)

    4. Prerenal azotemia

5. Serosanguineous peritoneal effusion characterized by lipid droplets, erythrocytes, and neutrophils (nonseptic exudate)
6. Hypocalcemia. Mechanism is unclear (see Chapter 11)
7. Transient or persistent hyperglycemia (diabetes mellitus)

B. Methemalbumin. Hemolysis of erythrocytes present in the hemorrhagic form of the disease may cause increase in this hemoglobin breakdown product (see Chapter 1).

LABORATORY DETECTION OF MALDIGESTION AND MALABSORPTION
Malabsorption may be secondary to maldigestion or intestinal lesions characterized by decreased absorptive surface area, death of epithelial cells, interference with venous or lymphatic drainage, or distention of the lamina propria with cells. Most of the testing for these syndromes has been done in the dog and, to a lesser extent, the horse.

I. Fecal examination
A. Fecal smears. Undigested or nonabsorbed materials can be detected microscopically in feces; special staining may be required.
1. Sudan-stained smears
a. Neutral fats (undigested) appear as orange globules on direct staining with Sudan III or IV.
(1) Control smears of feces from normal animals on the same diet should be examined.
(2) Normal feces contain very little or no neutral fat.
b. If 36% acetic acid is added to the feces-Sudan stain mixture and boiled, fatty acids (digested or split fats) appear as orange globules (form spicules on cooling). They do not stain without acid-heat treatment. Ten or more globules/high-power field is abnormal.
c. An increase in neutral fats indicates maldigestion caused by pancreatic insufficiency (Case 17), and an increase in digested fats is indicative of malabsorption (Case 18).
2. Iodine-stained smears
a. Starch appears as blackish blue structures with blue-green fringes
b. Increased starch may indicate amylase deficiency resulting from pancreatic insufficiency (Case 17).
3. Unstained smears
a. Undigested muscle fibers have blunt ends and prominent cross-striations.
b. Their presence in feces of animals on a meat diet indicates protease deficiency resulting from pancreatic insufficiency (Case 17).
B. Fecal proteases
1. The primary fecal proteases are of pancreatic origin and include trypsin, chymotrypsin, and carboxypeptidase A and B.

        a. Secretion takes place as the proenzyme, which is activated in the duodenum.

        b. Trypsinogen is activated to trypsin by enterokinase produced by the duodenal mucosa; trypsin activates the other proteases.

    2. Gelatin digestion tests

        a. The tube test is more sensitive than the X-ray film test.

        b. Failure to digest the gelatin or film emulsion indicates protease deficiency (Case 17).

        c. The test should be repeated because of daily fluctuation of protease levels in feces and the possible occurrence of false-negative and false-positive tests.

            (1) Absence of gelatin digestion in the presence of pancreatic protease secretion may occur because of trypsin inhibitors or complete inactivation of the enzyme in the intestine.

            (2) Digestion of gelatin in the absence of pancreatic protease may be caused by bacterial proteases.

C. Total fecal fat

    1. The test is performed on a portion of a 24-hour stool sample after weighing the entire sample.

    2. Normal amount of fat (neutral fat, free fatty acids, and soaps) excreted in dogs is less than 7 g/24 hours. Greater amounts indicate steatorrhea, which may be caused by either maldigestion or malabsorption.

II. Absorption and tolerance tests

    A. Fat absorption tests

        1. Normal fat absorption requires an adequate amount of pancreatic lipase and bile.

        2. Serum lipid levels are measured before and after a high fat meal; they are determined quantitatively or by measurement of plasma turbidity.

        3. Plasma turbidity test

            a. This qualitative test measures the appearance of plasma turbidity 2 to 3 hours following the oral administration of a fatty substance (1 ml corn oil/lb).

            b. Interpretation

                (1) The presence of plasma turbidity indicates fat is being digested and absorbed.

                (2) The absence of plasma turbidity indicates a lack of fat absorption. Causes are:

                    (a) Exocrine pancreatic insufficiency and failure of lipid digestion (Case 17)

                    (b) Bile insufficiency resulting in faulty emulsification of fat and reduced lipid digestion

                    (c) Intestinal malabsorption (Case 18)

                (3) If fat absorption does not occur, pancreatic enzymes may be added to a second fat meal and

incubated 30 minutes before feeding. The fat
absorption test is then repeated.
   (a)   Plasma turbidity indicates that the cause
         of the original absorption failure was
         maldigestion because of pancreatic
         insufficiency (Case 17).
   (b)   Continued absence of turbidity suggests
         intestinal malabsorption, bile
         insufficiency, or delayed gastric
         emptying.   .
    4.   Quantitative tests have measured absorption of ^{131}I- or
   ^{14}C-labeled triolein, ^{125}I-labeled oleic acid, and
   vitamin A.
B.   BT-PABA test (N-benzoyl-L-tyrosyl-p-aminobenzoic acid)
    1.   BT-PABA is a synthetic peptide that is cleaved by
      chymotrypsin, releasing PABA.
    2.   PABA is absorbed into the blood and excreted in the
      urine. Peak blood levels are at 2 to 3 hours after oral
      administration (16.7 mg/kg).
    3.   Low blood levels (less than 85 mg/dl) usually indicate
      pancreatic insufficiency. Occasionally there are
      minimal decreases in serum PABA in intestinal disease;
      but PABA is usually absorbed, even in cases of
      malabsorption syndrome.
C.   Starch tolerance test
    1.   Dietary starch is digested to disaccharides by
      pancreatic enzymes and to monosaccharides by brush
      border disaccharidases before absorption.
    2.   A failure to increase blood glucose levels after oral
      starch administration indicates maldigestion,
      malabsorption, or abnormal glucose metabolism.
D.   Oral D-xylose absorption test
    1.   Xylose is a five-carbon monosaccharide that is
      passively absorbed by the jejunum via the portal
      circulation and not the lymphatics.
    2.   It is poorly metabolized, rapidly excreted by the
      kidney, and not as subject as glucose to changes in the
      metabolic state.
    3.   Plasma concentrations are usually measured and are
      expected to peak 60 to 90 minutes after oral
      administration (0.5 g/kg as a 5% solution in the dog
      and 2 g/kg as a 20% solution in the horse).
    4.   A flat absorption curve may indicate reduced absorption
      as a result of intestinal disease, but delayed gastric
      emptying, vomiting, enteric bacterial overgrowth, or
      rapid transit may also delay or reduce absorption.
      Renal disease may give false high results, since the
      kidney is the excretory route.
    5.   This test has been successfully used in dogs and
      horses.
    6.   A combined BT-PABA and D-xylose tolerance test has been
      used to simultaneously test for both digestion and
      absorption.
E.   Oral glucose tolerance test (see Chapter 6)

1. Glucose requires no digestion, but plasma levels are affected by factors other than absorption; hormones associated with carbohydrate metabolism influence plasma levels.
2. A low plasma glucose curve may indicate malabsorption.

MISCELLANEOUS TESTS FOR SPECIFIC GASTROINTESTINAL DISORDERS

I. Laboratory detection of excessive enteric protein loss. Normally, a certain amount of plasma protein enters the gastrointestinal tract each day. It is digested to its constituent amino acids, which are almost completely reabsorbed and reanabolized to protein. Excessive protein loss is associated with mucosal ulceration, disorders or intestinal lymphatic drainage, and inflammatory diseases.
   A. ^{51}Cr-labeled albumin excretion. Labeled albumin is given intravenously, and the degree of protein loss determined by measuring the amount of radioactivity in the feces (Case 18). ^{51}Cr is split from albumin after its loss into the intestinal tract and is not absorbed; an increase in radioactivity indicates increased enteric albumin excretion.
   B. Serum protein concentration. Hypoproteinemia (panhypoproteinemia) in the absence of other possible causes (renal disease, liver disease, malnutrition, etc.) and associated with signs of enteric disease suggests enteric loss exceeding increased synthesis (see Chapter 6).

II. Gastric or ruminal content pH. A pH greater than 6 suggests intestinal reflux associated with colic or obstruction in horses. A pH less than 5 is found with rumen overload and lactic acid accumulation, and a pH greater than 7 occurs with urea toxicity and ammonia production.

III. Fecal tests
   A. Cytology
      1. Abnormal squamous cells in gastric washings or abdominal effusions in the horse are found with gastric squamous carcinoma.
      2. Intact neutrophils in Wright-stained fecal smears indicate inflammation of the colon and/or lower small intestine.
      3. Degenerate neutrophils, bacteria, and/or plant material in abdominal effusions are associated with intestinal rupture and peritonitis.
      4. Increased cell count and/or protein concentration in abdominal effusions are found in a variety of situations associated with equine colic.
      5. Pathogenic organisms may be found in rectal scrapings (e.g., Mycobacterium paratuberculosis, Histoplasma capsulatum, and Prototheca zopfi).
   B. Fecal occult blood. In animals not on a diet containing muscle (dietary myoglobin and hemoglobin may give a positive test), a positive test suggests gastrointestinal hemorrhage. Plant peroxidases may give a false positive test result.

IV. Urine tests
    A. Urine indican. Indicanuria occurs in intestinal obstruction
        (putrefaction of ingesta) in carnivores. Indican is
        produced from tryptophan by action of tryptophanase-
        producing bacteria in the gut lumen.
    B. Urine urobilinogen. High intestinal obstruction and
        complete bile duct obstruction can lead to an absence of
        urobilinogen in urine (see Chapter 7).

REFERENCES

Anderson NV: Veterinary gastroenterology. Philadelphia, Lea and Febiger, 1980.
Barton CL, Smith C, Troy G, et al: The diagnosis and clinicopathological features of
    canine protein-losing enteropathy. J Am Anim Hosp Assoc 14:85, 1978.
Batt RM: The molecular basis of malabsorption. J Small Anim Pract 21:555, 1980.
Batt RM, Mann LC: Specificity of the BT-PABA test for the diagnosis of exocrine pancreatic
    insufficiency in the dog. Vet Rec 108:303, 1981.
Boulton JR, Merritt AM, Cimprick RE, et al: Normal and abnormal xylose absorption in the
    horse. Cornell Vet 66:183, 1976.
Breukink HJ: Oral mono- and disaccharide tolerance tests in ponies. Am J Vet Res 35:1523,
    1974.
Brobst DF: Pancreatic function. In Kaneko JJ (ed): Clinical biochemistry of domestic
    animals, 3rd ed. New York, Academic Press, 1980.
Brobst DF, Ferguson AB, Carter JM: Evaluation of serum amylose and lipose
    activity in experimentally induced pancreatitis in the dog. J Am Vet Med Assoc
    157:1697, 1970.
Burrows C, Merritt AM, Chiapella AM: Determination of fecal fat and trypsin output in the
    evaluation of chronic canine diarrhea. J Am Vet Med Assoc 174:62, 1979.
Burrows LF: The assessment of canine gastrointestinal function: Recent advances and future
    needs. Baton Rouge, La, Proc 31st Gaines Vet Symp, 1981.
Cornelius LM: Laboratory diagnosis of acute pancreatitis and pancreatic adenocarcinoma.
    Vet Clin North Am 6:671, 1976.
Dietz HH, Nielsen K: Turnover of ^{131}I-labelled albumin in horses with gastrointestinal
    disease. Nord Vet Med 32:369, 1980.
Easley JR: Gastroenteritis and associated eosinophilia in a dog. J Am Vet Med Assoc
    161:1030, 1972.
Finco DR, Duncan JR, Schall WD, et al: Chronic enteric disease and hypoproteinemia in
    nine dogs. J Am Vet Med Assoc 163:262, 1973.
Finco DR, Stevens JB: Clinical significance of serum amylase activity in the dog. J Am Vet
    Med Assoc 155:1686, 1969.
Fittschen C, Bellamy JEC: Prednisone treatment alters the serum amylase and lipase
    activities in normal dogs without causing pancreatitis. Can J Comp Med 48:136, 1984.
Hardy RM, Stevens JB: Exocrine pancreatic diseases. In Ettinger SJ (ed): Textbook of
    veterinary internal medicine, Vol 2. Philadelphia, WB Saunders Co, 1975.
Hayden DW, Van Kruiningen HJ: Control values for evaluating gastrointestinal function in
    the dog. J Am Anim Hosp Assoc 12:31, 1976.
Hayden DW, Van Kruiningen, HJ: Lymphocytic-plasmacytic enteritis in German shepherd dogs.
    J Am Anim Hosp Assoc 18:89, 1982.
Heise KM: Lymphangiectasia and protein-losing enteropathy in a German shepherd dog. Vet
    Med Small Anim Clin 78:67, 1983.
Hill FWG: Malabsorption syndrome in the dog: A study of thirty-eight cases. J Small Anim
    Pract 13:575, 1972.
Hill FWG, Kidder DE, Frew J: A xylose absorption test for the dog. Vet Rec 87:250, 1970.
Hoenig M: Intestinal malabsorption attributed to bacterial overgrowth in a dog. J Am Vet
    Med Assoc 176:533, 1980.
Hoskins JD, Turk JR, Turk MA: Feline pancreatic insufficiency. Vet Med Small Anim Clin
    77:1745, 1982.
Jacobs KA, Bolton JR: Effect of diet on the oral glucose tolerance test in the horse. J Am
    Vet Med Assoc 180:884, 1982.
Jacobs KA, Normal P, Hodgson DRG, et al: Effect of diet on the oral d-xylose absorption
    test in the horse. Am J Vet Res 43:1856, 1982.
Kallfelz FA, Norrdin RW, Neal TW: Intestinal absorption of oleic acid ^{131}I and triolein
    [131]I in the differential diagnosis of malabsorption syndrome and pancreatic dysfunction
    in the dog. J Am Vet Med Assoc 153:46, 1968.
Loeb WF, McKenzie LD, Hoffsis GF: The carbohydrate digestion-absorption test in the horse:
    Technique and normal values. Cornell Vet 62:524, 1972.
Lorenz MD: Laboratory diagnosis of gastrointestinal disease and pancreatic insufficiency.
    Vet Clin North Am 6:662, 1976.
Marsh CL, Mebus CA, Underdahl NR: Loss of serum proteins via the intestinal tract in
    calves with infectious diarrhea. Am J Vet Res 30:163, 1969.

Merritt AM, Burrows CF, Cowgill L, et al: Fecal fat and trypsin in dogs fed a meat-base or cereal-base diet. J Am Vet Med Assoc 174:59, 1979.

Merritt AM, Kohn CW, Ramberg CF, et al: Plasma clearance of [^{51}Cr] albumin into the intestinal tract of normal and chronically diarrheal horses. Am J Vet Res 38:1769, 1977.

Meuten DF, Butler DG, Thomson GW, et al: Chronic enteritis associated with malabsorption and protein-losing enteropathy in the horse. J Am Vet Med Assoc 172:326, 1978.

Mulvany MH, Feinberg CK, Tilson DL: Clinical characterization of acute necrotizing pancreatitis. Compend Contin Educ Pract Vet 4:394, 1982.

Neuman NB: Acute pancreatic hemorrhage associated with iatrogenic hypercalcemia in a dog. J Am Vet Med Assoc 166:381, 1975.

Olson NC, Zimmer JF: Protein-losing enteropathy secondary to intestinal lymphangiectasia in a dog. J Am Vet Med Assoc 173:271, 1978.

Parent J: Effects of dexamethasone on pancreatic tissue and on serum amylase and lipase activities in dogs. J Am Vet Med Assoc 180:743, 1982.

Pearson EG, Baldwin BH: D-xylose absorption in the adult bovine. Cornell Vet 71:288, 1981.

Perman V, Stevens JB: Clinical evaluation of the acinar pancreas of the dog. J Am Ved Med Assoc 155:2053, 1969.

Roberts MC: Protein-losing enteropathy in the horse. Compend Contin Educ Pract Vet 5:550, 1983.

Roberts MC, Hill FWG: The oral glucose tolerance test in the horse. Equine Vet J 5:171, 1973.

Roberts MC, Norman P: A re-evaluation of the D(+) xylose absorption test in the horse. Equine Vet J 11:239, 1979.

Roberts MC, Pinsent PJN: Malabsorption in the horse associated with alimentary lymphosarcoma. Equine Vet J 7:166, 1975.

Rogers WA: Diseases of the exocrine pancreas. In Ettinger SJ (ed): Textbook of veterinary internal medicine, Vol 2, 2nd ed. Philadelphia, WB Saunders Co, 1983.

Rogers WA, Stradley RP, Sherding RG, et al: Simultaneous evaluation of pancreatic exocrine function and intestinal absorptive function in dogs with chronic diarrhea. J Am Vet Med Assoc 177:1128, 1980.

Schaer M: A clinicopathologic surgery of acute pancreatitis in 30 dogs and 5 cats. J Am Anim Hosp Assoc 15:681, 1979.

Simpson JW, Doxey DL: Quantitative assessment of fat absorption and its diagnostic value in exocrine pancreatic insufficiency. Res Vet Sci 35:249, 1983.

Strombeck DR: New method for evaluation of chymotrypsin deficiency in dogs. J Am Vet Med Assoc 173:1319, 1978.

Strombeck DR: Small animal gastroenterology. Davis, Calif, Stonegate Publishing, 1979.

Strombeck DR, Harrold D: Evaluation of 60-minute blood p-aminobenzoic acid concentration in pancreatic function testing of dogs. J Am Vet Med Assoc 180:419, 1982.

Tams TR, Twedt DC: Canine protein-losing gastroenteropathy syndrome. Compend Contin Educ Pract Vet 3:105, 1981.

Tennant BL, Hornbuckle WE: Gastrointestinal function. In Kaneko JJ (ed): Clinical biochemistry of domestic animals, 3rd ed. New York, Academic Press, 1980.

Van Kruiningen HJ: Giant hypertrophic gastritis of basenji dogs. Vet Pathol 14:19, 1977.

Williams DA, Batt RM: Diagnosis of canine exocrine pancreatic insufficiency by the assay of serum trypsin-like immunoreactivity. J Small Anim Pract 24:583, 1983.

9
Urinary System

URINALYSIS

The examination of urine is a very useful procedure to evaluate sick animals. Abnormalities in the urinalysis may reflect a variety of disease processes involving several different organs. It is not just a measure of renal and lower urinary tract problems. Components of the urinalysis include inspection of color, transparency, and odor; determination of solute concentration; chemical analysis and quantitation of select normal and abnormal constituents; and microscopic examination of urine sediment.

I. Physical characteristics
   A. Color
      1. Normal urine is yellow to amber with the depth of the color related to volume and concentration. Urochromes and urobilin are responsible for this color.
      2. Causes of abnormal color are listed below.
         a. Blood (hematuria) is red; the urine is cloudy and usually clears on centrifugation.
            (1) When red discoloration is most prominent at the beginning of urination, it suggests lower urinary tract or genital tract origin.
            (2) When red discoloration is most prominent at the end of urination it suggests urinary bladder origin.
         b. Bilirubin is dark yellow to brown and has a yellow foam.
         c. Hemoglobin and myoglobin are reddish brown.
         d. Porphyrins are colorless but give a pink fluorescence in acid urine when exposed to ultraviolet light.
         e. Various drugs discolor urine.
   B. Transparency
      1. Normal urine is clear when freshly voided, but it may become cloudy on standing as a result of precipitation of salts forming crystals.

153

2. Fresh normal horse urine is cloudy owing to calcium carbonate crystals and mucus (Case 13).
3. The cause of cloudy urine should always be identified microscopically. Causes include crystals, cells, blood, mucus, bacteria, casts, and sperm (see III. Sediment examination). Many of these causes are not pathologic.

C. Odor
1. Ammonia is formed by bacterial urease action. Its odor is particularly prominent in retained urine.
2. An acetone odor suggests ketosis.
3. Excretion of certain drugs gives characteristic odors to urine.

D. Volume
1. Control of urine volume
   a. Urine enters the proximal tubule at approximately the same osmolality as plasma.
   b. Obligatory reabsorption of water independent of body needs occurs in the proximal tubules. By osmotic action water follows sodium, glucose, and other solutes that are actively reabsorbed. Urine is iso-osmotic to plasma on entering the loop of Henle.
   c. The osmolality of the urine increases in the descending loop of Henle, which is highly permeable to water but rather impermeable to solute.
   d. The ascending loop of Henle is permeable to solute and the site of active chloride transport but rather impermeable to water. Fluid entering the distal tubule is hypo-osmotic to plasma.
   e. Water reabsorption in the distal and collecting tubules is in excess of solute. It is under the influence of antidiuretic hormone (ADH) and requires a hypertonic medulla. The major control of urine volume is at this level.
   f. Maintenance of the medullary hypertonicity is a function of the countercurrent multiplier system of the loop of Henle and vasa recta.
2. Methods of measurement
   a. The measurement of total amount of urine voided during 24 hours, using a metabolism cage, is the most accurate method.
   b. Estimation of volume may be made from the specific gravity or osmolality. Volume and specific gravity or osmolality are inversely related in health and most diseases. Exceptions are diabetes mellitus (both are high), acute renal disease, and terminal chronic renal disease (both may be low).
   c. Low urine creatinine (less than 50 mg/dl) and low solute (osmolality less than 500 mOsm/l or specific gravity less than 1.015) equal polyuria in the cow.
3. Causes of abnormal urine volume are listed in Table 9.1.

E. Solute concentration
1. Methods of measurement

TABLE 9.1. Causes of Abnormal Urine Volume
_____
Polyuria (increased volume)
  Acute renal disease (diuretic phase)
  Chronic renal disease
  Diabetes mellitus
  Hepatic failure
  Hyperadrenocorticism
  Hypercalcemia
  Hyperparathyroidism (cats)
  Nephrogenic diabetes insipidus
  Pituitary diabetes insipidus
  Postobstructive diuresis
  Primary renal glycosuria
  Psychogenic polydipsia
  Pyelonephritis
  Pyometra
Oliguria (reduced volume)
  Acute renal disease
  Dehydration
  Shock
  Terminal chronic renal disease
  Urinary tract obstruction
_____

    a. Osmolality (see Chapter 5)
        (1) The number of particles in the solution is the
             determining factor in this measurement of
             concentration.
        (2) Depression of freezing point or lowering of
             vapor pressure are the methods of measurement.
    b. Specific gravity (sp gr)
        (1) This measurement is dependent on particle size
             and weight as well as number.
        (2) It is a simple procedure and a valid
             reflection of the osmolality; therefore, it is
             the method most commonly used in clinical
             practice.
        (3) Refractometry and hydrometry are the usual
             methods of measurement.
  2. Interpretation (also see urine concentration tests)
    a. Sp gr can range from 1.001 to 1.065 in normal
        animals and up to 1.080 in the cat. This range
        includes values associated with renal
        abnormalities.
    b. A dog with a random sp gr greater than 1.030
        (greater than 1.035 in the cat) is presumed to have
        adequate concentrating ability. A sp gr greater
        than 1.025 (extrapolated from humans) has been used
        for other species.
    c. Interpretation of a low sp gr requires knowledge of
        the hydration status of the animal; ADH release and
        urine concentration should take place if there is
        greater than 3% dehydration.
    d. Isosthenuria is the maintenance of a constant urine
        osmolality in the range of the glomerular filtrate
        (sp gr of 1.008 to 1.012, "fixed" sp gr);
        concentration is not occurring (Case 14).
    e. Urine sp gr below 1.008 indicates some renal

function; solute is reabsorbed in excess of water.
    f. Most neonates except the calf do not have efficient
        concentrating mechanisms.

II. Chemical characteristics
    A. Protein
        1. Methods of measurement
            a. Reagent strip or acid precipitation tests are used
                to semiquantitate urine protein.
                (1) Reagent strips yield 1 to 4+ reactions that
                     are approximately equivalent to 30, 100, 300,
                     and 1000 mg protein/dl; precipitation tests
                     may also be graded 1 to 4+.
                (2) The small amount of protein normally present
                     in urine is not detected by these methods.
                (3) The reagent strip method is most sensitive for
                     albumin and not reliable for detection of
                     globulins and the Bence Jones paraprotein of
                     plasma cell myeloma.
            b. Quantitative tests are available to measure the
                total protein excretion in a 24-hour urine sample.
        2. Interpretation of a positive test (proteinuria)
            a. Amount of protein (1 to 4+) should be evaluated in
                light of the urine volume or sp gr to estimate the
                total amount being lost (Case 2). Measurement of
                total protein in a 24-hour volume of urine is
                better.
            b. False-positive reagent strip tests may occur in
                highly alkaline urine; confirm with acid
                precipitation tests.
            c. Occult blood test and sediment examination are
                necessary to determine the cause of proteinuria
                (Cases 3, 13, 15, 16).
            d. The following causes of proteinuria are listed in
                the order by which differentiation is best
                accomplished.
                (1) Hemorrhage into the urinary tract (Case 16)
                     (a) The urine occult blood test is positive,
                          and erythrocytes are observed in the
                          sediment.
                     (b) High urine protein values occur with
                          hemorrhage.
                     (c) Trauma, inflammation, and neoplasia are
                          common causes.
                (2) Inflammation within the urinary tract
                     (a) Leukocytes will be observed in the
                          sediment.
                     (b) Precise location of the inflammation is
                          difficult to detect on examination of
                          urine alone.
                     (c) Bacteria may be present.
                     (d) Protein concentration is seldom over 2+
                          unless the inflammation is hemorrhagic.
                          Hemorrhagic inflammation is difficult to
                          differentiate from traumatic hemorrhage
                          (Case 16).

        (3)   Renal disease (Cases 7, 14, 15)

            (a)   Lack of occult blood and an absence of significant cellular sediment are typical findings.

            (b)   Casts may or may not be present.

            (c)   Primary glomerular disease may cause very high values; the major component is albumin.

            (d)   Primary tubular disease gives low to moderate values; the major components are low molecular weight globulins that normally pass the glomerulus but are not reabsorbed by defective tubules.

            (e)   Usually proteinuria of renal origin is associated with both glomerular and tubular disease.

        (4)   Prerenal proteinuria (Cases 3, 13)

            (a)   Certain extrarenal factors may cause a transitory, mild proteinuria via increased glomerular permeability (e.g., fever, cardiac disease, central nervous system disease, shock, muscular exertion).

            (b)   A proteinuria owing to colostral proteins occurs in foals, calves, kids, and lambs under 40 hours of age.

            (c)   High concentrations of low molecular weight proteins in the blood may pass the glomerulus and overwhelm the resorptive capacity of the tubules, causing an overflow proteinuria (e.g., Bence Jones protein, hemoglobin monomers, and myoglobin).

B.   Glucose

   1.   Methods of measurement

      a.   Reagent strips employ the glucose oxidase method, which is specific for glucose. These methods are more sensitive than reduction methods.

      b.   The copper reduction tablet method semiquantitates glucose, but it is also positive with other reducing substances (e.g., lactose, galactose, pentose, ascorbic acid, conjugated gluconates, and salicylates).

   2.   Interpretation of a positive test (glucosuria)

      a.   Hyperglycemia (causes listed in Table 6.1) of sufficient magnitude to exceed the tubular transport capacity is the most common cause (Case 17). The resorptive capacity is exceeded when blood glucose values reach approximately 180 mg/dl or more (the bovine threshold is 100 mg/dl).

      b.   Decreased tubular reabsorption (normoglycemia) is a minor cause.

        (1)   Canine Fanconi-like syndrome and primary renal glucosuria are associated with defective absorption.

        (2)   Other types of renal disease rarely have

glucosuria; therefore, urine glucose is not a
reliable measurement of tubular disease.

C. Ketones
    1. Methods of measurement
        a. Reagent strip and tablet methods employ the
           nitroprusside reaction.
        b. The above methods detect acetone and acetoacetic
           acid but not betahydroxybutyric acid.
        c. False-negative reactions occur when the urine is
           not fresh.
    2. Interpretation of a positive test (ketonuria) (Case 17)
        a. Ketonuria is present before detectable ketonemia
           occurs (see Chapter 6).
        b. Ketonuria indicates excessive fat degradation
           and/or deficiency in carbohydrate metabolism and
           may occur in the following.
           (1) Ketosis of cattle
           (2) Pregnancy disease of ewes
           (3) Diabetes mellitus
           (4) Starvation
           (5) Low-carbohydrate, high-fat diets

D. Bilirubin (see Chapter 7)
    1. Methods of measurement
        a. Reagent strips utilize the diazotization method.
           Urine colors may interfere with the reading of this
           test.
        b. The tablet method uses a similar procedure but is
           more sensitive.
        c. These tests are most reactive with conjugated
           bilirubin and rather insensitive to free bilirubin.
        d. Bilirubin may be oxidized to biliverdin or
           hydrolyzed to free bilirubin on exposure to light;
           excessive delay in analysis results in a negative
           test.
    2. Interpretation of a positive test (bilirubinuria)
       (Case 11)
        a. It indicates obstruction to bile flow and
           regurgitation of conjugated bilirubin into the
           blood. A significant degree of hepatic disease can
           be present without the occurrence of bilirubinuria.
        b. Bilirubinuria can be detected when a concomitant
           rise in serum bilirubin is not present. This is
           especially true in the dog, which has a low renal
           threshold. Trace readings are common in health in
           this species, especially in concentrated urine.
        c. In potentially hyperbilirubinemic conditions
           bilirubinuria may precede hyperbilirubinemia.
        d. In cases of intravascular hemolysis and
           hemoglobinuria, tubular cell conjugation of free
           bilirubin may result in a positive urine test.

E. Occult blood (hemoglobin, myoglobin) test
    1. Methods of measurement. The commonly used reagent strip
       and tablet methods are based on the peroxidase
       properties of free hemoglobin or myoglobin and the
       subsequent oxidation of orthotoluidine to a blue-
       colored derivative.

2. Causes of a positive occult blood test and their differentiation (Cases 3, 13, 16)
   a. Hematuria is differentiated by the following.
      (1) Red, cloudy urine that usually clears on centrifugation
      (2) Erythrocytes in the sediment (enough will usually have lysed, releasing hemoglobin to give a positive test)
      (3) Absence of clinical or laboratory evidence of anemia or muscle disease.
      (4) Evidence of urinary tract disease (usually lower tract)
   b. Hemoglobinuria is differentiated by the following.
      (1) Red to brown urine that does not clear on centrifugation
      (2) Absence of erythrocytes in the sediment. Erythrocytes in very low sp gr urine (less than 1.008) may all lyse, thus masking a hematuria.
      (3) Reddish discoloration of the plasma (hemoglobinemia). Plasma will be discolored before hemoglobinemia is sufficient to exceed the "renal threshold" and cause hemoglobinuria.
      (4) Evidence of anemia, particularly an intravascular hemolytic type
      (5) Absence of clinical or laboratory evidence of muscle disease
      (6) Addition of saturated ammonium sulfate, which will precipitate and remove the color caused by hemoglobin but not myoglobin. Spectrophotometric tests are better for differentiating between these two compounds.
   c. Myoglobinuria is characterized by the following.
      (1) Brownish urine that does not clear on centrifugation
      (2) Absence of erythrocytes in the sediment
      (3) Clear, normal-colored plasma. Myoglobin does not bind significantly to serum proteins and is excreted in the urine before reaching levels that discolor the plasma.
      (4) Absence of clinical or laboratory evidence of an anemia
      (5) Clinical or laboratory evidence of muscle disease
F. Urobilinogen (see Chapter 7)
   1. Methods of measurement
      a. Urobilinogen generates a cherry red color in Ehrlich's reagent; the method is semiquantitative.
      b. Reagent strip tests are semiquantitative; the absence of urobilinogen cannot be detected by this method.
      c. Urobilinogen may be catabolized to urobilin in the bladder or on standing, causing a false-negative reaction; a fresh sample is essential.

       2. Interpretation of findings
          a. Urobilinogen is formed in the gut from conjugated bilirubin by the action of intestinal bacteria and absorbed into the portal blood. Some is excreted into the urine, but most is recycled through the liver.
          b. Its presence in urine indicates a patent bile duct.
          c. Absence of urobilinogen may indicate complete bile duct obstruction; but because of its instability and diurnal variation in excretion, many normal animals have no detectable urobilinogen in their urine.
          d. Increased concentration may occur in hemolytic disease and diseases with reduced functional hepatic mass. In the latter, bile flow persists; but less reabsorbed urobilinogen is removed from the portal blood by the liver.
          e. The correlation between urine urobilinogen concentration and hepatobiliary disease is poor in animals.
    G. Hydrogen ion concentration (pH)
       1. Methods of measurement
          a. A variety of reagent strips impregnated with chemical indicators are available for the determination of pH.
          b. A fresh sample is necessary because urine becomes alkaline on standing owing to loss of CO_2 and conversion of urea to ammonia by bacteria.
       2. Interpretation
          a. Urine pH is the result of renal regulation of blood bicarbonate and H^+ levels, but it should not be used alone to evaluate acid base status.
          b. Diet affects pH.
             (1) A lower pH occurs with high–protein diets (meat and milk in carnivores and nursing animals) and complete anorexia in herbivorous animals.
            (2) A higher pH occurs with a vegetable diet (herbivores).
          c. Cystitis and other causes of urine retention yield higher urine pH because of bacterial catabolism of urea to ammonia.
          d. Urine pH determines the type of crystals and uroliths that may form in urine.
          e. Therapy may affect urine pH, or pH may affect efficiency of certain therapeutic agents.
    H. Nitrite. This test has been used to screen for certain bacteria that reduce nitrates. It has not proved to be a reliable test in animals.

III. Sediment examination
    A. Principles
       1. Examine unstained sediment, using reduced light to furnish contrast.
       2. Stains are available for use but are not necessary.

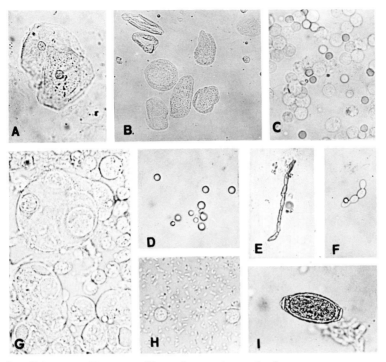

Fig. 9.1. Urinary sediment: cells and organisms. A. Squamous epithelial cells, B. transitional epithelial cells, C. erythrocytes and leukocytes, D. fat droplets (in focus), E. fungal hypha, F. yeast, G. transitional carcinoma cells, H. bacterial rods and leukocytes, I. Capillaria plica egg. (Unstained, ×240.) (From Duncan JR, Prasse KW: Clinical examination of urine. Vet Clin North Am 6:647, 1976.)

      3. The quantity of sediment is related to urine volume; therefore, values obtained from sediment examination should be evaluated in light of the urine sp gr.

      4. The method of collection influences the type and amount of sediment present because of variation in extraurinary contamination and iatrogenic hemorrhage.

B. Epithelial cells (Fig. 9.1)

      1. Squamous epithelial cells are large with irregular, angular margins and small nuclei. They desquamate from the urethra and vagina or prepuce and are of no diagnostic significance.

      2. Transitional epithelial cells are oval, spindled, or caudate and originate from the proximal urethra, urinary bladder, ureter, and renal pelvis. They may occur in groups, especially in catheterized samples, but are of little diagnostic importance unless neoplastic.

      3. Renal epithelial cells are small, round, slightly larger than leukocytes, and derived from the tubules. They are usually degenerate and difficult to identify and differentiate from leukocytes.

C. Erythrocytes (Fig. 9.1)
    1. Erythrocytes are round, slightly refractile, lack
        internal structure, and resemble fat droplets (fat
        droplets float to a different plane of focus and vary
        in size).
    2. More than 4 to 5 erythrocytes/high-power field (HPF)
        indicate hemorrhage (hematuria), which may be traumatic
        or inflammatory in nature (Case 16) (see IIE. Occult
        blood test).
    3. Erythrocytes may often appear crenated in concentrated
        urine (high sp gr).
    4. Erythrocytes may lyse or become ballooned ghost cells
        in dilute urine (sp gr less than 1.008).
    5. Oval, yeast-type fungi are similar to erythrocytes, but
        they are more variable in size and may be budding.
D. Leukocytes (Fig. 9.1)
    1. These cells are round and granular, larger than
        erythrocytes, and smaller than epithelial cells. They
        degenerate in old urine and may lyse in hypotonic or
        alkaline urine.
    2. More than 5 to 8 leukocytes/HPF indicate a urogenital
        tract inflammation (pyuria) that may or may not be
        septic (Case 16).
    3. Leukocytes are frequently associated with bacteriuria,
        but significant bacteriuria may occur without pyuria.
E. Casts (Fig. 9.2) (Cases 9, 13)
    1. General features of casts
        a. Casts are elongated structures composed of a matrix
            of mucoprotein (Tamm-Horsfall protein) produced by
            the distal tubules.
        b. They are formed in distal tubules where urine is
            more acidic; they may dissolve in alkaline urine.
        c. Structures present in the tubule at the time of
            formation may be embedded in the cast.
        d. Although casts indicate some tubular change, they
            tell nothing of its severity. They can be observed
            in apparently normal individuals.
        e. Casts tend to be discharged into urine
            intermittently and may or may not be observed in a
            single urinalysis.
        f. The absence of casts does not rule out renal
            disease; only a few casts may be observed during
            severe, chronic generalized renal disease.
    2. Types of casts
        a. Hyaline casts are colorless, homogeneous, semi-
            transparent, and difficult to detect even with
            reduced light. They are composed mostly of
            mucoprotein.
        b. Granular casts are the most common type observed
            and are composed of mucoprotein, plasma proteins,
            and occasionally tubular debris.
        c. Epithelial casts are similar to granular casts but
            contain cells that have desquamated from the
            tubules.
        d. Waxy casts are wide structures without granular
            contents and usually have broken or square ends.

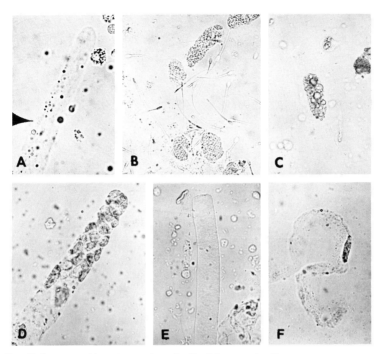

Fig. 9.2. Urinary sediment: casts. A. Hyaline cast, B. granular casts and spermatozoa, C. fatty cast, D. cellular cast and
fat droplets (out of focus), E. waxy cast, F. mucous thread.
(Unstained, ×240.) (From Duncan JR, Prasse KW: Clinical
examination of urine. Vet Clin North Am 6:647, 1976.)

They evolve from degenerating cellular and granular
casts and indicate a chronic tubular lesion.

   e. Fatty casts contain fat globules derived from
degenerating tubular epithelial cells. They are the
most common type found in cats because of high
lipid content of the tubular epithelial cells of
this species.

   f. Erythrocyte casts indicate renal hemorrhage or
inflammation.

   g. Leukocyte casts indicate renal inflammation.

F. Mucus (Fig. 9.2)

   1. Mucus occurs as narrow, twisted, ribbonlike,
homogeneous threads and signifies urethral irritation
or genital secretions.

   2. Mucus is normal in horse urine (Case 13).

G. Fat (Figs. 9.1, 9.2)

   1. Fat droplets are highly refractile, variable-sized
spheres that are out of focus with other sediment
because they rise to the surface. They may be stained
with Sudan III.

   2. Fat is usually of no pathologic significance in urine.

H. Bacteria (Fig. 9.1)

   1. Identifying features

      a. Bacterial rods occur singly or in chains.

      b. Cocci are difficult to identify unstained unless

present in chains because small crystals and debris resemble them.

    c. Wright- or Gram-stained preparations can be used to substantiate bacteria in questionable cases.

    2. Significance of bacteriuria

        a. Greater than 30,000 bacteria/ml must usually be present before visual detection is possible.

        b. Urine is normally sterile only until midurethra; therefore, bacteria present in catheterized and voided samples may represent contamination from the lower urogenital tract.

        c. Quantitative and qualitative urine cultures are required to accurately assess clinically significant bacteriuria.

I. Sperm (Fig. 9.2)

J. Parasitic structures that may occur in urine include *Stephanurus* dentatus, *Dioctophyma* renale, and *Capillaria* plica eggs (Fig. 9.1) and microfilaria of *Dirofilaria* immitus.

K. Fungi (Fig. 9.1). Segmented hyphae or budding yeasts may be found; they are contaminants.

L. Crystals (Fig. 9.3)

    1. Precipitation of solutes depends on pH of the urine and solubility and concentration of the crystalloid.

    2. Crystals are identified by their shape, color, and solubility in acid or alkali.

    3. They seldom have clinical significance; therefore, tedious identification is not worthwhile.

    4. Crystals with possible pathologic significance are:

        a. Ammonium biurate, which can occur with portal venous-systemic shunting or other liver diseases (Case 12)

        b. Tyrosine, which may be associated with liver disease

        c. Cystine caused by altered protein metabolism (i.e., congenital cystinuria of dogs)

        d. Sulfonamide crystals, which may form with excessive treatment

        e. Oxalates, which occur in ethylene glycol and certain plant toxicities; they also may be normal.

        f. Hippuric acid crystals, which may also occur in ethylene glycol toxicity

        g. Triple phosphate (struvite) crystals, which are associated with some calculi but are more often present in alkaline urine unassociated with calculi

MEANS OF EVALUATING RENAL FUNCTION

I. Urine concentration tests

    A. Rationale

        1. Dehydration increases plasma osmolality, which stimulates the release of ADH by the pituitary. ADH acts on the collecting tubule epithelial cells, causing resorption of water and an increase in urine sp gr.

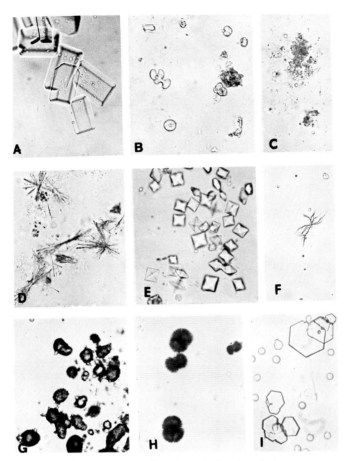

Fig. 9.3. Urinary sediment: crystals. A. Triple phosphates, B. calcium carbonate, C. amorphous urates or phosphates, D. tyrosine, E. calcium oxalate, F. bilirubin, G. ammonium biurate, H. sulfonamide, I. cystine. (Unstained, ×240.) (From Duncan JR, Prasse KW: Clinical examination of urine. Vet Clin North Am 6:647, 1976.)

2. Clinical indications include the following.
    a. Polydipsia and polyuria with urine sp gr less than 1.030 in the dog, 1.035 in the cat, and 1.025 in the horse and cow, and not associated with azotemia
    b. Repeated random urine sample with sp gr in the isosthenuric or low range in the nonazotemic animal
3. Contraindications to the above include the following.
    a. Azotemia or uremia. A diagnosis of renal disease is already established if azotemia accompanies a dilute urine. Prerenal azotemia is associated with concentrated urine.
    b. Dehydration. Maximal stimulation for ADH release is already in effect.
    c. Severe debilitation
B. Types of concentration tests
    1. Abrupt water deprivation test

        a. The animal is abruptly deprived of water and the urine sp gr monitored. The test is halted if adequate concentrating ability (sp gr greater than 1.030 in the dog, 1.035 in the cat, and 1.025 in the cow and horse) is demonstrated, 5 to 7% of the body weight is lost, or undesirable signs develop.

        b. In the cow, 3 to 4 days of water restriction are required for maximum concentration because of the large rumen reservoir of water.

    2. Gradual water deprivation test

        a. The animal is progressively deprived of increasing amounts of water until it is completely withheld; the rules of the abrupt test are then followed.

        b. This test is suggested to be of value when polyuria is associated with medullary washout of solute. In this situation medullary hypertonicity must be reestablished before the tubules can respond to ADH and the abrupt test.

        c. Diseases causing polyuria associated with medullary washout include psychogenic water consumption and hyperadrenocorticism (Case 20).

    3. Pitressin concentration test

        a. In lieu of water deprivation, an exogenous source of ADH (pitressin) is given to stimulate water reabsorption and urine concentration.

        b. This test may be used when water deprivation is a risk to the patient. It has been used primarily in the dog.

        c. Concentrating ability appears to be better after water deprivation than after injection of pitressin.

C. Interpretation of concentration tests

    1. A urine sp gr greater than 1.030 in the dog, 1.035 in the cat, and 1.025 in the horse and cow indicates adequate urine concentration.

    2. Causes of abnormal concentration tests are:

        a. Renal disease

            (1) Approximately two-thirds of the nephrons are nonfunctional before abnormal concentrating ability can be demonstrated (Cases 10, 14).

            (2) Impaired concentrating ability usually occurs before increased blood urea nitrogen (BUN) or serum creatinine. In the cat, and in the early stage of primary glomerular disease in any species (Case 15), azotemia may precede concentration abnormalities.

        b. Pituitary diabetes insipidus

            (1) Pituitary disease causes a lack of ADH secretion. The renal tubules are normal but are not stimulated to reabsorb water.

            (2) The sp gr is usually in the 1.001 to 1.007 range because the animal can reabsorb solute.

            (3) These animals will respond to the pitressin concentration test.

        c. Nephrogenic diabetes insipidus. The tubules are

refractory to ADH stimulation, but other renal
function tests are normal.

    d. Diseases that cause polyuria and medullary washout
        (e.g., hyperadrenocorticism). The gradual
        deprivation test is indicated.

II. Blood urea nitrogen
    A. Basic concepts of urea metabolism
        1. Small quantities of urea are ingested.
        2. The majority is synthesized in the liver from ammonia
            that is either formed from protein catabolism or
            absorbed from the large intestine.
        3. Urea is not found in feces because it is absorbed or
            metabolized.
        4. Once urea enters the vascular system, it passively
            diffuses throughout the total body water compartment.
            Approximately 90 minutes are required for
            equilibration. Therefore, BUN and serum urea nitrogen
            are the same.
    B. Urea excretion
        1. The kidney is the most important route of urea
            excretion.
            a. Urea concentration in the glomerular filtrate is
                the same as in the blood. This is a process of
                simple filtration and does not require energy.
                Diminished glomerular filtration causes high BUN
                concentration.
            b. Urea passively diffuses with water from the tubular
                lumen back into the blood.
                (1) The amount of absorption is inversely related
                     to the rate of urine flow through the tubules.
                (2) At the highest urine flow rate, approximately
                     40% of the urea is reabsorbed. If urine flow
                     is decreased, more is reabsorbed (up to 60% or
                     more), adding to the blood urea concentration.
                (3) Urea absorption from collecting ducts is
                     needed to maintain medullary hypertonicity.
        2. Gastrointestinal tract excretion is another route.
            a. This route is futile in simple-stomached animals,
                since nearly all the ammonia formed by intestinal
                bacterial degradation of urea is used to
                resynthesize urea in the liver.
            b. In the ruminant the ammonia formed can be utilized
                in the synthesis of amino acids and thereby effect
                excretion of urea.
            c. Ruminants on a low-protein diet reabsorb most of
                the urea (90%) filtered by the glomerulus; most of
                this endogenous urea enters the rumen where it
                eventually contributes to the synthesis of protein.
            d. Transfer of urea from blood to rumen occurs
                normally, but above a certain blood concentration
                very little increase in transfer occurs. Rumen
                catabolism does not have a marked effect in
                lowering the degree of azotemia.
    C. Methods of measurement

   1. Reagent strips that employ urease may be used to
       semiquantitate BUN concentration, but the method is not
       accurate.
   2. Chromatographic strips are based on ammonia release,
       which produces color change allowing semiquantitation
       of BUN concentration.
   3. Colorimetric methods are quantitative.
D. Interpretation of increased BUN concentration (azotemia)
   1. Prerenal azotemia (Case 4)
       a. Increased protein catabolism secondary to small
           bowel hemorrhage, necrosis, starvation, prolonged
           exercise, infection, fever, and corticosteroids may
           cause a mild BUN increase via increased hepatic
           synthesis of urea.
       b. Decreased renal perfusion (reduced glomerular
           filtration) can cause azotemia and occurs with
           shock, dehydration, and cardiovascular disease.
       c. High-protein diet seldom causes significant
           increase in BUN in normal animals, but it may
           precipitate a rise in animals with occult renal
           disease.
       d. Azotemia, whether prerenal or renal, is often
           associated with electrolyte and acid base
           disorders, particularly in the cow.
       e. Factors causing pre- or postrenal azotemia may
           eventually cause renal azotemia.
       f. In most species prerenal azotemia is a more
           frequent occurrence than renal azotemia.
       g. Urine solute concentration (sp gr and osmolality)
           is high, urine osmolality/plasma osmolality ratio
           is high, and urine sodium concentration is low
           (less than 10 mEq/1).
   2. Renal azotemia (Cases 9, 13, 14, 15, 23, 25)
       a. Renal azotemia occurs after approximately 75% of
           the nephrons are nonfunctional. BUN value approxi-
           mately doubles each time the remaining functional
           mass is halved; therefore, modest increases at this
           stage are highly significant.
       b. Concentrating ability usually has already
           been affected by the time azotemia develops;
           low urine solute concentration and low urine
           osmolality/plasma osmolality ratio occur. Cats
           are an exception to this rule; some concentrating
           ability persists after azotemia develops.
       c. Urine/plasma urea and urine/plasma creatinine
           ratios are low.
       d. Moderate BUN levels are more significant in the
           horse than in other species.
       e. BUN values do not increase proportionally to
           creatinine in the ruminant because of rumen
           excretion of urea (Case 23).
       f. Single BUN determinations are not reliable
           prognostic indicators. It is best to use serial
           evaluation, noting progressive increases in spite
           of therapy.

3. Postrenal azotemia (obstruction or leakage) (Case 16)
    a. Clinical signs (oliguria, anuria) and physical and radiologic examination are usually sufficient to differentiate this cause of azotemia.
    b. The urine specific gravity may be in the isosthenuric range.
    c. BUN values should return to normal in several days after relief of obstruction or repair of rupture.
E. Causes of decreased BUN concentration are low-protein diet, hepatic insufficiency, and anabolic steroids.

III. Serum creatinine
A. Basic concepts of metabolism
    1. Small quantities may be ingested in diets containing muscle tissue.
    2. Most creatinine originates endogenously from non-enzymatic conversion of creatine that stores energy in muscle as phosphocreatine.
    3. A rather constant amount of creatine is converted to creatinine daily; creatinine is not reutilized.
    4. The creatine pool is influenced by muscle mass, which may be altered by muscle disease, generalized wasting, and conditioning (training).
    5. Creatinine is distributed throughout the body water but diffuses slower than urea (4 hours are required for equilibration).
B. Creatinine excretion
    1. Renal excretion
        a. Creatinine is freely filtered through the glomerulus. Tubular reabsorption does not occur.
        b. A small amount is secreted by proximal tubules.
    2. Degradation by enteric organisms is another excretion route. Creatinine is not present in feces nor is there evidence for recycling.
C. Interpretation of increased serum creatinine concentration
    1. Creatinine concentration is not significantly affected by diet and catabolic factors.
    2. Reduced renal perfusion affects creatinine similarly to BUN; therefore, prerenal azotemia is characterized by increased BUN and creatinine.
    3. Creatinine gives information similar to that of BUN in renal disease and postrenal obstruction or leakage (Cases 13, 14, 15, 16).
    4. Most treatments have less effect on lowering serum creatinine than on lowering BUN. Creatinine is not affected by urine flow as is BUN and diffuses more slowly between fluid compartments than does urea. Therefore, diuresis and dialysis facilitate the excretion of less creatinine than urea.
    5. Noncreatinine chromagens may result in false high values. Ketones are the most significant of these interfering compounds.

IV. BUN/creatinine ratio
A. This ratio has been suggested to be of value in the

differential diagnosis of azotemia because of differences in tubular reabsorption and diffusion rates and effects of diet and protein metabolism between the two compounds.
B. Clinical experience has shown that there are too many variables for the ratio to be used as a diagnostic parameter in veterinary medicine.

V. Clearance tests. The ideal substance for a renal clearance test should be exclusively cleared and not reabsorbed by the kidney and not subject to metabolism or excretion by extrarenal routes. All clearance tests are affected by decreased renal perfusion.
   A. Endogenous creatinine clearance
      1. A 20-minute test is usually performed. The volume of urine formed during the period is measured, and concurrent urine and serum creatinine concentrations are determined.
      2. It is used as a measurement of glomerular filtration rate (GFR) because blood levels are rather constant, most creatinine is filtered by the glomerulus, and tubular reabsorption does not occur.
      3. Inaccuracies in estimation of GFR are related to tubular secretion of creatinine, extrarenal excretion, and measurement of noncreatinine chromagens.
         a. Clearance = [urine creatinine (mg/dl) × urine volume (ml/min)]/[serum creatinine (mg/dl)].
         b. The results are expressed as ml/min/kg.
   B. Inulin clearance for measuring GFR and p-aminohippuric acid clearance for measuring renal plasma flow are more accurate tests but are available only at large research centers.
   C. Sulfanilate clearance
      1. Sodium sulfanilate is eliminated from the blood primarily by glomerular filtration.
      2. A half-time for clearance is calculated from blood samples collected at intervals over a 90-minute period after intravenous injection of sodium sulfanilate (20 mg/kg).
      3. This test is suggested to be of value in the dog for detecting decreases in renal function before development of azotemia or concentration abnormalities.
   D. Phenolsulfonphthalein (PSP) clearance
      1. PSP injected intravenously binds to albumin and is excreted primarily by the kidneys via tubular secretion. However, at the dosages used, blood levels do not reach the tubular maximum. Blood flow to the tubules is the major factor causing abnormal values.
      2. Methods of measurement
         a. The excretion test measures the percent PSP excreted in the urine during a 20-minute period following intravenous injection (6 mg).
         b. The clearance procedure determines the plasma half-time over a 60-minute period following intravenous injection (1 mg/kg).
      3. Approximately two-thirds of the nephrons are nonfunctional before an abnormal value occurs.

E.   Urine electrolyte clearance ratios (fractional clearances)
1.   These tests measure renal function by determining the clearance of a particular electrolyte.
2.   Electrolyte clearance may be quantified by comparing with the clearance of endogenous creatinine (% creatinine clearance). This procedure simultaneously measures the electrolyte and creatinine concentration in a single urine and serum sample. The formula is: % creatinine clearance = [urinary electrolyte (mEq/l)/serum electrolyte (mEq/l)] × [serum creatinine (mg/dl)/urinary creatinine (mg/dl)] × 100.
3.   Fractional clearances of Na^+, K^+, P, or Ca^{++} have been used in animals (fractional clearance of Ca is unreliable in the horse because of crystallization of $CaCO_4$ in the urine of this species).
4.   Variability in intake and nonurinary excretion results in a variability in clearance ratios of normal animals. This has limited their use in the detection of renal disease.

VI.   Miscellaneous alterations occurring in renal disease
A.   Progressive nonregenerative anemia occurs in chronic renal disease (Cases 14, 15).
B.   Hyperphosphatemia is associated with decreased GFR (Cases 13, 14, 15, 16). Hyperphosphatemia is less significant in the cow because the kidney is not the major excretory route.
C.   Hyperkalemia is associated with oliguria or anuria and acidosis in renal failure (Case 16).
D.   Metabolic acidosis may be associated with renal failure in the dog and cat (Case 14). Cows have a normal acid base status or metabolic alkalosis (Case 23).
E.   Hypercalcemia is common in the horse because the kidney is a major excretory route. Hypocalcemia is usual in the cow (Case 23), and in the dog and cat normocalcemia or slight hypocalcemia is the rule.
F.   Hypochloridemia is a consistent finding in the cow (Case 23).
G.   Increased sodium loss into the urine occurs during the diuretic phase of acute renal disease.
H.   Hypercholesterolemia is associated with primary glomerular disease and the nephrotic syndrome (Case 15).
I.   Hyperamylasemia and hyperlipasemia may be associated with renal failure in the dog.

REFERENCES

Asheim, A.: Pathogenesis of renal damage and polydipsia in dogs with pyometra. J Am Vet Med Assoc 147:736, 1965.
Barlough JE, Osborne, CA, Stevens, JB: Canine and feline urinalysis: Value of macroscopic and microscopic examinations. J Am Vet Med Assoc 178:61, 1981.
Barsanti JA, Finco, DR: Protein concentration in urine of normal dogs. Am J Vet Res 40:1583, 1979.
Barsanti JA, Finco DR: Laboratory finding in urinary tract infections. Vet Clin North Am 9:729, 1979.
Behr MJ, Hackett RP, Bentinck-Smith J, et al: Metabolic abnormalities associated with rupture of the urinary bladder in neonatal foals. J Am Vet Med Assoc 178:263, 1981.
Bloedow AG: Familial renal disease in samoyed dogs. Vet Rec 108:167, 1981.

Bovee KC: Urine osmolarity as a definitive indicator of renal concentrating capacity. J
    Am Vet Med Assoc 155:30, 1969.
Bovee KC: The uremic syndrome. J Am Anim Hosp Assoc 12:189, 1976.
Bovee KC, Joyce T: Clinical evaluation of glomerular function: 24-hour creatinine
    clearance in dogs. J Am Anim Hosp Assoc 17:488, 1979.
Bovee KC, Joyce T, Blazer-Yost B, et al: Characterization of renal defects in dogs with a
    syndrome similar to the Fanconi syndrome in man. J Am Vet Med Assoc 174:1094, 1979.
Bovee KC, Segal S: Canine cystinuria and cystine calculi. Proc 21st Gaines Vet Symp, 1971.
Breitschwerdt EB: Clinical abnormalities of urine concentration and dilution. Compend
    Contin Educ Pract Vet 3:414, 1981.
Breitschwerdt EB, Verlander JW, Hribernik TN: Nephrogenic diabetes insipidus in three
    dogs. J Am Vet Med Assoc 179:235, 1981.
Brobst DF, Grant BD, Hilbert BJ, et al: Blood biochemical changes in horses with prerenal
    and renal disease. J Equine Med Surg 1:171, 1977.
Brobst DF, Lee HA, Spencer GR: Hypercalcemia and hypophosphatemia in a mare with renal
    insufficiency. J Am Vet Med Assoc 173:1370, 1978.
Brobst DF, Parish SM, Torbeck RL, et al: Azotemia in cattle. J Am Vet Med Assoc 173:481,
    1978.
Buoro IBJ, Atwell RB: Urinalysis in canine dirofilariasis with emphasis on proteinuria.
    Vet Rec 112:252, 1983.
Campbell JR, Watts C: Blood urea in the bovine animal. Vet Rec 87:127, 1970.
Carlson GP, Kaneko JJ: Simultaneous estimation of renal function in dogs, using sodium
    sulfanilate and sodium iodohippurate-^{131}I. J Am Vet Med Assoc 158:1229, 1971.
Carlson GP, Kaneko JJ: Sulfanilate clearance in clinical renal disease in the dog. J Am
    Vet Med Assoc 158:1235, 1971.
Coffman J: Clinical chemistry and pathophysiology of horses: Percent creatinine clearance
    ratios. Vet Med Small Anim Clin 75:671, 1980.
Cowgill LD: Diseases of the kidney. In Ettinger SJ (ed): Textbook of veterinary internal
    medicine, Vol 2, 2nd ed. Philadelphia, WB Saunders Co, 1983.
DiBartola SP: Acute renal failure. Pathophysiology and management. Compend Contin Educ
    Pract Vet 2:952, 1980.
DiBartola SP, Spaulding GL, Chew DJ, et al: Urinary protein excretion and immunopathologic
    findings in dogs with glomerular disease. J Am Vet Med Assoc 177:73, 1980.
Divers TJ: Chronic renal failure in horses. Compend Contin Educ Pract Vet 5:S310, 1983.
Divers TJ, Crowell WA, Duncan JR, et al: Acute renal disorders in cattle: A retrospective
    study of 22 cases. J Am Vet Med Assoc 181:694, 1982.
Duncan JR, Prasse, KW: Clinical examination of the urine. Vet Clin North Am 6:647, 1976.
Easley JR, Breitschwerdt, EB: Glucosuria associated with renal tubular dysfunction in
    three basenji dogs. J Am Vet Med Assoc 168:938, 1976.
Finco DR: Simultaneous determination of phenolsulfonphthalein excretion and endogenous
    creatinine clearance in the normal dog. J Am Vet Med Assoc 159:336, 1971.
Finco DR: Kidney function. In Kaneko JJ (ed): Clinical biochemistry of domestic animals,
    3rd ed. New York, Academic Press, 1980.
Finco DR, Barsanti JA: Mechanism of urinary excretion of creatinine by the cat. Am J Vet
    Res 43:2207, 1982.
Finco DR, Duncan JR: Evaluation of blood urea nitrogen and serum creatinine concentrations
    as indicators of renal dysfunction: A study of 111 cases and a review of related
    literature. J Am Vet Med Assoc 168:593, 1976.
Finco DR, Rowland GN: Hypercalcemia secondary to chronic renal failure in the dog: A
    report of four cases. J Am Vet Med Assoc 173:990, 1978.
Grauer GF: The differential diagnosis of polyuric-polydipsic diseases. Compend Contin Educ
    Pract Vet 3:1079, 1981.
Grossman BS, Brobst DF, Kramer JW, et al: Urinary indices for differentiation of prerenal
    azotemia and renal azotemia in horses. J Am Vet Med Assoc 180:284, 1982.
Haber MH: Urinary sediment: A textbook atlas. Chicago, American Society of Clinical
    Pathologists, 1981.
Hardy RM, Osborne CA: Water deprivation test in the dog: Maximal normal values. J Am Vet
    Med Assoc 174:479, 1979.
Hoyer JR, Seiler MW: Pathophysiology of Tamn-Horsfall protein. Kidney Int 16:279, 1979.
Hurvitz AI, Kehoe JM, Capra JD, et al: Bence Jones proteinemia and proteinuria in a dog.
    J Am Vet Med Assoc 159:1112, 1971.
Koterba AM, Coffman JR: Acute and chronic renal disease in the horse. Compend Contin Educ
    Pract Vet 3:461, 1981.
Kramer JW, Bistline D, Sheridan P, et al: Identification of hippuric acid crystals in the
    urine of ethylene glycol intoxicated dogs and cats. J Am Vet Med Assoc 184:584, 1984.
Loeb WF, Knipling GD: Glucosuria and pseudoglucosuria in cats with urethral obstruction.
    Mod Vet Pract 52:40, 1971.
Madewell BR, Osborne CA, Rorrdin RA, et al: Clinicopathologic aspects of diabetes
    insipidus in the dog. J Am Anim Hosp Assoc 11:497, 1975.

Mulnix JA, Rijnberk A, Hendriks HJ: Evaluation of a modified water-deprivation test for
    diagnosis of polyuric disorders in dogs. J Am Vet Med Assoc 169:1327, 1976.
O'Brien TD, Osborne CA, Yano BL, et al: Clinicopathologic manifestations of progressive
    renal disease in Lhasa apso and Shih Tzu dogs. J Am Vet Med Assoc 180:658, 1982.
Orita Y, Ueda N, Aoki K, et al: Immunofluorescent studies of urinary casts. Nephron
    19:19, 1977.
Osbaldiston GW, Moore WE: Renal function tests in cattle. J Am Vet Med Assoc 159:292,
    1971.
Osborne CA: Urologic logic-diagnosis of renal disease. J Am Vet Med Assoc 157:1656, 1970.
Osborne CA, Finco DR, Low, DG: Pathophysiology of renal disease, renal failure, and
    uremia. In Ettinger SJ (ed): Textbook of veterinary internal medicine, Vol 2, 2nd ed.
    Philadelphia, WB Saunders Co, 1983.
Osborne CA, Johnson KH, Perman V, et al: Renal amyloidosis in the dog. J Am Vet Med Assoc
    153:669, 1968.
Osborne CA, Johnson KH, Perman V: Amyloid nephrotic syndrome in the dog. J Am Vet Med
    Assoc 154:1545, 1969.
Osborne CA, Low DG, Finco DR: Reversible versus irreversible renal disease. J Am Vet Med
    Assoc 155:2062, 1969.
Osborne CA, Low DG, Finco DR: Canine and feline urology. Philadelphia, WB Saunders Co,
    1972.
Osborne CA, Polzin DJ: Azotemia: A review of what's old and what's new. Part I. Definition
    of terms and concepts. Compend Contin Educ Pract Vet 5:497, 1983.
Osborne CA, Polzin DJ: Azotemia: A review of what's old and what's new. Part II.
    Localization. Compend Contin Educ Pract Vet 5:561, 1983.
Osborne CA, Stevens JB: Handbook of canine and feline urinalysis. St. Louis, Ralston
    Purina Co, 1981.
Osborne CA, Stevens JB, Lees GE, et al: Clinical significance of bilirubinuria. Compend
    Contin Educ Pract Vet 2:897, 1980.
Ross LA, Finco DR: Relationship of selected clinical renal function tests to glomerular
    filtration rate and renal blood flow in cats. Am J Vet Res 42:1704, 1981.
Senior DF: Acute renal failure in the dog: A case report and literature review. J Am Anim
    Hosp Assoc 19:837, 1983.
Stuart BP, Phemister RD, Thomassen RW: Glomerular lesions associated with proteinuria in
    clinically healthy dogs. Vet Pathol 12:125, 1975.
Tennant B, Bettleheim P, Kaneko JJ: Paradoxic hypercalcemia and hypophosphatemia
    associated with chronic renal failure in the horse. J Am Vet Med Assoc 180:630, 1982.
Traver DS, Salem C, Coffman JR, et al: Renal metabolism of endogenous substances in the
    horse: Volumeteric vs. clearance methods. J Equine Med Surg 1:378, 1977.
Ward PCJ: Renal dysfunction 1. Urea and creatinine. Postgrad Med 69(5):93, 1981.
Ward PCJ: Renal dysfunction 2. Proteinuria. Postgrad Med 69(6):91, 1981.

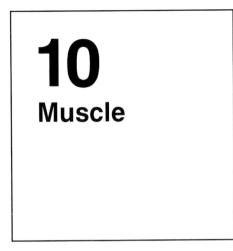

10
Muscle

SERUM ENZYMES OF MUSCLE ORIGIN

Muscle diseases characterized by degeneration or necrosis may be detected with clinical chemistry techniques. Muscular atrophy, neoplasia, and ischemic injury without associated necrosis usually will not cause biochemical changes.

I. Enzyme characteristics
   A. Creatine phosphokinase (CK, CPK)
      1. CK catalyzes the transfer of a high-energy phosphate bond from adenosine triphosphate (ATP) to creatine in resting muscle and the reverse when muscle works and consumes more ATP.
      2. CK is a dimeric enzyme with isoenzyme types CK_1 (BB), CK_2 (MB), and CK_3 (MM).
         a. The isoenzymes can be separated and the proportion of each composing total serum CK activity determined. Electrophoretically, CK_1 is the most anodal of the three isoenzymes.
         b. CK_1 (BB) is found in brain, peripheral nerves, cerebrospinal fluid, and viscera. It is not found in serum, even during neurologic disease.
         c. CK_2 (MB) is found in cardiac muscle, and minute amounts may be in various skeletal muscles.
         d. CK_3 (MM) is found in skeletal and cardiac muscle.
      3. Falsely high serum CK activity may occur in serum containing hemolyzed erythrocytes, excess bilirubin, and muscle fluids derived during difficult venipuncture.
      4. Extremely high serum CK activity may be reported in certain animals with degenerative muscle disease. Dilution of serum, which is necessary in the laboratory in these cases, may elute or dilute naturally occurring CK inhibitors; the CK activity is greatly potentiated.
      5. Serum CK activity in healthy dogs varies with age. One-day-old pups may have five times more activity than adults. Adult levels are reached by 7 months of age. Old dogs have lower values.

175

6. The plasma half-life of CK is short (approximately 4 hours in cattle, less than 2 hours in horses).
7. Serum CK activity is considered to be specific for muscle if the causes of false high activity are excluded.

B. Lactate dehydrogenase (LDH)
1. LDH catalyzes the reversible reaction of L-lactate to pyruvate in all tissues.
2. LDH is a tetrameric enzyme with isoenzyme types LDH_1 (H_4), LDH_2 (H_3M_1), LDH_3 (H_2M_2), LDH_4 (H_1M_3), and LDH_5 (M_4).
    a. The isoenzymes can be separated and the proportion of each composing total serum LDH activity determined. Electrophoretically, LDH_1 is the most anodal of the five isoenzymes.
    b. LDH_1 (H_4) is the principal isoenzyme in cardiac muscle and kidney and (in cattle and sheep) in the liver. It may be called hydroxybutyrate dehydrogenase. It is heat stable, whereas LDH_{2-5} are inactivated in serum heated at $65^{\circ}C$ for 30 minutes.
    c. LDH_5 (M_4) is the principal isoenzyme in skeletal muscle and erythrocytes.
    d. All tissues contain various amounts of the five LDH isoenzymes. Species differ in the amounts of isoenzymes found in their serum in health.
3. Most LDH in normal canine serum may originate from imperceptible hemolysis. Hemolyzed serum has high total LDH activity. In spite of high erythrocyte LDH activity, hemolyzed serum from horses causes little change in total LDH activity.
4. Total serum LDH activity decreases with age in cattle and dogs. Certain old dogs have unexplained high serum LDH activity.
5. Serum LDH activity is tissue nonspecific, although muscle, liver, and erythrocytes may be the major sources of high activity.

C. Aspartate aminotransferase (AST, GOT)
1. AST catalyzes the transamination of L-aspartate and alpha ketoglutarate to oxaloacetate and glutamate. It is found in almost all tissues.
2. The plasma half-life of AST is longer than CK, being approximately 12 hours in dogs, shorter in cats, 18 hours in swine, and probably longer in horses and cattle.
3. Serum AST activity is tissue-nonspecific, but muscle and liver (see Chapter 7) may be considered the major sources.

II. Diagnostic significance of CK, LDH, and AST
A. Increased serum CK, LDH, and AST activity occurs with degenerative or necrotizing muscle injury (Case 13). Diseases are listed in Table 10.1.
1. The magnitude of increased serum activity of the muscle

TABLE 10.1   Diseases with High Serum Enzyme Activity (CK, LDH, AST)
             of Muscle Origin
_____
Inflammatory myopathies
  Infectious
    Clostridial myositis, nonspecific infections
  Noninfectious
    Immune-mediated polymyositis (dogs), eosinophilic myositis
    (dogs, cattle)
Traumatic myopathies
  Accidental, postoperative, postcardiac resuscitation, downer
  animals, CNS diseases (especially with seizures), secondary to joint
  diseases
Degenerative myopathies
  Inherited or congenital
    Irish terrier myopathy, greyhound cramp, myotonia (dogs), Labrador
    retriever myopathy, congenital myopathies in lambs and calves
  Metabolic, toxic, or unknown cause
    Hyperadrenocorticism (dogs), hypothyroidism (dogs), copper
    poisoning (sheep), monensin-induced myocardial degeneration
    (horse), Cassia occidentalis (coffee weed) poisoning (cattle),
    equine rhabdomyolysis (paralytic myoglobinuria, azoturia, Monday
    morning disease, tying-up syndrome), transport myopathy (cattle,
    sheep, swine), malignant hyperthermia associated with halothane
    anesthesia (horses, swine), porcine stress syndrome
  Nutritional
    Vitamin E/selenium deficiency (calves, lambs, yearling cattle,
    foals, horses, swine, dogs)
Ischemic myopathies
  Bacterial endocarditis, dirofilariasis, aortic thrombosis
_____

enzymes does not correlate with the extent of muscle
injury.

2. CK is the most sensitive indicator.
   a. Increased serum CK activity occurs within a few
      hours after the onset of injury and reaches maximum
      values in 6 to 12 hours (Case 13).
   b. If the injury is not progressive, serum CK values
      return to normal 24 to 48 hours after further
      injury ceases.
   c. Persistent high serum CK activity indicates
      continuing disease.

3. LDH activity may parallel CK activity, but the
   magnitude of change is less dramatic. Maximal activity
   is reached within 48 to 72 hours and returns to normal
   values more slowly than does CK or AST after cessation
   of tissue damage.

4. AST activity increases more slowly than the activities
   of CK and LDH, and the change may persist several days
   after cessation of muscle injury.

5. Increased AST and/or LDH activity with concomitant
   normal CK activity may indicate muscle injury that
   occurred in previous days, liver disease, or some other
   nonspecific tissue injury.

B. Certain serum CK and LDH isoenzymes may have tissue
   specificity.
   1. Skeletal muscle degeneration increases the proportions
      of CK_3 (MM) and LDH_5 (M_4).
   2. Cardiac muscle degeneration increases the proportions

of CK_2 (MB) and LDH_1 (H_4); CK_3 (MM) would also increase.

3. LDH_1 (H_4) increases in hemolytic disease.

C. Serum CK activity is very sensitive to minor muscle injury. Certain events unrelated to primary muscle disease may cause high values.

1. Placement of electrodes for electromyography increases serum CK activity, but usually not out of the reference range.

2. Intramuscular injections increase serum CK activity. The more irritating drugs or drug vehicles cause the most dramatic changes. Injections up to 1 week previously should be considered as possible cause for high CK activity.

3. Strenuous exercise in dogs and horses increases serum CK activity. Physical training minimizes the postexercise increase.

4. Shipment of animals may cause high serum CK activity.

D. Central nervous system (CNS) disease may cause increased serum CK activity generally owing to muscle trauma; isoenzyme CK_3 (MM) would be increased. Cerebrospinal fluid CK activity also may increase with CNS disease (see Chapter 12).

E. Lymphosarcoma in cattle is associated with high serum LDH activity in about 70% of the cases. The origin of the activity is unknown. Values overlap between normal and affected cattle. Cattle with persistent lymphocytosis have normal serum LDH activity.

OTHER CHANGES IN MUSCLE DISEASE

I. Myoglobinuria. Myoglobin is released from degenerating or necrotic muscle. It readily passes the glomerulus into the urine because of its low molecular weight and lack of significant binding to serum proteins. Detection and significance are discussed in Chapter 7.

II. Hyperkalemia. Intracellular potassium concentration is much higher than extracellular fluid levels. Because of the mass of cells involved compared with other tissues, massive degeneration or necrosis of muscle causes hyperkalemia. Other causes of this change relate to disorders of acid base and electrolyte balance discussed in Chapter 5.

REFERENCES

Argiroudis SA, Kent JE, Blackmore DJ: Observations on the isoenzymes of creatine kinase in equine serum and tissues. Equine Vet J 14:317, 1982.
Beatty EM, Doxey DL: Lactate dehydrogenase and creatine kinase isoenzyme levels in the tissues and serum of normal lambs. Res Vet Sci 35:325, 1983.
Cardinet GH: Skeletal muscle. In Kaneko JJ, Cornelius CE (eds): Clinical biochemistry of domestic animals, Vol 2. New York, Academic Press, 1971.
Cardinet GH, Littrell JF, Freedland RA: Comparative investigations of serum creatine phosphokinase and glutamic-oxalacetic transaminase activities in equine paralytic myoglobinuria. Res Vet Sci 8:219, 1967.
Chrisman CL: Diseases of peripheral nerves and muscles. In Ettinger SJ (ed): Textbook of veterinary internal medicine, Vol 2. Philadelphia, WB Saunders Co, 1975.

Coffman J: Enzymology, Part 2. Vet Med Small Anim Clin 74:1791, 1979.

DiBartola SP, Tasker JB: Elevated serum creatine phosphokinase: A study of 53 cases and a review of its diagnostic usefulness in clinical veterinary medicine. J Am Anim Hosp Assoc 13:744, 1977.

Dorner JL, Hoffman WE, Lock TF: Effects of in vitro hemolysis on equine serum chemical values. Am J Vet Res 42:1519, 1981.

Freedland RA, Kramer JW: Use of serum enzymes as aids to diagnosis. Adv Vet Sci Comp Med 14:61, 1970.

Geiser D: The azoturia tying-up syndrome. Vet Med Small Anim Clin 70:710, 1975.

Gerber H: The clinical significance of serum enzyme activities with particular reference to myoglobinuria. Proc Am Assoc Equine Pract, Philadelphia, 1968.

Greene CE, Lorenz MD, Munnell JF, et al: Myopathy associated with hyperadrenocorticism in the dog. J Am Vet Med Assoc 174:1310, 1979.

Hammel EP, Raker CW: Myopathies. In Calcott EV, Smithcors JF (eds): Equine medicine and surgery, 2nd ed. Wheaton, Ill, American Veterinary Publications, 1972.

Hansen MA: Plasma transaminase activity in myopathies of horses. Nord Vet Med 22:617, 1970.

Hayes MA, Russell RG, Babiuk LA: Sudden death in young dogs with myocarditis caused by parvovirus. J Am Vet Med Assoc 174:1197, 1979.

Indrieri RJ, Holliday TA, Kleen CL: Critical evaluation of creatine phosphokinase in cerebrospinal fluid of dogs with neurologic disease. Am J Vet Res 41:1299, 1980.

Johnson BD, Perce RB: Unique serum isoenzyme characteristics in horses having histories of rhabdomyolysis (tying up). Equine Pract 3(4):24, 1981.

Kornegay JN, Gorgacz EJ, Dawe DL, et al: Polymyositis in dogs. J Am Vet Med Assoc 176:431, 1980.

Koterba A, Carlson GP: Acid-base and electrolyte alterations in horses with exertional rhabdomyolysis. J Am Vet Med Assoc 180:303, 1982.

Krum SH, Cardinet GH, Anderson BC, et al: Polymyositis and polyarthritis associated with systemic lupus erythematosus in a dog. J Am Vet Med Assoc 170:61, 1977.

Lannek N, Lindberg P: Vitamin E and selenium deficiencies (VESD) of domestic animals. Adv Vet Sci Comp Med 19:127, 1975.

Littlejohn A, Blackmore DJ: Blood and tissue content of the isoenzymes of lactate dehydrogenase in the thoroughbred. Res Vet Sci 25:118, 1978.

Loeb WF, Nagode LA, Frajola WJ: The distribution of four enzymes between canine serum and erythrocytes. Enzymol Biol Clin 7:215, 1966.

Osborne BE, Dent NJ: Electrocardiography and blood chemistry in the detection of myocardial lesions in dogs. Food Cosmet Toxicol 11:265, 1973.

Owen R, Moore JN, Hopkins JB, et al: Dystrophic myodegeneration in adult horses. J Am Vet Med Assoc 171:343, 1977.

Rich LJ, Dunavant ML: Serum enzymes in bovine practice. Bovine Pract 5:8, 1972.

Spangler WL, Muggli FM: Seizure-induced rhabdomyolysis accompanied by acute renal failure in a dog. J Am Vet Med Assoc 172:1190, 1978.

Strauss HD, Roberts R: Plasma MB creatine kinase activity and other conventional enzymes. Arch Intern Med 140:336, 1980.

Thoren-Tolling K, Jonsson L: Creatine kinase isoenzymes in serum of pigs having myocardial and skeletal muscle necrosis. Can J Comp Med 47:207, 1983.

Thornton JR, Lohni MD: Tissue and plasma activity of lactic dehydrogenase and creatine kinase in the horse. Equine Vet J 11:235, 1979.

Walden-Mease E, Klein LV, Rosenburg H, et al: Malignant hyperthermia in a halothane-anesthetized horse. J Am Vet Med Assoc 179:896, 1981.

Wilson JW: Serum creatine phosphokinase in the canine. J Am Anim Hosp Assoc 12:522, 1976.

Wilson TM, Morrison HA, Palmer NC, et al: Myodegeneration and suspected selenium/vitamin E deficiency in horses. J Am Vet Med Assoc 169:213, 1976.

PARATHYROID GLAND, CALCIUM, PHOSPHORUS, MAGNESIUM
Parathyroid function is integrated with thyroid parafollicular cell function and vitamin D metabolism in the regulation of calcium and phosphorus homeostasis. Altered serum calcium and phosphorus concentrations are often encountered coincidentally during screening with chemistry profiles and in animals showing clinical signs of altered calcium metabolism. Magnesium abnormalities are of most concern in ruminants.

I. Basic concepts
    A. Parathormone (PTH)
        1. Commercially available radioimmunoassay for PTH has been successfully used on canine samples.
        2. PTH is produced by the parathyroid gland in response to hypocalcemia and, perhaps, hypomagnesemia. Because hyperphosphatemia causes reciprocal decrease in serum calcium, increased serum phosphorus indirectly stimulates PTH release.
        3. The net effect of PTH is increased serum calcium, decreased serum phosphorus, and increased renal excretion of phosphorus. PTH promotes the following.
            a. Calcium reabsorption from bone
            b. Phosphorus excretion by the kidney
            c. Accelerated formation of the active form of vitamin D (1,25-dihydroxycholecalciferol) by the kidney
            d. Calcium absorption from the gut and reabsorption by renal tubules (both are minor functions of PTH)
    B. Calcitonin (thyrocalcitonin). Assay techniques are available only for research purposes.
        1. Calcitonin is produced by thyroid parafollicular cells (C cells) in response to hypercalcemia.
        2. In concert with PTH, calcitonin regulates blood calcium concentration within precise limits and tempers the PTH resorptive action on bone.
    C. Metabolically active vitamin D. Assay techniques are available only for research purposes.

1. Hydroxylation of vitamin D to 25-hydroxycholecalciferol occurs in the liver and to 1,25-dihydroxycholecalciferol occurs under PTH regulation in the kidney.
2. It promotes calcium absorption by intestinal mucosa and may facilitate PTH action on bone.

D. Calcium
1. Methods of measurement
   a. Most methods are colorimetric and measure total serum calcium (i.e., ionized, protein bound, and complexed forms). False high values occur with lipemia. Results are usually reported as mg/dl, but some laboratories report mEq/l; values differ.
   b. Special electrodes are required to measure ionized calcium, the biologically active form. Samples must be maintained anaerobically at 37°C, which greatly increases the difficulty.
   c. An estimate of ionized calcium can be determined using colorimetric methods on protein-free ultrafiltrates of plasma.
   d. Differentiation of diseases causing abnormal serum calcium can be facilitated by measuring urinary calcium excretion.
      (1) The same assay methods are used.
      (2) A 24-hour urine collection is made, and the amount of calcium excreted per 24 hours is determined.
      (3) A simpler method is to determine the fractional clearance of calcium on samples of serum and urine collected at the same time. Fractional clearance of calcium = [urine Ca^{++} (mg/dl)/serum Ca^{++} (mg/dl)] × [serum creatinine (mg/dl)/urine creatinine (mg/dl)].
2. Total serum calcium is approximately 50% ionized; 40% is protein-bound, especially to albumin; and 10% is complexed with anions such as citrate or phosphate.
   a. Only ionized calcium is biologically active in bone formation, neuromuscular activity, cellular biochemical processes, and blood coagulation.
      (1) In all species except cattle, clinical manifestations of decreased serum ionized calcium relate to increased neuromuscular excitability; cattle get flaccid paralysis.
      (2) Signs of increased serum ionized calcium are associated with decreased neuromuscular excitability, renal calcinosis, and bone disorders.
   b. The proportion of ionized calcium is affected by acid base balance.
      (1) Alkalosis decreases ionized calcium level. Severely affected animals may show neuromuscular signs concomitant with normal total serum calcium.
      (2) Acidosis increases the ionized calcium level.

    c. Ionized calcium is almost always increased in hypercalcemic conditions.

    d. The protein-bound fraction and total serum calcium decrease in hypoalbuminemia, but ionized calcium remains normal.

      (1) Although hypocalcemia is found in hypoalbuminemic conditions, clinical signs of hypocalcemia do not occur.

      (2) In hypoalbuminemic dogs, measured serum calcium can be adjusted with a correction formula to rule out the possibility of a true or functional hypocalcemia: adjusted Ca^{++} (mg/dl) = measured Ca^{++} (mg/dl) $- 0.4$[serum protein (g/dl)] $+ 3.3$. In most cases of hypoalbuminemia the adjusted calcium level will be normal.

3. Serum calcium concentration usually represents a balance between bone formation and bone reabsorption and is regulated by PTH, 1,25-dihydroxycholecalciferol, and calcitonin.

    a. Hypocalcemia or hypercalcemia usually indicates hormonal imbalance. Exceptions are acid base imbalance and hypoalbuminemia as described above.

    b. Dietary intake of calcium seldom affects the serum level directly.

      (1) Reduced intake of calcium (or magnesium) is accommodated by increased PTH activity, and normocalcemia occurs.

      (2) Increased intake of calcium is balanced by exogenous fecal loss and urinary excretion.

    c. Reduced renal excretion causes hypercalcemia in horses, rarely in other species.

E. Phosphorus

1. Colorimetric methods measure inorganic phosphate that is present in bodily fluids as $HPO_4^=$, PO_4^-, H_2PO_4, and phosphate ions. Because of the differing valences, results are expressed as mg/dl.

    a. Hemolyzed serum causes false high phosphorus concentration.

    b. Young animals have higher values than adults.

    c. Urinary excretion over 24 hours or fractional renal clearance determination may help evaluate phosphorus metabolism. Fractional clearance of phosphorus is determined in the same way as described above for calcium.

2. Phosphorus, in its various anionic forms, functions with phosphoric acid as a buffer in bodily fluids, but acid base balance is evaluated by measuring components of the bicarbonate buffer system instead of the phosphate buffer system (see Chapter 5).

3. Serum phosphorus primarily is regulated by the kidneys where phosphaturia occurs when the tubular reabsorption maxima is exceeded.

        a. PTH may enhance phosphaturia by decreasing tubular reabsorption.

        b. Dietary intake of phosphorus may directly affect the serum phosphorus concentration.

        c. Abnormal serum phosphorus is caused by altered dietary levels, decreased renal excretion, and the hormonal imbalances that affect serum calcium.

  F. Magnesium

    1. Colorimetric methods are used to measure serum or urine magnesium concentration.

    2. Serum magnesium is dependent on dietary intake and regulated by mineralocorticoids, thyroxine, and PTH.

    3. Abnormal magnesium metabolism and associated diseases are described primarily in ruminants.

II. Laboratory abnormalities in calcium, phosphorus, and magnesium

  A. Hypercalcemia. Concomitant hypoalbuminemia and the associated decrease in serum calcium may mask the severity of hypercalcemia in the following diseases (see earlier discussion).

    1. Primary hyperparathyroidism is caused by functional parathyroid neoplasms or idiopathic hyperplasia.

        a. Serum PTH concentration is high in affected dogs.

        b. Increased urinary excretion of calcium and decreased urinary excretion of phosphorus seem to conflict with the known effects of PTH; but hypercalcemia and hypophosphatemia are usually marked, which explains the associated urinary findings.

        c. Serum magnesium varies.

        d. Hypophosphatemia is severe, but serum phosphorus may increase after renal calcinosis and insufficiency develop.

        e. Bone lesions, soft-tissue mineralization, and increased serum alkaline phosphatase activity may occur.

    2. Pseudohyperparathyroidism is a common cause of hypercalcemia in dogs and also has been described in cats and horses (Case 9).

        a. A variety of neoplasms may produce a PTH-like peptide, a vitamin D-like steroid, a prostaglandin, or osteoclast-activating factor, any of which may cause hypercalcemia and hypophosphatemia.

        b. Neoplasms that have been associated with pseudohyperparathyroidism include canine lymphosarcoma, anal sac apocrine gland carcinoma, pancreatic carcinoma, mammary gland carcinoma, nasal adenocarcinoma, squamous cell carcinoma, seminoma, and epidermoid carcinoma; equine lymphosarcoma and gastric carcinoma; and feline lymphosarcoma.

        c. Hypophosphatemia is severe, but serum phosphorus may increase following the onset of renal calcinosis and insufficiency.

        d. Urinary excretion of calcium is increased and that

of phosphorus is decreased for reasons similar to
that of primary hyperparathyroidism.
   e.   Bone lesions, soft-tissue mineralization, and
        increased serum alkaline phosphatase activity are
        mild.
3.   Hypervitaminosis D is an uncommon cause of
     hypercalcemia.
   a.   Iatrogenic hypervitaminosis D occurs in over-
        supplemented, large breeds of dogs and in horses.
        Cats that have eaten the ornamental plant jessamine
        may be affected.
   b.   Hyperphosphatemia may occur before the development
        of renal disease.
   c.   Urinary excretion of calcium and phosphorus is
        decreased.
   d.   Soft-tissue mineralization is severe, but bone
        lesions are mild.
4.   Osteolytic metastatic tumors in bone (such as
     lymphosarcoma, myeloma, osteosarcoma, or certain
     carcinomas) may cause hypercalcemia secondary to marked
     reabsorption of bone. Serum phosphorus may be normal or
     increased.
5.   Other causes of hypercalcemia and proposed mechanisms
     (if known) are as follows.
   a.   Ingestion of plants (Cestrum sp. and Solanum sp.)
        in herbivores causes hypercalcemia, parathyroid
        atrophy, and soft-tissue mineralization. Serum
        calcium decreases as the disease progresses.
   b.   Renal disease in horses causes hypercalcemia,
        apparently by decreased urinary excretion.
   c.   Occasionally, canine renal disease causes
        hypercalcemia. Proposed mechanisms include
        decreased degradation of PTH, more plasma calcium-
        citrate complexing, exaggerated responsiveness to
        vitamin D, and soft-tissue calcium mobilization
        following therapeutic diuresis.
   d.   Canine adrenal insufficiency may be associated with
        hypercalcemia. The proposed mechanism is increased
        renal tubular reabsorption of calcium.
   e.   Certain granulomatous disorders (e.g., canine
        blastomycosis) have been associated with
        hypercalcemia. In humans, the proposed mechanism is
        hyperreactivity to vitamin D.
   f.   Miscellaneous disorders in which hypercalcemia has
        been seen include severe hypothermia,
        hypervitaminosis A, septic osteomyelitis, and
        hyper- and hypothyroidism. Mechanisms are unknown.
B.   Hypocalcemia. Hypoalbuminemia (in all species) and alkalosis
     (especially in ruminants) are common causes of hypocalcemia
     that must be differentiated in each case (see earlier
     discussion) (Cases 12, 15, 18). Hypocalcemic diseases are
     listed below.
   1.   Hypoparathyroidism is described in dogs and may be
        caused by surgical removal, atrophy secondary to canine
        distemper virus infection, lymphocytic parathyroiditis,

or idiopathic PTH unresponsiveness.
  a. Serum PTH concentration is low in affected dogs.
  b. Serum phosphorus is normal or increased.
  c. Urinary excretion of calcium is increased and that
     of phosphorus is decreased.
  d. Serum magnesium is usually normal.
2. Nutritional hyperparathyroidism secondary to dietary
   calcium deficiency, hypovitaminosis D, or dietary
   phosphorus excess is an uncommon cause of hypocalcemia.
  a. Serum phosphorus is normal or decreased in dietary
     calcium lack or hypovitaminosis D, but it is normal
     or increased in dietary phosphorus excess.
  b. Urinary excretion of calcium is decreased and that
     of phosphorus is increased.
3. Hypocalcemia may occur in some cases of renal disease
   (except in the horse) despite compensatory PTH activity
   to maintain normocalcemia (Case 14, 15).
  a. Mechanisms are decreased renal hydroxylation of
     vitamin D, soft-tissue calcification, reciprocal
     decrease in serum calcium secondary to
     hyperphosphatemia, and skeletal resistance to the
     effects of PTH.
  b. The change occurs in acute and chronic renal
     disease.
  c. Postrenal urinary obstruction in cats may cause a
     similar calcium and phosphorus pattern.
  d. Uremic acidosis may temper the severity of
     hypocalcemia because the proportion of ionized
     calcium in serum is increased.
4. Parturient paresis in cattle (milk fever) is caused by
   hypocalcemia. Puerpural tetany (eclampsia) in the
   bitch, mare, or ewe is similar.
  a. In the cow the disease accompanies the sudden
     calcium demand of lactation, particularly after
     high-calcium diets were fed in the dry period,
     which depressed PTH secretion and secretory
     potential for quick response to negative calcium
     balance.
  b. Affected cows are usually hypophosphatemic.
5. Hypomagnesemic tetany in ruminants has concomitant
   hypocalcemia in about 75% of the cases. Differentiation
   from milk fever can be accomplished by measuring urine
   magnesium.
  a. Urine is nearly devoid of magnesium in affected
     cattle.
  b. Normal cattle or cows with milk fever have about 50
     mg magnesium/dl urine.
6. Acute pancreatitis in dogs causes hypocalcemia in
   approximately 50% of the cases.
  a. Hypocalcemia may be a late change in necrotizing
     pancreatitis because ionized calcium is bound to
     free fatty acids in necrotic fat.
  b. Another proposed mechanism is increased glucagon
     release, which directly decreases ionized calcium
     or increases calcitonin secretion.

   7. Other uncommon causes of hypocalcemia are ethylene
      glycol toxicity in dogs or cats; intestinal
      malabsorption in dogs; transport tetany in sheep;
      blister beetle toxicosis in horses; idiopathic, acute
      hypocalcemic tetany in horses; and hypercalcitonism
      secondary to thyroid C-cell tumors in bulls.
C. Hyperphosphatemia
   1. The most common mechanism of hyperphosphatemia is
      decreased glomerular filtration rate associated with
      the causes of prerenal, renal, and postrenal azotemia
      (Cases 14, 15, 16, 23).
   2. Other causes are secondary to disturbances of calcium
      metabolism and are described with the disorders of
      hyper- or hypocalcemia above.
      a. Hyperphosphatemia that accompanies hypercalcemia
         and precedes renal insufficiency may occur with
         hypervitaminosis D.
      b. Hyperphosphatemia that accompanies hypocalcemia
         occurs with hypoparathyroidism and dietary
         phosphorus excess-induced nutritional secondary
         hyperparathyroidism.
D. Hypophosphatemia
   1. This is an uncommon laboratory finding. The cause is
      often undetermined.
   2. Primary hyperparathyroidism and pseudohyper-
      parathyroidism cause hypophosphatemia (see description
      under hypercalcemia above). Other hypercalcemic
      disorders are associated with either normal serum
      phosphorus or increased phosphorus secondary to renal
      calcinosis and insufficiency.
   3. Nutritional secondary hyperparathyroidism caused by
      dietary lack of calcium or hypovitaminosis D is
      associated with normal or decreased serum phosphorus.
   4. Other causes of hypophosphatemia are milk fever in
      cattle, malabsorption, canine Fanconi-like syndrome,
      and starvation.
E. Hypermagnesemia. This may occur in herbivores with renal
   failure.
F. Hypomagnesemia. This occurs in calves, adult cattle, and
   sheep.

THYROID FUNCTION
     The thyroid hormones, thyroxine (T4) and triiodothyronine (T3),
increase metabolism of most cells and stimulate growth in the young.
They induce DNA translation, which results in greater activity in
cell synthesis, oxidative phosphorylation, and membrane transport of
electrolytes.

I. Basic concepts
   A. Secretion and transport of T4 and T3
      1. Over 90% of secreted thyroid hormone is T4 and less
         than 10% is T3.
         a. T3 is three- to four-fold more stimulatory to cells
            than T4, but both function at the cellular level.

          b. One-third of all T4 deiodinates to T3, which accounts for 80% of serum T3 concentration.

          c. A failing thyroid gland preferentially makes T3, so in developing hypothyroidism, T4 is expected to decrease earlier than T3 decreases.

          d. The regulation of thyroid hormone secretion is by the pituitary gland through the thyroid-stimulating hormone (TSH), which stimulates thyroid secretion. Negative feedback control of TSH secretion is mediated by thyroid hormone, principally T3.

    2. Greater than 99% of thyroid hormone is bound to albumin and globulins in plasma.

          a. Dogs lack a protein with high affinity for binding thyroid hormone comparable to thyroxine-binding globulin in man. This may be the reason canine serum T4 concentration is much lower than human serum T4, an important difference related to T4 measurement (see below).

          b. T3 has less protein-binding affinity and more readily enters cells. This may partly account for the ratio of serum T4/T3 concentrations, about 25:1 compared with the secretion T4/T3 ratio of 9:1.

          c. Unbound thyroid hormone, called "free thyroxine," accounts for less than 1% of the plasma hormone level.

B. Measurement of serum T4

    1. Commercial human assays by radioimmunoassay (RIA) or competitive protein-binding (CPB) techniques are used for canine, feline, and equine samples.

          a. Human assay kits usually have standard curves in the range of 1 to 30 μg/dl. Assay of animal samples using such a standard curve is inaccurate because their values are often below this range.

          b. The human assay kits are accurate if the laboratory prepares standard curves that range from 0.1 to 10 μg/dl (equivalent to 10 to 100 ng/ml and covering the expected range of values in dogs, cats, and horses).

    2. T4 measured by RIA or CPB is total serum T4, including protein-bound and free thyroxine.

          a. Hypoproteinemic conditions cause decreased serum T4, although the animal may be euthyroid.

          b. Drugs (such as corticosteroids, nonsteroidal antiinflammatory agents, OPDDD, and others) decrease the affinity of thyroid hormone for plasma protein, which may enhance cellular uptake of hormone and increase the proportion of free thyroxine. Greater free thyroxine causes feedback inhibition of TSH release. These combined effects are a low serum T4 concentration, although the animal is euthyroid (Case 20).

C. Measurement of serum T3. RIA or CPB commercial human assay kits are used.

    1. As with T4 assay, laboratories must be sure that standard curves are adjusted to suit the expected range of animal values.

2. Drugs (see discussion for T4 measurement) also decrease serum T3 concentration.

3. T3 measurement for thyroid function offers no advantage over the use of T4 measurement alone.

II. Hypothyroidism
   A. Direct assessment with serum T4 or T3 measurement
      1. Hypothyroidism causes low serum T4 or T3 value in dogs, horses, and other species.
         a. A major problem occurs in the diagnosis of canine hypothyroidism. As many as 20% of tested dogs have low T4 or T3 values but are euthyroid. Causes may be hypoproteinemia, current drug therapy, concurrent disease (hyperadrenocorticism), or others (Case 20).
         b. Low T4- or T3-euthyroid dogs can be differentiated from hypothyroid dogs by the TSH stimulation test: T4 or T3 is measured immediately before and 8 hours after administering 5 units TSH/20 lb (10 units max.) intramuscularly; or before and 4 hours after 0.1 units TSH/lb (5 units max.) intravenously. A commonly practiced rule of thumb is that serum T4 or T3 concentration should at least double after TSH stimulation, and failure to do so confirms hypothyroidism.
      2. Recent treatment with thyroid hormone may complicate diagnosis of hypothyroidism. Therapy should be discontinued for 1 to 2 weeks before testing by serum T4 or T3 measurement and TSH stimulation.
      3. An occasional observation in dogs is simultaneous low T3 and normal T4 concentrations. This pattern is not consistent with canine hypothyroidism. The change is equated with the human "low T3 syndrome," which is characterized by T4 deiodination to inactive reverse T3 rather than active T3; it occurs in euthyroid sick individuals.
      4. Primary and secondary hypothyroidism in dogs are usually differentiated by their clinical mani-festations. Daily TSH stimulation tests over 3 to 8 consecutive days will result in eventual increase in T4 or T3 concentration in cases of secondary hypo-thyroidism, whereas primary hypothyroidism consistently fails to respond.
   B. Other laboratory findings in hypothyroidism
      1. Free thyroxine (free T4), when measured directly after dialysis, is useful to differentiate euthyroid-low T4 caused by hypoproteinemia or drug-induced reduction in protein binding from hypothyroidism.
         a. Both total and free T4 are reduced in hypothyroidism, and free T4 is normal or increased in euthyroid-low T4 patients.
         b. Direct measurement of free T4 after dialysis is usually not practiced in commercial laboratories. They substitute a test called "free T4 index" which is a product of total T4 concentration and T3-resin uptake value; T3-resin uptake is invalid on canine

samples, so the free T4 index is invalid in dogs.
2. Serum cholesterol is increased in about two-thirds of
hypothyroid dogs. Values in excess of 500 mg/dl plus
clinical signs consistent with hypothyroidism may be
diagnostic.
3. Nonregenerative anemia occurs in about one-fourth of
hypothyroid dogs.
4. Serum CK activity is increased in about one-tenth of
hypothyroid dogs.

III. Hyperthyroidism. Serum T4 and T3 may be increased in dogs with
either clinical or suspected hyperthyroidism owing to thyroid
neoplasia or hyperplasia. Both T4 and T3 serum concentrations
are usually increased in hyperthyroid cats.

ENDOCRINE PANCREAS
In addition to its digestive functions, the pancreas secretes
hormones that regulate glucose, lipid, and protein metabolism. Two
diseases, diabetes mellitus and hyperinsulinism associated with
neoplasia of the islets of Langerhans, require laboratory evaluation
for diagnosis and therapeutic management. These diseases occur most
often in the dog and cat and only rarely in other domestic species.

I. Basic concepts of endocrine pancreatic hormones
   A. Metabolic effects of insulin
      1. Beta cells of the islets of Langerhans secrete insulin
         under the stimulus of hyperglycemia and to a lesser
         extent other hormones and amino acids.
      2. Insulin target organs are primarily liver, skeletal
         muscle, and fat. Erythrocytes, neurons, and renal
         tubular cells (glucose reabsorption) do not require
         insulin.
      3. Insulin promotes anabolic metabolism of carbohydrates,
         fats, proteins, and nucleic acids by potentiating the
         cellular uptake of glucose, other monosaccharides, some
         amino acids, fatty acids, K^+, and Mg^{++}.
   B. Metabolic effects of glucagon
      1. Alpha cells of the islets of Langerhans secrete
         glucagon in response to hypoglycemia or increases in
         plasma concentration of certain amino acids.
      2. The two major effects of glucagon are to promote
         hepatic glycogenolysis and gluconeogenesis, thereby
         increasing blood glucose concentration.
   C. Metabolic activity of other hormones that oppose the
      effects of insulin
      1. Glucocorticoids antagonize insulin effects by promoting
         hepatic gluconeogenesis and lipolysis and by inhibiting
         muscular protein synthesis and utilization of insulin
         by insulin-responsive cells.
      2. Catecholamines increase hepatic glycogenolysis.
      3. Growth hormone inhibits utilization of insulin by
         insulin-responsive cells.
      4. Delta cells of the islets of Langerhans produce
         somatostatin, which is inhibitory to glucagon and
         insulin secretion.

      5.   Progesterone, secreted in high levels during late estrus and metestrus, may cause excess growth hormone release and thereby antiinsulin effects.

II. Laboratory assessment of the endocrine pancreas
    A. Serum insulin
        1.   Certain commercial radioimmunoassay kits for measuring human insulin have been validated for canine, bovine, and equine insulin.
            a.   Reference values may vary between laboratories.
            b.   Serum insulin is stable over several days at refrigerator temperatures.
        2.   Functional islet cell tumor and hyperinsulinism may be detected by measuring serum insulin.
            a.   The diagnostic sensitivity is greatly increased by determining the amount of insulin relative to the blood glucose concentration. In humans, serum insulin is usually zero when blood glucose is less than 30 mg/dl. The relationship between serum insulin and glucose is expressed as the "amended insulin/glucose ratio," which equals: [serum insulin (μU/ml) $\times$ 100]/[blood glucose (mg/dl) $-$ 30].
            b.   Dogs suspected of having hyperinsulinism should be tested as follows.
                (1)   Determine blood glucose concentration before fasting. If hypoglycemic, determine serum insulin on the same sample and calculate the amended insulin glucose ratio.
                (2)   If the nonfasting blood glucose is within normal limits, fast the dog and measure glucose every 2 hours. If hypoglycemia develops within 8 hours, measure serum insulin on the first sample in which blood glucose is low and calculate the ratio.
                (3)   Ratios less than 30 are considered normal for dogs, and increased values indicate hyperinsulinism.
        3.   Diagnosis of diabetes mellitus by serum insulin alone is unreliable, but diagnosis is made by determining persistent hyperglycemia or glucose intolerance (described below). Once diagnosis is made, diabetes mellitus can be divided into types on the basis of serum insulin response patterns during intravenous glucose tolerance testing (IGTT), which is described in Chapter 6.
            a.   Type I diabetes mellitus is characterized by a very low baseline serum insulin and no insulin response to the glucose injection.
            b.   Type II is characterized by normal or even increased baseline serum insulin and no insulin response to the glucose injection.
            c.   Type III is characterized by a normal baseline serum insulin and a normal or delayed increase in serum insulin in response to the glucose injection.
    B. Blood glucose

1. The laboratory measurement of blood glucose, various sample management factors that affect the result, and the general interpretation of hyperglycemia and hypoglycemia are described in Chapter 6.
2. The primary effects of hyperinsulinism are hypoglycemia and hypokalemia, which produce certain clinical signs.
    a. In animals in which hyperinsulinism is suspected, blood glucose should always be measured without fasting to avoid inducing a hypoglycemic seizure.
    b. Frequently, the animal may have eaten, and although a hypoglycemia history was evident, the concentration is within normal limits.
    c. Diagnosis is enhanced by calculating the amended insulin glucose ratio as described above.
3. The primary effects of insulin lack or insulin unresponsiveness (diabetes mellitus) are persistent hyperglycemia and glucosuria with osmotic diuresis (Case 17).
    a. A wide variety of other causes of hyperglycemia (see Chapter 6) do not result in persistent hyperglycemia.
    b. On rare occasions diabetes mellitus may be suspected when blood glucose in increased but the concentration is still below the renal threshold. Glucose intolerance can be determined with the IGTT (test protocol and response curves are described in Chapter 6).
    c. Glucose intolerance may also occur in hyperadrenocorticism, hyperthyroidism, hyperpituitarism, and hepatic insufficiency; hyperadrenocorticism and diabetes mellitus are frequently concomitant.
        (1) In diabetic dogs with sustained hyperglycemia and glucosuria despite insulin therapy, hyperadrenocorticism can be diagnosed by plasma cortisol testing (described later in this chapter).
        (2) In dogs with hyperadrenocorticism, concomitant diabetes mellitus is suspected if blood glucose values approach and/or exceed renal threshold values despite treatment for hyperadrenocorticism.
C. Other laboratory findings in disorders of the endocrine pancreas
    1. Hyperinsulinism. The amended insulin glucose ratio (described above) has replaced older procedures such as the glucagon, insulin, epinephrine, and tolbutamide tolerance tests; these tests are not recommended because severe hypoglycemia and seizures may occur. Hypokalemia is characteristic with hyperinsulinism, but other findings are nonspecific.
    2. Diabetes mellitus
        a. Ketonemia, ketonuria, and ketoacidosis occur (see Chapter 6).
        b. Lipemia is common (see Chapter 6).

     c. Osmotic diuresis produces progressive dehydration
       and electrolyte loss.
     d. Proteinuria may occur.
     e. Glycosylated hemoglobin (HbA_1) develops gradually,
       and the concentration may be used as a time-
       averaged index of blood glucose; as more knowledge
       is gained, HbA_1 concentration may prove useful to
       monitor effectiveness of treatment for diabetes
       mellitus.

ADRENAL CORTEX
     Two primary syndromes affect this gland, hyperadrenocorticism
(Cushing's syndrome) and adrenal insufficiency. Hyperadrenocorticism
is separated into two types, pituitary-dependent or adrenal-
dependent, which are treated differently. Laboratory objectives are
to confirm the diagnosis and to distinguish between the types of
hyperadrenocorticism.

  I. Basic concepts
    A. Glucocorticoids, regulation of secretion and function
       1. The glucocorticoids (cortisol, corticosterone, and
          cortisone) are secreted by the zona fasciculata and
          zone reticularis.
       2. Secretion is stimulated by the adrenocorticotropic
          hormone (ACTH), which is released from the anterior
          pituitary under stimulation of corticotropin-releasing
          hormone (CRH) from the hypothalamus. Glucocorticoid
          secretion is circadian in some species, but not in
          cats.
       3. Cortisol inhibits release of CRH, suppressing ACTH
          secretion, which forms the feedback regulation of
          plasma cortisol concentration. Exogenous gluco-
          corticoids also suppress ACTH secretion.
       4. The general effects of glucocorticoids are glucose
          sparing and hyperglycemia. They have many other
          actions, including suppression of wound healing,
          inflammation, and immunologic responsiveness.
    B. The mineralocorticoid, regulation of secretion and function
       1. Aldosterone, the mineralocorticoid, is secreted by the
          zona glomerulosa. Regulation is by several complex
          mechanisms that involve ACTH, renin, direct stimulation
          by rising serum K^+ concentration, and possibly
          declining serum Na^+ concentration.
       2. In the kidney, the primary target organ of aldosterone,
          tubular Na^+ reabsorption and tubular K^+ excretion are
          promoted. Similar effects may occur in skin and other
          tissues.
    C. The zona reticularis secretes androgens, estrogens, and
      proestrogens, which may relate to certain clinical features
      of adrenocortical disease.

 II. Laboratory evaluation of the adrenal cortex
    A. Plasma cortisol measurement
       1. Most laboratories use a RIA procedure that has been

validated for dogs, cats, and horses.
2. Of the endogenous glucocorticoids, only cortisol is measured; corticosterone and cortisone do not react.
3. Of commonly used therapeutic glucocorticoids, only prednisolone will cross-react with the cortisol-RIA test. Whatever the blood concentration of prednisolone is at the time of sampling, about 60% will be additive to the cortisol measured.
4. Resting or baseline cortisol values of some animals with hyperadrenocorticism overlap with those having normal adrenocortical activity. Consequently, cortisol values after stimulation with exogenous ACTH or after administration of dexamethasone to suppress endogenous ACTH are used in conjunction with baseline values for diagnosis of adrenocortical dysfunction (Case 20).

B. ACTH stimulation test
1. Samples for plasma cortisol assay are collected before and after ACTH administration.
   a. In the dog and cat, 1 IU ACTH gel/lb body weight is given intramuscularly. In the horse, 1 IU/kg is given; an alternative in the horse is 100 IU synthetic ACTH given intravenously.
   b. The post-ACTH sample is collected at 2 hours in the dog and horse and at 1 hour in the cat; these times approximate peak cortisol concentrations after ACTH administration.
2. Animals with normal adrenocortical activity are expected to increase plasma cortisol concentration two- to threefold after ACTH administration.
   a. A lesser or no response to ACTH indicates adrenocortical atrophy.
   b. Responses greater than normal, called exaggerated responses, indicate adrenocortical hyperplasia (pituitary-dependent hyperadrenocorticism) or adrenal tumor responsive to ACTH stimulation (Case 20).
   c. A few cases of pituitary-dependent hyperadreno- corticism and about half the adrenal neoplasms in dogs yield a normal response to ACTH stimulation. If these animals happen to have baseline cortisol levels within normal limits, the diagnosis, hyper- adrenocorticism, is not confirmed; the dexametha- sone suppression test is required.

C. Low-dose dexamethasone suppression test
1. This test is used primarily to substantiate the diag- nosis of hyperadrenocorticism in an affected animal that fails to be confirmed by the ACTH-stimulation test.
2. Samples for cortisol assay are collected before and after administration of dexamethasone.
3. Dosages of dexamethasone are:
   a. 0.01 μg/kg body weight in the dog, intravenously
   b. 0.1 mg/kg body weight in the cat, orally
   c. 40 μg/kg body weight in the horse, intramuscularly; an alternative is 10 mg, intramuscularly.

4. The postdexamethasone sample is collected after 8 hours in all species or after 3 hours in horses in which the 10-mg dose is given.

5. Animals with normal pituitary-adrenal cortex function respond to dexamethasone by a marked decrease in plasma cortisol concentration at 8 hours after injection.

    a. Some interpret a normal response to be greater than 50% decrease in baseline cortisol value. .

    b. In the dog and horse, postdexamethasone values are often less than 10 ng/ml.

6. In most cases of pituitary-dependent and in all cases of adrenal-dependent hyperadrenocorticism, low-dose dexamethasone fails to suppress the plasma cortisol concentration (Case 20).

D. High-dose dexamethasone suppression test

1. In animals in which hyperadrenocorticism has been confirmed by either the ACTH-stimulation test or the low-dose dexamethasone suppression test, this test is used to aid differentiation of pituitary-dependent and adrenal-dependent hyperadrenocorticism.

2. Samples for cortisol assay are collected before and after administration of dexamethasone.

3. The dose in dogs is 1.0 mg/kg body weight intramuscularly, and the postdexamethasone sample is collected after 8 hours; an alternative is 0.1 to 1 mg/kg intravenously, the sample collected after 4 hours.

4. In adrenal-dependent hyperadrenocorticism, dexamethasone at any dosage will not suppress cortisol levels because ACTH secretion has been suppressed maximally by high endogenous cortisol concentration.

5. In pituitary-dependent hyperadrenocorticism, the threshold for glucocorticoid feedback inhibition of ACTH is higher than normal.

    a. The high dose will suppress plasma cortisol below 50% of the baseline value in most affected dogs (Case 20).

    b. A few dogs with pituitary-dependent hyperadrenocorticism fail to suppress, and these may be misdiagnosed as adrenal-dependent hyperadrenocorticism.

    c. Horses with pituitary-dependent hyperadrenocorticism (the lesion is usually in the pars intermedia, which may not be under CRH control) fail to suppress at any dose of dexamethasone; therefore, the test is of limited value in this species.

E. ACTH assay by RIA

1. Sample management difficulty precludes routine clinical use of ACTH assay. Heparinized plasma must be collected in cold, plastic syringes and tubes, separated in a refrigerated centrifuge, and kept frozen until assayed.

2. Plasma ACTH concentrations are normal or increased in dogs with pituitary-dependent hyperadrenocorticism.

3. Concentrations are low in dogs with adrenal-dependent hyperadrenocorticism.

III. Summary laboratory findings in diseases of the adrenal cortex

A. Hyperadrenocorticism
   1. Indirect findings include the following.
      a. Lymphopenia and eosinopenia
      b. Neutrophilia or, in protracted cases, normal neutrophil number
      c. High serum alkaline phosphatase activity (in dogs)
      d. Hyperglycemia, usually lower than the renal threshold in dogs; glucosuria is common in the horse
   2. Direct findings in pituitary-dependent hyperadrenocorticism include the following.
      a. Normal or high baseline plasma cortisol concentration
      b. Exaggerated response to ACTH stimulation; a few affected dogs have a normal response
      c. Failure to suppress the plasma cortisol value with low-dose dexamethasone in the horse and in most affected dogs
      d. Suppression of plasma cortisol value with high-dose dexamethasone in most affected dogs. A few affected dogs and all affected horses fail to suppress.
      e. Bilateral adrenocortical hyperplasia
   3. Direct findings in adrenal-dependent hyperadrenocorticism include:
      a. Normal or high baseline plasma cortisol concentration
      b. Either a normal or an exaggerated response to ACTH stimulation
      c. Failure to suppress plasma cortisol value with any dose of dexamethasone
      d. Neoplasm in the adrenal cortex with contralateral adrenocortical atrophy
   4. Direct findings in iatrogenic hyperadrenocorticism include:
      a. Normal or low baseline plasma cortisol value
      b. No response to ACTH stimulation
      c. Bilateral adrenocortical atrophy
B. Adrenal insufficiency (hypoaldosteronism)
   1. Indirect findings include:
      a. Hyponatremia and hyperkalemia from renal loss of Na^+ and retention of K^+ because of deficiency of aldosterone
         (1) Na^+/K^+ ratio of less than 23:1 is very suggestive; some believe less than 26:1 may be suggestive of the disease.
         (2) Normal serum Na^+ and K^+ values do not rule out hypoaldosteronism.
      b. Variably, hypocalcemia or hypercalcemia, hypoglycemia or hyperglycemia, lymphocytosis or lymphopenia
   2. Direct findings include:
      a. Normal or low baseline plasma cortisol value
      b. No response to ACTH stimulation
      c. No lesion or adrenocortical atrophy

NEUROHYPOPHYSIS AND HYPOPHYSIS

Disorders of these endocrine organs are usually manifested in abnormality of target organ function (e.g., thyroid or adrenal cortex). An exception is diabetes insipidus; the laboratory evaluation of this syndrome is described in Chapter 9.

REFERENCES

Allen WM, Davies DC: Milk fever, hypomagnesemia, and the downer cow syndrome. Br Vet J 137:435, 1981.

Anderson JH, Brown RE: Serum thyroxine (T4) and triiodothyronine (T3) uptake values in normal adult cats as determined by radioimmunoassay. Am J Vet Res 40:1493, 1979.

Anderson JJB, Dorner JL: Total serum thyroxine in thyroidectomized beagles using ^{125}I-labeled thyroxine and comparison of T-3 and T-4 tests. J Am Vet Med Assoc 159:750, 1971.

Atkins CE, Hill JR, Johnson RK: Diabetes mellitus in the juvenile dog: A report of four cases. J Am Vet Med Assoc 175:362, 1980.

Beglinger RE, Siegel ET: Double antibody radioimmunoassay of insulin in canine serum. Am J Vet Res 33:2149, 1972.

Belshaw BE, Rijnberk A: Radioimmunoassay of plasma T4 and T3 in the diagnosis of primary hypothyroidism in dogs. J Am Anim Hosp Assoc 15:17, 1979.

Braithwaite GD: Calcium and phosphorus metabolism in ruminants with special reference to parturient pariesis. J Dairy Res 43:501, 1976.

Capen CC, Belshaw BE, Martin SL: Endocrine disorders. In Ettinger SJ (ed): Textbook of veterinary internal medicine, Vol 2. Philadelphia, WB Saunders Co, 1975.

Capen CC, Martin SL: Hyperinsulinism in dogs with neoplasia of the pancreatic islets. Pathol Vet 6:309, 1969.

Carrillo JM, Burk RL, Bode C: Primary hyperparathyroidism in a dog. J Am Vet Med Assoc 174:67, 1979.

Chastain CB: Canine hypothyroidism. J Am Vet Med Assoc 181:349, 1982.

Chastain CB, Hill BL, Nichols CE: Excess triiodothyronine production by a thyroid adenocarcinoma in a dog. J Am Vet Med Assoc 177:172, 1980.

Chastain CB, Mitten RW, Kluge JP: An ACTH-hyperresponsive adrenal carcinoma in a dog. J Am Vet Med Assoc 172:586, 1978.

Chen CL, Riley AM: Serum thyroxine and triiodothyronine concentrations in neonatal foals and mature horses. Am J Vet Res 42:1415, 1981.

Coffman JR: Calcium and phosphorus physiology and pathophysiology. Vet Med Small Anim Clin 75:93, 1980.

Cohn DV, Hamilton JW: Newer aspects of parathyroid chemistry and physiology. Cornell Vet 66:271, 1976.

Cotton RB, Cornelius LM, Theran P: Diabetes mellitus in the dog: A clinico-pathologic study. J Am Vet Med Assoc 159:863, 1971.

David DS: Calcium metabolism in renal failure. Am J Med 58:48, 1975.

Deem-Morris D, Garcia MC: Thyroid stimulating hormone (TSH) response test in normal horses. Proc Am Coll Vet Intern Med, 1982.

DeLucia HF: The kidney as an endocrine organ involved in the function of vitamin D. Am J Med 58:39, 1975.

Drazner FH: Hypercalcemia in the dog and cat. J Am Vet Med Assoc 178:1252, 1981.

Eiler H, Goble D, Oliver J: Adrenal gland function in the horse: Effects of cosyntropin (synthetic) and corticotropin (natural) stimulation. Am J Vet Res 40:724, 1979.

Eiler H, Oliver J: Combined dexamethasone suppression and cosyntropin (synthetic ACTH) stimulation test in the dog: New approach to testing of adrenal gland function. Am J Vet Res 41:1243, 1980.

Eiler H, Oliver J, Goble D: Adrenal gland function in the horse: Effect of dexamethasone on hydrocortisone secretion and blood cellularity and plasma electrolyte concentrations. Am J Vet Res 40:727, 1979.

Eiler H, Oliver J, Goble D: Combined dexamethasone-suppression cosyntropin (synthetic ACTH) stimulation test in the horse: A new approach to testing of adrenal gland function. Am J Vet Res 41:430, 1980.

Feldman EC: Effect of functional adrenocortical tumors on plasma cortisol and corticotropin concentrations in dogs. J Am Vet Med Assoc 178:832, 1981.

Feldman EC: Comparison of ACTH response and dexamethasone suppression as screening tests in canine hyperadrenocorticism. J Am Vet Med Assoc 182:506, 1983.

Feldman EC: Distinguishing dogs with functioning adrenocortical tumors from dogs with pituitary-dependent hyperadrenocorticism. J Am Vet Med Assoc 183:195, 1983.

Feldman EC, Bohannon NV, Tyrell B: Plasma adrenocorticotropin levels in normal dogs. Am J Vet Res 38:1643, 1977.

Feldman EC, Nelsen RW: Insulin-induced hyperglycemia in diabetic dogs. J Am Vet Med Assoc 180:1432, 1982.

Finn JP, Martin CL, Manns JG: Feline pancreatic islet cell hyalinosis associated with diabetes mellitus and lowered serum insulin concentrations. J Small Anim Pract 11:607, 1970.

Ganong WF, Alpert LC, Lee TC: ACTH and the regulation of adrenocortical secretion. N Engl J Med 209:1006, 1974.

Gershwin LJ: Familial canine diabetes mellitus. J Am Vet Med Assoc 167:479, 1975.

Gosselin SJ, Capen CC, Martin SL, et al: Biochemical and immunological investigations on hypothyroidism in dogs. Can J Comp Med 44:158, 1980.

Grain E, Walder EJ: Hypercalcemia associated with squamous cell carcinoma in a dog. J Am Vet Med Assoc 181:165, 1982.

Gribble DH: The endocrine system. In Catcott EJ, Smithcors JF (eds): Equine medicine and surgery, 2nd ed. Wheaton, Ill, American Veterinary Publications, Inc, 1972.

Halliwell REW, Schwartzman RM, Hopkins L, et al: The value of plasma corticosteroid assays in the diagnosis of Cushing's disease in the dog. J Small Anim Pract 12:453, 1971.

Hause WR, Stevens S, Meuten DJ, et al: Pseudohyperparathyroidism associated with adenocarcinomas of anal sac origin in four dogs. J Am Anim Hosp Assoc 17:373, 1981.

Hoge WR, Lund JE, Blakemore JC: Response to thyrotropin as a diagnostic aid for canine hypothyroidism. J Am Anim Hosp Assoc 10:167, 1974.

Holzworth J, Theran P, Carpenter SL, et al: Hyperthyroidism in the cat: Ten cases. J Am Vet Med Assoc 176:345, 1980.

Irvine CHG, Evans MJ: Hypothyroidism in foals. NZ Vet J 25:354, 1977.

Johnson RK: Insulinoma in the dog. In Kirk RW (ed): Current veterinary therapy V. Philadelphia, WB Saunders Co, 1974.

Johnston SD, Mather EC: Canine plasma cortisol (hydrocortisone) measured by radioimmunoassay: Clinical absence of diurnal variation and results of ACTH stimulation and dexamethasone suppression tests. Am J Vet Res 39:1766, 1978.

Johnston SD, Mather EC: Feline plasma cortisol (hydrocortisone) measured by radioimmunoassay. Am J Vet Res 40:190, 1979.

Joyce JR, Pierce KR, Romane WM, et al: Clinical study of nutritional secondary hyperparathyroidism in horses. J Am Vet Med Assoc 158:2033, 1971.

Juan D: Hypocalcemia. Arch Intern Med 139:1166, 1979.

Kallfelz FA: Observations on thyroid gland function in dogs: Response to thyrotropin and thyroidectomy and determination of thyroid secretion rate. Am J Vet Res 34:535, 1973.

Kaneko JJ: Thyroid function. In Kaneko JJ (ed): Clinical biochemistry of domestic animals, 3rd ed. New York, Academic Press, 1980.

Koterba A, Carlson GP: Acid-base and electrolyte alterations in horses with exertional rhabdomyolysis. J Am Vet Med Assoc 180:303, 1982.

Krook L, Wasserman RH, Shively JN, et al: Hypercalcemia and calcinosis in Florida horses: Implication of the shrub Cestrum diurnum as the causative agent. Cornell Vet 65:26, 1975.

Kruth SA, Feldman EC, Kennedy PC: Insulin-secreting iselt cell tumors: Establishing a diagnosis and the clinical course for 25 dogs. J Am Vet Med Assoc 181:54, 1982.

Larson PR: Tests of thyroid function. Med Clin North Am 59:1063, 1975.

Legendre AM, Merkley DF, Carrig CB, et al: Primary hyperparathyroidism in a dog. J Am Vet Med Assoc 168:694, 1976.

Legendre AM, Walker M, Buyukmihci N, et al: Canine blastomycosis: A review of 47 clinical cases. J Am Vet Med Assoc 178:1163, 1981.

Ling GV, Lowenstine LJ, Kaneko JJ: Serum thyroxine (T-4) and triiodothyronine (T-3) uptake values in normal adult cats. Am J Vet Res 35:1247, 1974.

Ling GV, Lowenstine LJ, Pulley LT, et al: Diabetes mellitus in dogs: A review of initial evaluation, immediate and long-term management, and outcome. J Am Vet Med Assoc 170:521, 1977.

Lorenz MD, Cornelius LM: Laboratory diagnosis of endocrinological disease. Vet Clin North Am 6:687, 1976.

Lorenz MD, Stiff ME: Serum thyroxine content before and after thyrotropin stimulation in dogs with suspected hypothyroidism. J Am Vet Med Assoc 177:78, 1980.

Lowe JE, Baldwin BH, Foote RH, et al: Equine hypothyroidism: The long-term effects of thyroidectomy on metabolism and growth in mares and stallions. Cornell Vet 64:276, 1974.

Lucas MJ, Huffman EM, Johnson LW: Clinical and clinicopathologic features of transport tetany of feedlot lambs. J Am Vet Med Assoc 181:381, 1982.

Mahaffey EA, Cornelius LM: Glycosylated hemoglobin in diabetic and nondiabetic dogs. J Am Vet Med Assoc 180:635, 1982.

Meuten DJ, Chew DJ, Capen CC, et al: Relationship of serum total calcium to albumin and total protein in dogs. J Am Vet Med Assoc 180:63, 1982.

Meuten DJ, Cooper BJ, Capen CC, et al: Hypercalcemia associated with an adenocarcinoma derived from the apocrine glands of the anal sac. Vet Pathol 18:454, 1981.

Meyer DJ, Terrell TG: Idiopathic hypoparathyroidism in a dog. J Am Vet Med Assoc 168:858, 1976.

Moise NS, Reimers TJ: Insulin therapy in cats with diabetes mellitus. J Am Vet Med Assoc 182:158, 1983.

Mostaghni K, Ivoghli B: Diabetes mellitus in the bovine. Cornell Vet 67:24, 1977.

Mulnix JA: Adrenal cortical disease in dogs. Scope 19:12, 1975.

Mundy GR, Ibbotson KJ, D'Souza SM, et al: The hypercalcemia of cancer: Clinical implications and pathogenic mechanisms. N Engl J Med 310:1718, 1984.

Nafe LA, Patnaik AK, Lyman R: Hypercalcemia associated with epidermoid carcinoma in a dog. J Am Vet Med Assoc 176:1253, 1980.

Nesbitt GH, Izzo J, Peterson L, et al: Canine hypothyroidism: A retrospective study of 108 cases. J Am Vet Med Assoc 177:1117, 1980.

Nurmio P, Roine K, Kokkola P: Observations on non-parturient hypocalcemia in cattle. Nord Vet Med 26:483, 1974.

Olsen PN, Bowen RA, Husted PW, et al: Effect of storage on concentrations of hydrocortisone (cortisol) in canine serum and plasma. Am J Vet Res 42:1618, 1981.

Osborne CA, Stevens JB: Pseudohyperparathyroidism in the dog. J Am Vet Med Assoc 162:125, 1973.

Pedersen NC: Nutritional secondary hyperparathyroidism in a cattery associated with the feeding of a fad diet containing horsemeat. Feline Pract 13(6):19, 1983.

Peterson ME, Drucker WD: Advances in the diagnosis and management of canine Cushing's syndrome. Proc 31st Gaines Vet Symp, 1981.

Peterson ME, Feinman JM: Hypercalcemia associated with hypoadrenocorticism in sixteen dogs. J Am Vet Med Assoc 181:802, 1982.

Peterson ME, Gilbertson SR, Drucker WD: Plasma cortisol response to exogenous ACTH in 22 dogs with hyperadrenocorticism caused by adrenocortical neoplasia. J Am Vet Med Assoc 180:542, 1982.

Peterson ME, Nesbitt GH, Schaer M: Diagnosis and management of concurrent diabetes mellitus and hyperadrenocorticism in thirty dogs. J Am Vet Med Assoc 178:66, 1981.

Phillips RW, Knox KL, Pierson RE, et al: Bovine diabetes mellitus. Cornell Vet 61:114, 1971.

Reimers TJ: Radioimmunoassays and diagnostic tests for thyroid and adrenal disorders. Compend Contin Educ Pract Vet 4:65, 1982.

Reimers TJ, Cowan RG, Davidson HP, et al: Validation of radioimmunoassays for triiodothyronine, thyroxine, and hydrocortisone (cortisol) in canine, feline, and equine sera. Am J Vet Res 42:2016, 1981.

Reimers TJ, Cowan RG, McCann JP, et al: Validation of a rapid solid-phase radioimmunoassay for canine, bovine, and equine insulin. Am J Vet Res 43:1274, 1982.

Richards MA: The diabetes insipidus syndrome in dogs. In Kirk RW (ed): Current veterinary therapy V. Philadelphia, WB Saunders Co, 1974.

Rogers W, Straus J, Chew D: Atypical hypoadrenocorticism in three dogs. J Am Vet Med Assoc 179:155, 1981.

Santen RJ, Samojlik E, Demers L, et al: Adrenal of male dog secretes androgens and estrogens. J Physiol 239:E109, 1980.

Schaer M: A clinical survey of thirty cats with diabetes mellitus. J Am Anim Hosp Assoc 13:23, 1977.

Schryver HF, Hintz HF, Lowe JE: Calcium and phosphorus in the nutrition of the horse. Cornell Vet 64:495, 1974.

Sherding RG, Meuten DJ, Chew DJ, et al: Primary hypoparathyroidism in the dog. J Am Vet Med Assoc 176:439, 1980.

Siegel ET, Kelly DF, Berg P: Cushing's syndrome in the dog. J Am Vet Med Assoc 157:2081, 1970.

Simesen MG: Calcium, phosphorus, and magnesium metabolism. In Kaneko JJ (ed): Clinical biochemistry of domestic animals, 3rd ed. New York, Academic Press, 1980.

Spangler WL, Gribble DH: Vitamin D intoxicant and the pathogenesis of vitamin D nephropathy in the dog. Am J Vet Res 40:73, 1979.

Strafuss AC, Njoku CO, Blauch B, et al: Islet cell neoplasm in four dogs. J Am Vet Med Assoc 159:1008, 1971.

Straus E, Johnson GF, Yalow RS: Canine Zollinger-Ellison syndrome. Gastroenterology 72:380, 1977.

Tasker JB, Whiteman CE, Martin BR: Diabetes mellitus in the horse. J Am Vet Med Assoc 149:393, 1966.

Thomas CL, Adams JC: Radioimmunoassay of equine serum for thyroxine: Reference values. Am J Vet Res 39:1239, 1978.

Wilkinson JS: Pituitary and adrenal function. In Kaneko JJ (ed): Clinical biochemistry of domestic animals, 3rd ed. New York, Academic Press, 1980.

Willard MD, Schall WD, McCaw DE, et al: Canine hypoadrenocorticism: Report of 37 cases and review of 39 previously reported cases. J Am Vet Med Assoc 180:59, 1982.

Willard MD, Schall WD, Nachreiner RF, et al: Hypoadrenocorticism following therapy with o,p-DDD for hyperadrenocorticism in four dogs. J Am Vet Med Assoc 180:638, 1982.

Wilson JW, Harris SG, Moore WD, et al: Primary hyperparathyroidism in a dog. J Am Vet Med Assoc 164:942, 1974.

Wilson JW, Hulse DA: Surgical correction of islet cell adenocarcinoma in a dog. J Am Vet Med Assoc 164:603, 1974.

Wilson MG, Nicholson WE, Holscher MA, et al: Propiolipomelanocortin peptides in normal pituitary, pituitary tumor, and plasma of normal and Cushing's horses. Endocrinology 110:941, 1982.

Wilson RB, Bronstad DC: Hypercalcemia associated with nasal adenocarcinoma in a dog. J Am Vet Med Assoc 182:1246, 1983.

12
Cytology

BODY CAVITY EFFUSIONS

I.   Parameters evaluated
   A.   Physical and chemical
      1.   Color
         a.   Normal fluid is clear and colorless to slightly yellow.
         b.   Varying shades of red may indicate free hemoglobin or erythrocytes.
         c.   A green color is caused by bile.
         d.   A white fluid may indicate chyle or cells (pseudochylous).
      2.   Transparency. Turbidity correlates roughly with the number of cells present. Flecks or strands may indicate fibrin.
      3.   Protein. A concentration greater than 3 g/dl usually indicates inflammation, but greater values may occur in some transudative processes (e.g., congestive heart failure).
      4.   Bilirubin, urea, triglyceride, amylase. Concentrations of these substances greater than those observed in serum may indicate leakage from bile ducts or gallbladder, urinary bladder, thoracic duct or abdominal lymphatics, or pancreatic acinar cells or ducts respectively.
   B.   Cytologic
      1.   Total nucleated cell count
         a.   Methods for enumeration are the same as for the white blood cell (WBC) count.
         b.   Values may be erroneous because cell clumping and fragmentation are common in effusions.
      2.   Cytomorphology and cell differentiation
         a.   Direct smears are useful to evaluate cellularity in lieu of the nucleated cell count.
         b.   Sediment smears from a centrifuged sample are

201

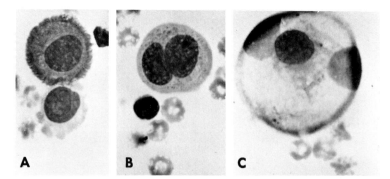

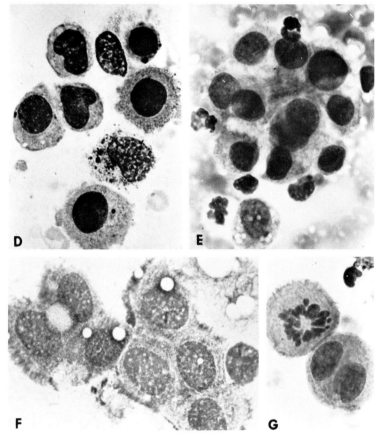

Fig. 12.1. Transudates or modified transudates. A. Basophilic
mesothelial cell with eosinophilic brush border; B. binucleated
mesothelial cell, small lymphocyte, and erythrocytes; C. vacuo-
lated mesothelial cell cluster and erythrocytes; D. mesothelial
cells in various stages of reactivity; E. aggregate of mesothelial cells and nondegenerate neutrophils; F. mesothelial cell
sheet collected by pleural imprint; G. one mitotic and one
trinucleated mesothelial cell. (Wright's stain, ×1200.) (From
Prasse KW, Duncan JR: Laboratory diagnosis of pleural and
peritoneal effusions. Vet Clin North Am 6:625, 1976.)

necessary to concentrate enough cells for cytologic
study in effusions of low cellularity.
   c. The edges or feathered end of smears contain the
       larger cells and should be examined.
   3. Gram-stained smears. Bacteria are observed with
       Wright's stain, but their characterization may be
       facilitated by Gram staining.

II. Cells found in effusions
   A. Mesothelial cell (Fig. 12.1)
       1. Mesothelial cells line the pleural, pericardial, and
           peritoneal cavities; they undergo hypertrophy and
           hyperplasia and desquamate during periods of fluid
           accumulation in the cavities.
       2. Hypertrophied mesothelial cells are characterized by:
           a. Large size (12 to 30 μm)
           b. Deep blue cytoplasm
           c. Red hairlike cytoplasmic processes (occasionally
               occurs as a drying artifact)
           d. Single or multiple, round to oval nuclei with one
               or more nucleoli. Mitoses may be observed.
           e. Clusters of cells that must be differentiated from
               neoplastic cell clusters (see Table 12.1)
   B. Macrophage (Figs. 12.2, 12.3). These large cells (15 to 50
       μm) initially resemble the blood monocyte. The cytoplasm
       becomes vacuolated and may contain varying-sized granules
       and have evidence of phagocytosis (i.e., intracytoplasmic
       erythrocytes, neutrophils, cell debris, or organisms).
       Bacteria are uncommon in macrophages.
   C. Neutrophil (Figs. 12.1, 12.2, 12.3)
       1. Nondegenerate neutrophil
           a. Nuclei are characterized by intact membranes and
               densely aggregated chromatin.

TABLE 12.1. Cytomorphologic Criteria for Malignancy
General criteria
   Large cell size: often the first feature observed
   Aggregates of cells
   Monomorphism: belong to the same cell line
   Pleomorphism: variability in cell size and shape
Nuclear criteria
   High nuclear/cytoplasmic ratio: large nuclei
   Anisokaryosis: variability in nuclear size
   Multinucleation of individual cells
   Normal or abnormal mitotic figures
   Nuclear molding or deformation by adjacent cells
   Nucleoli enlarged or variable in size or shape
   Thickened nuclear membrane (requires Papanicolaou stain)
   Nuclear chromacenters vary in size or shape (requires
      Papanicolaou stain)
Cytoplasmic criteria
   Hyperchromasia
   Cytoplasmic inclusions: phagocytosed materials (cells, cell
      debris) or secretory products (mucin, melanin)
   Source: Prasse KW and Duncan JR: Diagnosis of pleural and
peritoneal effusions. Vet. Clin. North Am. 6:625, 1976.

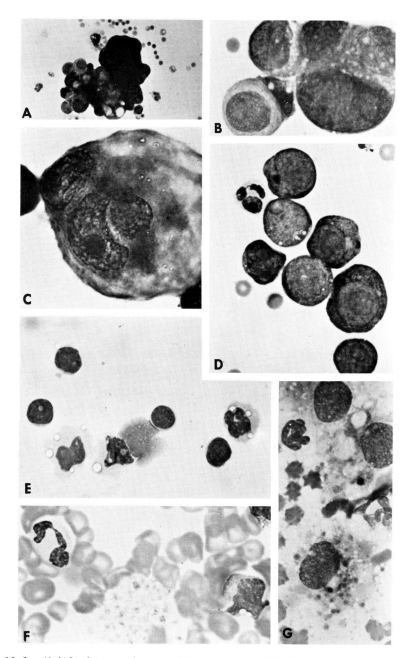

Fig. 12.2. Modified transudates and hemorrhagic effusions.
A. Low magnification of neoplastic cell aggregate; B. adenocarcinoma cell aggregate illustrating anisokaryosis; C. adenocarcinoma cell aggregate illustrating nuclear molding and giant
nucleolus; D. neoplastic lymphocytes, a nondegenerate neutrophil, and erythrocytes (feline thymic lymphosarcoma); E. small
lymphocytes and nondegenerate neutrophils with a smudged cell
and several lipid droplets (feline chylothorax); F. active
hemorrhagic effusion with erythrocytes, leukocytes, and a large
platelet aggregate; G. chronic or resolving hemorrhagic effusion with macrophages containing erythrocytes and hemosiderin,
nondegenerate neutrophils, and free erythrocytes. (Wright's
stain, ×1200.) (From Prasse KW, Duncan JR: Laboratory diagnosis
of pleural and peritoneal effusions. Vet Clin North Am 6:625,
1976.)

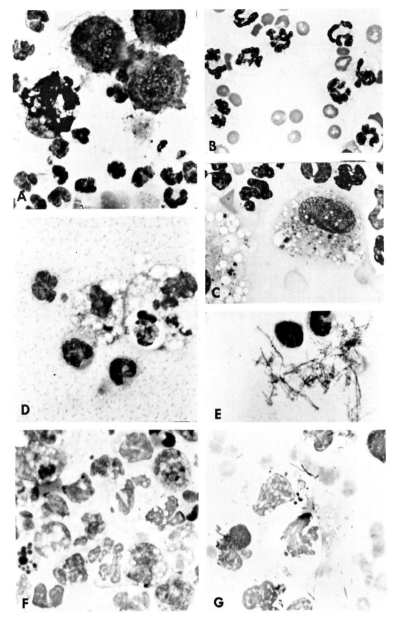

Fig. 12.3.   Exudates. A. Nonseptic exudate — bile-induced
peritonitis with three basophilic mesothelial cells, a macrophage filled with biliary pigment, and nondegenerate neutrophils; B. nonseptic exudate with nondegenerate neutrophils and
erythrocytes; C. nonseptic exudate with nondegenerate neutrophils and macrophages; D. macrophages containing phagocytosed
cell debris, nondegenerate neutrophils, and a uniformly
dispersed proteinic precipitate in the background (feline
infectious peritonitis); E. two nondegenerate neutrophils (one
very pyknotic and rounded) and beaded branching filamentous
bacteria compatible with Actinomyces sp.; F. septic exudate
with numerous karyolytic (degenerate) neutrophils, occasional
pyknotic and karyorrhectic neutrophils, and macrophages;
G. septic exudate from intestinal-perforation peritonitis with
degenerate neutrophils, one small lymphocyte, and a variety of
bacteria. (Wright's stain, ×1200.) (From Prasse KW, Duncan JR:
Laboratory diagnosis of pleural and peritoneal effusions.
Vet Clin North Am 6:625, 1976.)

        b.   They predominate in transudates and exudates in which the etiology is of low toxicity.

    2. Degenerate neutrophil

        a.   Degenerate neutrophils are swollen and characterized by karyolysis (i.e., swollen nuclear lobes), loss of nuclear membrane, and homogeneous, pink-staining chromatin). Cytoplasm may be vacuolated. Karyolysis may not be as obvious in new methylene blue (NMB)-stained preparations.

        b.   Autolysis or mechanical damage during preparation causes similar changes.

        c.   These cells are characteristic of septic inflammation with potent toxin production. When present, one should search for bacteria and culture the fluid.

  D. Other cells commonly found in effusions include eosinophils, lymphocytes, plasma cells, mast cells, and erythrocytes.

III. Types of effusions

  A. Transudate

    1. Mechanisms of transudation are lowered plasma osmotic pressure, increased capillary hydrostatic pressure, and lymphatic obstruction.

    2. Characteristics

        a.   Colorless, clear fluid

        b.   Low protein concentration, less than 3.0 g/dl

        c.   Low cellularity, less than 500 cells/μl. Healthy horses may have up to 9,000 cells/μl.

        d.   Nondegenerate neutrophils, monocytes, and basophilic mesothelial cells. In the case of hydrothorax of feline cardiac disease, the small lymphocyte is the principal cell.

    3. Examples and causes

        a.   Hydrothorax and ascites of hypoproteinemia (Case 18). Effusions usually do not occur until the serum albumin concentration is less than 1.0 g/dl.

        b.   Hydrothorax of right heart failure. Some effusions of feline cardiac disease take a pseudochylous appearance (discussed in IIIB2c).

        c.   Ascites of chronic hepatic disease (Case 12). The modern theory is that a primary sodium retention by renal tubules expands the extracellular fluid compartment and together with presinusoidal obstruction of portal venous flow leads to a low-protein ascites. Portal vein obstruction alone will not cause ascites.

  B. Modified transudate

    1. General characteristics

        a.   This effusion occurs by transudative mechanisms and is modified by the addition of protein and/or cells.

        b.   Cells originate from a hyperplastic mesothelial lining, neoplasms communicating with the cavity, congested venules, or obstructed lymphatics.

    c. This is usually a transitory stage and may progress to a nonseptic exudative process because degenerating cells and serum protein components are chemotactic for neutrophils and monocytes.

    d. There is no clear-cut separation of a modified transudate and nonseptic exudate. Placing an effusion in the modified transudate category merely suggests that the process at the time is primarily noninflammatory.

2. Examples and their characteristics

    a. Ascites of congestive heart failure (Case 7)

        (1) Pink to red sometimes slightly turbid fluid due to diapedesis of erythrocytes

        (2) Protein concentration of 2.5 to 5.0 g/dl. Protein-rich hepatic lymph weeps from liver capsule as a result of postsinusoidal stasis.

        (3) Cell count of 300 to 5,500/μl

        (4) Variable numbers of erythrocytes, nondegenerative neutrophils, basophilic mesothelial cells, macrophages, and occasionally eosinophils (dirofilariasis) and lymphocytes.

    b. Chylous effusion from leakage of thoracic duct or other lymphatic channels

        (1) White to pink turbid fluid

        (2) Inaccurate protein values owing to interference by lipids if refractometry is used

        (3) Cell count usually less than 10,000/μl

        (4) Small lymphocytes predominate with variable numbers of nondegenerate neutrophils and erythrocytes. Lysed cells are common in fluids rich in lymphocytes.

        (5) Sudanophilic droplets (chylomicra). These droplets are refractile with NMB stain.

        (6) High triglyceride levels (higher than serum)

        (7) Fluid clears on alkalinization and ether extraction, but no change occurs with alkalinization alone.

    c. Effusion associated with feline cardiac disease

        (1) Some are chylous, and others are pseudochylous and characterized by:

            (a) Whitish turbid fluid

            (b) Triglyceride levels lower than serum

            (c) Absence of Sudan staining

            (d) Failure to clear with ether but some clearing on alkalinization

        (2) Some have clear fluid.

        (3) The cell count is variable, usually less than 8,000 cells/μl.

        (4) Small lymphocytes usually predominate. Some macrophages and neutrophils. Erythrophagia may be evident.

        (5) Protein concentration is variable, and refractometric values may be inaccurate if the fluid is turbid.

      d. Lymphosarcoma
         (1) The fluid is usually whitish and turbid.
         (2) Protein concentration and cell counts are variable.
         (3) Immature lymphocytes predominate; cell counts are usually less than $10,000/\mu l$.

      e. Carcinoma
         (1) Neoplastic cells often lodge in and occlude lymphatics. In these cases there is high protein concentration (3 to 6 g/dl) and low cell counts (less than $10,000/\mu l$), but neoplastic cells are not commonly observed.
         (2) In some instances, carcinoma cells may leak from lymphatics or proliferate on the serosal surface and desquamate into the fluid. The most common tumors exfoliating cells are ovarian carcinomas, pancreatic carcinomas, and gastric squamous carcinomas of the horse.
         (3) Hyperplasia of mesothelial cells usually occurs, and clusters of basophilic mesothelial cells may be observed that must be differentiated from carcinoma cells (see Table 12.1).

      f. Mesothelioma
         (1) Numerous clusters of malignant tumor cells are observed. They are difficult to differentiate from basophilic mesothelial cell clusters.
         (2) Histologic sections are usually needed for a definitive diagnosis.

C. Exudate
    1. This effusion is a consequence of increased vascular permeability and inflammation.
    2. Characteristics
      a. White, yellow, or pink turbid fluid
      b. Protein concentration greater than 3 g/dl
      c. High cell count, greater than $3,000/\mu l$. In the horse greater than 5,000 cells/μl are needed before an exudate is suspected.
      d. Neutrophils predominate, with variable numbers of macrophages, eosinophils, lymphocytes, basophilic mesothelial cells, and erythrocytes depending on the type and severity of the irritant and duration of the process.
    3. The exudate may be classified according to the general character of the cause.
      a. Nonseptic exudate
         (1) This type of effusion is caused by nonmicrobial irritants such as bile, urine, and sterile foreign bodies. It may develop as the result of components of the effusion in modified transudates (e.g., chylomicra, cells, protein).
         (2) Neutrophils in nonseptic exudates are nondegenerate because the causative irritants and their products are not toxic.

b. Septic exudate
    (1) This type of effusion is caused by micro-
         organisms, but the causative organism is not
         always visible in cytological preparations of
         the exudate.
    (2) Neutrophils are usually degenerate owing to
         the action of toxins elaborated by the
         organisms. Degenerate neutrophils are a key to
         search for the presence of bacteria.
    (3) Some septic exudates have unique
         characteristics.
         (a) Exudates of feline infectious peritonitis
              are very high in protein, primarily beta
              and gamma globulin. Neutrophils are
              nondegenerate, and a characteristic
              granular protein precipitate is evident
              on the background of stained smears.
              Fluids may have a greenish tint and
              relatively low cell counts compared to
              other exudates (Case 22).
         (b) Exudates caused by <u>Nocardia</u> or
              <u>Actinomyces</u> spp. are characterized by
              microcolonies of pleomorphic, fila-
              mentous, sometimes branching, beaded rods
              (seen when a granule from the sediment is
              smeared). Neutrophils around the colony
              are degenerate, while those distant from
              the colony are nondegenerate. Therefore,
              smears of fluid without colonies will
              have a nonseptic cytologic appearance.
D. Hemorrhagic effusions (Fig. 12.2)
    1. Hemorrhagic effusions are usually caused by trauma,
        surgery, infarction of the intestine, or neoplasia.
    2. Types and characteristics
        a. Recent hemorrhage (within several hours)
            (1) Clear supernatant fluid and red sediment.
                 Packed cell volume greater than 5% usually
                 indicates frank hemorrhage.
            (2) Protein and cell count values less than those
                 of peripheral blood
            (3) Intact erythrocytes
            (4) Leukocytes of similar morphology and
                 distribution as those in peripheral blood
            (5) Platelets and platelet aggregates that lyse
                 rapidly
        b. Longstanding or resolving hemorrhage
            (1) Erythrocytes and leukocytes that appear older
                 (hypersegmented) and distorted. Supernatant
                 fluid may be pink because of hemolysis or
                 may be xanthochromic.
            (2) Absence of platelets
            (3) Macrophages with phagocytized erythrocytes and
                 blood pigments. Hemosiderin stains bluish
                 green or black with Romanowski stains.

E. Equine abdominocentesis
    1. Collection of abdominal fluid in this species can be
        used as a diagnostic aid even though significant
        effusion may not be present.
    2. Results are used in concert with history and physical
        examination in rendering a prognosis and formulating a
        therapeutic plan in equine abdominal crises.
    3. Healthy horses have been reported to have up to 9,000
        cells/μl, predominantly nondegenerate neutrophils and
        some macrophages, in abdominal fluid. Therefore,
        inflammation cannot be determined with certainty until
        the nucleated cell count is greater than 9,000/μl.
        However, inflammation is a strong possibility with any
        count over 5,000 cells/μl.
    4. The highest counts occur with septic peritonitis and
        necrosis of the intestinal wall.
    5. The normal protein concentration is usually less than
        1.5 g/dl. Increase in protein can occur with
        thromboembolism and strangulation of vessels in
        addition to inflammation.

CEREBROSPINAL FLUID (CSF)

I. Physical characteristics
    A. Color
        1. Normal CSF is clear and colorless.
        2. Bright red CSF, which clears on centrifugation,
            indicates iatrogenic or very recent hemorrhage.
        3. Yellowish CSF (xanthochromia) indicates bilirubin. Free
            bilirubin is produced 48 hours following hemorrhage
            into the CSF, or conjugated bilirubin may pass the
            blood-brain barrier in severely icteric animals.
    B. Turbidity. Cells, usually over 500/μl, cause turbid CSF.
        Fibrinogen may also be present, resulting in clots in the
        fluid. An anticoagulant should be used in these cases.

II. Chemical constituents
    A. Protein
        1. The usual tests for serum protein are too insensitive
            to detect the small amount of protein usually present
            in CSF (see Chapter 6).
        2. Qualitative tests (Pandy, Nonne-Apelt) detect the
            presence of large molecular weight proteins
            (globulins).
        3. Urinary protein reagent strips may be used to grossly
            detect protein. An elevated protein would usually be
            represented on the reagent strip as 100 mg/dl or more.
        4. CSF protein concentration is increased in inflammation,
            hemorrhage, and malacia. It is accompanied by an
            increase in CSF cell count in inflammation and
            hemorrhage; but in noninflammatory degenerative or
            malacic disease, CSF protein may be increased without
            an increase in cells (albuminocytologic dissociation)
            (e.g., tumors, vascular lesions, sometimes canine
            distemper).

B. Glucose
1. CSF glucose concentration is dependent on blood glucose concentration; both should be measured concurrently. CSF glucose is normally 60 to 80% of the blood glucose level.
2. CSF glucose/blood ratio is decreased in pyogenic infections of the central nervous system (CNS) but normal in hypo- and hyperglycemic states.
C. Electrolytes
1. CSF electrolytes should always be measured concurrently with blood electrolytes. Some are normally higher (Na^+, Cl^-, Mg^{++}) and others lower (Ca^{++}, K^+) than in the blood.
2. CSF sodium is increased (greater than 160 to 200 mEq/1) in water deprivation syndrome of swine.
D. Enzymes. Aspartate aminotransferase, lactate dehydrogenase, and creatine phosphokinase (CK) activity may be increased in a variety of CNS diseases. It is difficult to determine if the enzyme leaked into the CSF from damaged CNS tissue or came from the plasma through an altered blood-brain barrier. CK has a specific brain isoenzyme (see Chapter 10).
III. Cytologic examination. Analysis should take place within 30 minutes after collection because cells autolyse rapidly. Cells may be preserved by prefixing in an equal volume of 90% ethanol.
A. Total nucleated cell count
1. CFS may be plated directly on a hemocytometer, or if the count is high, a special diluting fluid is used.
2. Increased counts (pleocytosis) are associated with meningeal lesions. A differential cell count should be done.
B. Differential cell count
1. Methods. Because of the relatively low cell counts observed in CSF, some form of concentration must be used. These include:
a. Slow centrifugation and direct smearing of the sediment after suspending in a few drops of homologous serum
b. Sedimentation using glass or plastic cylinders
c. Membrane filtration
d. Cytocentrifugation
C. Interpretation
1. Normal CSF contains less than 8 cells/μl, which are predominantly mononuclear (lymphocytes and monocytes).
2. Neutrophilic pleocytosis characterizes bacterial meningitis and encephalitis (listeriosis is an exception).
3. A mononuclear cell pleocytosis suggests viral inflammation.
4. Mycotic and protozoal diseases often have a mixed cellular reaction.
5. Eosinophils in varying numbers have been observed in some parasitic diseases, cryptococcosis, and prototothecosis.
6. Neoplastic cells are infrequently observed but may be evident when the meninges are infiltrated.

SYNOVIAL FLUID
        Except for positive culture results, no laboratory test has
complete specificity for any form of arthritis. Analysis of synovial
fluid can provide data that may confirm or support a tentative
diagnosis formulated from history and physical examination.

I.   Physical and chemical characteristics
     A.   Volume
          1.   The amount of fluid varies among the different-sized
               joints and animal species.
          2.   The small volume obtained in some normal and diseased
               joints, particularly from smaller animals, requires
               that priorities be established in terms of tests
               performed.
          3.   In general, the volume is increased in inflammatory
               diseases and hydrarthrosis and normal or only slightly
               increased in degenerative diseases.
     B.   Appearance
          1.   Synovial fluid is clear and colorless in most species;
               equine fluid is pale yellow.
          2.   Blood in synovial fluid is red if fresh and amber if
               old.
          3.   Turbidity indicates cells, therefore inflammation.
          4.   Flocculent material may be associated with cartilage
               degeneration.
          5.   Normal fluid does not clot (no fibrinogen) but may gel
               (thixotropism) on standing.
     C.   Viscosity
          1.   The quality and quantity of hyaluronic acid, produced
               by synovial lining cells, is responsible for the
               viscosity of the fluid.
          2.   Viscosity may be quantitated with a viscometer or
               estimated from the length of the string each drop makes
               before separating from the tip of the needle (normal is
               2 cm or more).
          3.   Decreased viscosity is caused by:
               a.   Dilution of hyaluronic acid by effusion into the
                    joint (e.g., inflammation and hydrarthrosis).
               b.   Severe synovitis resulting in decreased production
                    and incomplete polymerization of hyaluronic acid by
                    synovial cells.
               c.   Degradation of hyaluronic acid by bacterial
                    hyaluronidase.
     D.   Mucin clot test
          1.   This qualitative test grades the clot found after
               adding a few drops of synovial fluid to a 7N acetic
               acid solution.
          2.   A good clot is tight and ropy and the solution clear;
               while a poor clot is loose and friable with many flecks
               in the solution.
          3.   Decreased quality of the clot is caused by the same
               conditions that reduce viscosity except the dilutional
               effect of effusions is not as great.
          4.   EDTA may decrease the quality of the mucin clot.
     E.   Hyaluronic acid. This compound may be measured directly and

the absolute quantity determined. The procedure does not measure quality or degree of polymerization of the acid.
F. Protein. Increases in protein concentration occur with inflammatory effusions. Refractometry is not an accurate way of measurement.

II. Cytologic examination (Fig. 12.4)
A. Nucleated cell count. WBC counting techniques are employed, but diluting fluids containing acetic acid cannot be used. Counts are subject to greater error than with blood because of the viscosity of the fluid.
B. Microscopic examination
1. Direct or sediment smears may be used. Thin smears may be difficult to obtain with viscid fluids.
2. Filtration techniques may be used to isolate articular cartilage fragments. The zone or depth from which the fragment is derived can be determined from morphologic characteristics. The number and depth of origin of fragments relates to the severity of damage.

III. Interpretation
A. Normal. Monocytes, macrophages, lymphocytes, synovial lining cells, and neutrophils are found in normal synovial fluid, but fewer than 10% of the cells are neutrophils. Nucleated cell counts are usually less than 500 cells/μl; counts may be slightly higher in the dog (up to 3,000/μl have been reported).
B. Septic inflammation. The highest cell counts are found with bacterial infections and may be greater than 100,000

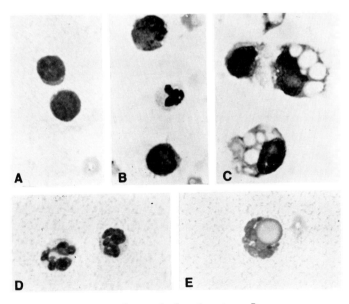

Fig. 12.4. Synovial fluid cytology. A. Lymphocytes, B. monocytes and neutrophil, C. macrophages, D. neutrophils, E. Lupus erythematosus cell. (Wright's stain, ×1000.)

cells/μl. Neutrophils predominate but may not be of
degenerate morphology because of the protective effect of
hyaluronate. Fluid is of reduced viscosity, and the mucin
clot test is of poor quality.

C. Nonseptic inflammation (usually immune-mediated, e.g.,
rheumatoid arthritis, lupus erythrematosus). Cell counts
are increased but usually less than in septic arthritis.
Neutrophils predominate, and viscosity and mucin clot
quality are variable.

D. Degenerative joint disease. Cell counts are normal or only
slightly increased (less than 5,000 cells/μl) and predominantly mononuclear. Macrophages and synovial lining cells
may be in increased proportions, and cartilage fragments
may be observed. Viscosity is high, and mucin clot quality
is good.

E. Trauma. The fluid is discolored by blood components and may
clot. The nucleated cell count is only slightly increased
and usually less than 25% neutrophils. Lipid droplets and
cartilage fragments may be observed with fractures. Mucin
clot quality is good and viscosity high unless there is
marked effusion.

VAGINAL FLUID
    This section pertains primarily to the dog. History of vulvar
swelling, attraction of males, vaginal discharge (amount, color, and
duration), and previous cycle (when and duration) should always be
acquired before an opinion is formulated after cytologic examination.

  I. Method of collection. After cleaning the labia, a moist cotton
swab, blunt pipette, or glass rod is inserted past the vaginal
sphincter into the vagina to collect cells. A smear is made and
stained with Wright's or NMB stain. Trichrome stains may
facilitate identification of cornified cells.
 II. Characteristics of the stages of the estrous cycle (Fig. 12.5)
      A. Anestrus
          1. History includes:

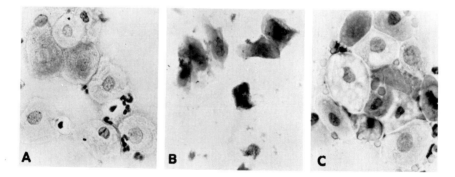

Fig. 12.5. Vaginal cytology (canine). A. Proestrus — noncor-
nified epithelial cells and neutrophils, B. estrus — cornified
epithelial cells and absence of neutrophils, C. metestrus — non-
cornified epithelial cells and neutrophils. (NMB stain, ×1200.)

        a. Estrus more than 2 to 3 weeks previously
        b. Absence of vulvar swelling, discharge, or
            attraction of males
    2. Cytologic findings are:
        a. Superficial and intermediate, noncornified squamous
            epithelial cells characterized by large, round,
            vesicular nuclei and voluminous cytoplasm with
            smooth rounded borders
        b. Nondegenerate neutrophils in small numbers
        c. Absence of erythrocytes

B. Proestrus
    1. History includes:
        a. Vulvar swelling
        b. Red vulvar discharge
        c. Attraction of males
    2. Cytologic findings are:
        a. Superficial and intermediate, noncornified squamous
            epithelial cells. Cornified cells may appear in the
            later stages.
        b. Numerous erythrocytes (may be trapped on cotton
            swab and not evident on the smear)
        c. Neutrophils decreasing in number during the period

C. Estrus
    1. History includes:
        a. Signs of proestrus 1 to 2 weeks previously
        b. Swollen vulva
        c. Red vulvar discharge becoming white toward the end
            of the period
        d. Acceptance of the male
    2. Cytologic findings are:
        a. Superficial, cornified squamous epithelial cells
            characterized by angular cytoplasmic margins and
            much folding. The nuclei are pyknotic, or the cell
            may be anucleate.
        b. Absence of neutrophils
        c. Abundant erythrocytes early but decreased number
            toward the end of the period
        d. Lack of debris
        e. Bacteria in some cases

D. Metestrus
    1. History includes:
        a. Signs of estrus 1 to 2 weeks previously
        b. Reduction in vulvar swelling
        c. Decrease in whitish vulvar discharge
    2. Cytologic findings are:
        a. Parabasal and intermediate noncornified
            squamous epithelial cells. Parabasal cells are
            round with bluish cytoplasm. Some have foamy
            cytoplasm, and others contain leukocytes and are
            referred to as metestrus cells.
        b. Numerous neutrophils
        c. Absence of erythrocytes
        d. Debris early in the period because of the breakdown
            of the cornified epithelial cells characteristic of
            estrus

III. Characteristics of vaginitis and metritis
  A. History
    1. Mild vulvar swelling is observed with a white to pink vulvar discharge.
    2. Evidence of a sequential estrous cycle is lacking, but the animal may have cycled recently.
  B. Cytology
    1. A large number of neutrophils, some in clumps, occur with noncornified epithelial cells. It may be difficult to differentiate inflammation from proestrus or metestrus.
    2. Neutrophils associated with superficial, cornified epithelial cells indicate inflammation because the two cell types do not normally occur together.
    3. The presence of bacteria is not diagnostic of inflammation since organisms may be observed during estrus.
    4. Mucus may be present in cases of mucometria.

TRANSTRACHEAL ASPIRATION BIOPSY

I. Method of collection. Washing of the bronchial tree is accomplished by insertion of a catheter or tube into the trachea at the ventral larynx (small animals) or between tracheal rings (large animals). Several milliliters of sterile saline without preservative (amount depending on size of animal) are injected. When the animal coughs, suction is immediately applied. Sediment from the aspirate is smeared on a slide. Cells lyse easily because of the lack of protective protein.

II. Contents of transtracheal washings (Fig. 12.6)
  A. Epithelial cells
    1. Ciliated epithelial cells are cuboidal or columnar with polar nuclei. The cells may lose their cilia during preparation or because of irritation. Cells from tracheal washings are very fragile and easily lysed.
    2. Goblet cells may be observed but only in small numbers.
    3. Neoplastic epithelial cells are large, occur individually or in clusters, and fit the criteria for malignancy listed in Table 12.1. They are uncommon because most tumors in animals are metastatic into the pulmonary interstitium and do not communicate with an open bronchus. Some primary tumors will exfoliate into an air passage.
  B. Exudative cells
    1. Neutrophils are nondegenerate or degenerate and may contain bacteria.
    2. Eosinophils are difficult to discern in thick areas of the smear; they often lyse, releasing their granules over the smear.
    3. Macrophages are present in different functional states. They may be small and cuboidal or very large with abundant vacuolated cytoplasm. Phagocytized residue may

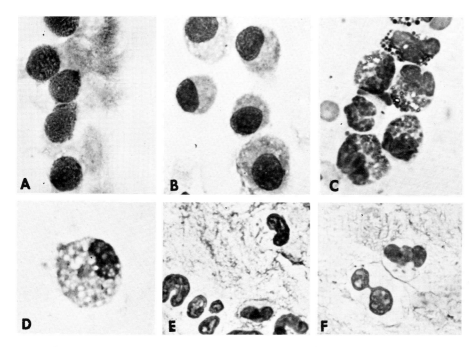

Fig. 12.6. Cytology of transtracheal aspiration. A. Ciliated epithelial cells, B. alveolar macrophages, C. eosinophils, D. activated alveolar macrophage, E, F. neutrophils containing bacteria (note mucus in the background). (Wright's stain, ×1200.)

        be evident (e.g., cellular debris, hemosiderin, carbon). Multinucleated cells are common in the horse.

C. Miscellaneous cells. Mast cells, lymphocytes, and plasma cells may occasionally be observed in small numbers.

D. Miscellaneous materials
  1. Pathogens including bacteria, fungi, and parasitic eggs or juveniles may be seen. Some parasite forms may float to the surface and be more numerous in the supernatant than in the sediment.
  2. Plant material and nonpathogenic fungal hyphae or spores (usually pigmented) are occasionally observed from normal herbivores. In some cases they may suggest aspiration pneumonia or reduced mucociliary clearance if accompanied by exudative cells.
  3. Mucus appears as pale pinkish blue fibrillar strands or amorphous sheets.

III. Types of findings
A. Normal washings. Small amounts of mucus and a few neutrophils, macrophages, and epithelial cells are observed.
B. Exudates
  1. Catarrhal exudate is characterized by excess mucus and a mild increase in neutrophils and macrophages.

        2. Mucopurulent exudate is composed of excess mucus and many neutrophils that are degenerate in septic conditions. Bacteria or fungi may be observed.

        3. Eosinophilic or mixed exudates characterize some allergic and parasitic conditions.

  C. Neoplasia. Neoplastic disease may be identified by finding tumor cells, but these cells are infrequently found in animals.

  D. Congestion and/or hemorrhage. Abundant erythrocytes and macrophages exhibiting erythrophagia or cytoplasmic hemosiderin suggest this process. Staining for iron is helpful.

  E. Oral contamination. Occasionally, the catheter may be misdirected or displaced by coughing, and the washing is obtained from the pharynx. Squamous cells coated with bacteria characteristic of the oral cavity are observed (e.g., <u>Simonsiella</u> sp.).

SOLID TISSUE CYTOLOGY

  I. Methods of collection

    A. Tissue imprints

        1. Touch imprints are made of freshly excised surfaces.

        2. If the excised surface is very bloody or moist, it should be blotted with paper prior to imprinting to remove excess fluid.

    B. Fine-needle tissue aspiration

        1. Tissue is immobilized as close to the skin surface as possible.

        2. A 20- to 22-gauge needle attached to a 10- to 12-ml dry syringe is placed into the tissue in several directions maintaining suction with the syringe. Aspirate may or may not appear in the syringe, but the needle will contain sufficient tissue for smears.

        3. Release suction before removing the needle from the tissue to prevent contaminating the needle contents with cells from surrounding tissues and skin and losing contents into the syringe.

        4. Gently express needle contents onto a slide and make a smear no matter how small the aspirate.

    C. Tissue scrapings. This method is used on lesions that are difficult to imprint or aspirate or yield too few cells by other methods.

    D. Smears of exudates and excretions

        1. Fluid exudates or excretions may be smeared as with blood.

        2. More viscid or particulate material may require gentle dragging across the slide with forceps or "squashing" between two slides and smearing.

  II. Lymph nodes (Fig. 12.7)

    A. Normal lymph node. The cytology is similar to that of a reactive or hyperplastic lymph node. The main difference is that hyperplastic lymph nodes are enlarged.

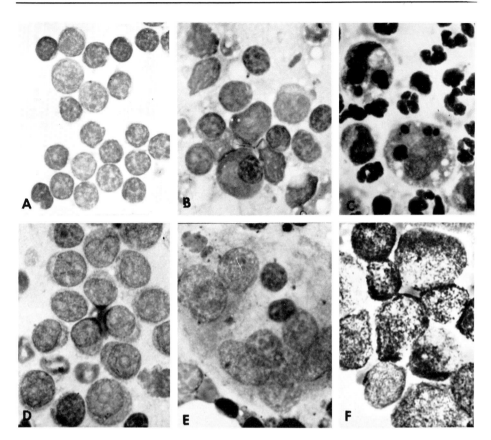

Fig. 12.7. Lymph node cytology. A. Small lymphocytes from a
normal lymph node; B. small lymphocytes, large lymphocyte,
and plasma cell from a hyperplastic lymph node; C. neutrophils
and macrophages from a case of lymphadenitis; D. immature
lymphocytes from a case of lymphosarcoma; E. squamous carcinoma
cells metastatic to a lymph node; F. malignant mast cells
metastatic to a lymph node. (Wright's stain, ×1200.)

    B.   Benign lymphoid hyperplasia (Case 4)
        1.   Characteristics
            a.   Small lymphocytes are the predominant cells.
                Their nuclei are approximately the size of canine
                erythrocytes, and the entire cell is smaller than a
                neutrophil. Many are lysed during preparation;
                therefore, smudge cells are common.
            b.   Variable numbers of large lymphocytes, mature and
                immature plasma cells, and macrophages may give the
                aspirate a mixed cellular appearance. Mitoses can
                be found.
        2.   The cause of benign hyperplasia is antigenic
            stimulation. Antigens are derived via afferent
            lymphatics or blood.
    C.   Lymphosarcoma (Case 9)
        1.   A uniform population of immature lymphocytes gives a

homogeneous appearance. These cells are characterized
by large size (equivalent to neutrophils or larger),
large nuclei (larger than canine erythrocytes) with
dispersed chromatin and prominent nucleoli, and
abundant basophilic cytoplasm.
2. Macrophages containing cell debris may be present in
small numbers.
3. Mitoses may be observed, but they can also be present
in hyperplastic lymph nodes.
4. Cytoplasmic fragments free among the cells are
numerous. These may also be observed in smaller numbers
in hyperplastic lymph nodes.
D. Lymphadenitis
1. Cytology is variable depending on the etiology.
Neutrophils (degenerate or nondegenerate), eosinophils,
or macrophages may predominate.
2. Cytologic features of benign lymphoid hyperplasia may
also be present unless abscessation has occurred.
3. The common causes are bacterial, fungal, or parasitic
organisms, which may be observed in the cytologic
preparation.
E. Metastatic neoplasia
1. The presence of cells not normally in lymph nodes
(epithelial cells) or an increased number of cells that
should occur in only small numbers (mast cells)
indicates metastatic neoplasia.
2. Metastasis is often focal, and the neoplastic cells are
easily missed on aspiration, resulting in the cytologic
appearance of a normal or hyperplastic node.

III. Subcutaneous and skin lesions (Fig. 12.8). The first objective
in cytologic evaluation of a skin lesion is to differentiate
between inflammatory and noninflammatory conditions. Noninflammatory lesions can then be separated into neoplastic and non-

Fig. 12.8. Cytology of the skin. A. Nondegenerate (dark
nuclei) and degenerate (light nuclei) neutrophils aspirated
from an abscess — intracellular bacterial rods are visible in
some of the degenerate neutrophils; B. degenerate neutrophils
from an abscess — karyolysis (swollen, light-staining nuclei)
and pyknosis and karyorrhexis (dark-staining nuclei) are
observed; C. large cells from a salivary cyst — the small, dark,
round cells are nondegenerate neutrophils, which are difficult
to distinguish from lymphocytes because salivary mucus causes
overstaining; D. aspirate from an epidermal cyst illustrating
keratinized cells, cholesterol crystals, and fat droplets;
E. lipid-laden epithelial cells aspirated from hyperplastic
sebaceous glands; F. large fat cells aspirated from a lipoma;
G. epithelial cells from a squamous carcinoma; H. epithelial
cells from a perianal adenoma; I. round cells from a histiocytoma; J. transmissible venereal tumor cells characterized by
coarse chromatin, large nucleoli, and cytoplasmic vacuoles;
K. cutaneous lymphosarcoma cells (some cells contain nucleoli);
L. cells from a mast cell tumor (note dark granules);
M. spindle-shaped connective tissue cells aspirated from a
fibrosarcoma. (Wright's stain, ×1200.) (From Duncan JR, Prasse
KW: Cytologic examination of the skin and subcutis. Vet Clin
North Am 6:637, 1976.)

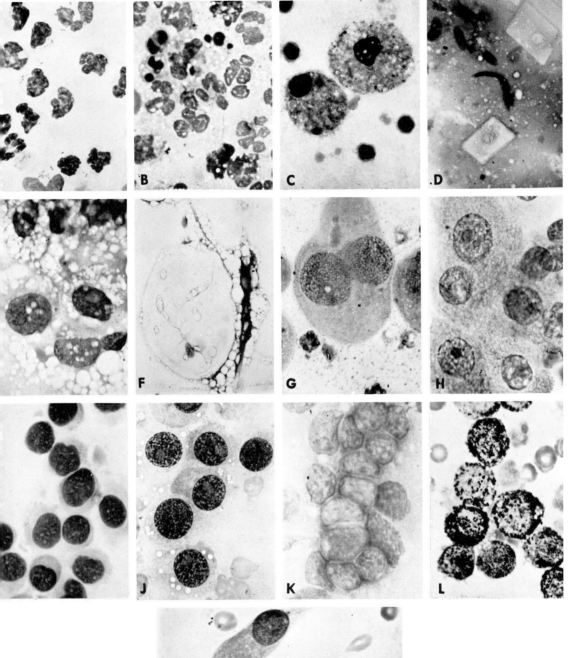
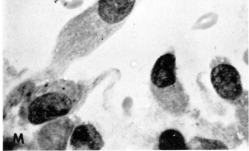

neoplastic types. Some lesions may not yield diagnostic
information.

A. Inflammatory lesions
    1. A preponderance of inflammatory cells (neutrophils,
        macrophages, eosinophils, lymphocytes, and plasma
        cells) places the lesion in this category.
    2. The inflammatory cell type predominating characterizes
        the inflammation (purulent, eosinophilic,
        granulomatous) and may suggest the type of etiology.
    3. The etiologic agent may be observed.

B. Noninflammatory, nonneoplastic lesions
    1. Keratin-producing lesions
        a. Epidermal cysts and certain benign skin tumors
            (e.g., trichoepithelioma, intracutaneous cornifying
            epithelioma) produce keratin.
        b. The lesion yields a whitish, flocculent material
            composed of epithelial cells, keratin, lipid
            droplets, debris, and occasionally cholesterol
            crystals.
        c. Ruptured cysts cause inflammation, and neutrophils
            and macrophages may be mixed with the cyst
            contents.
    2. Sebaceous hyperplasia. These papillary lesions are
        composed of large cells with abundant bluish,
        vacuolated cytoplasm. The nuclei are oval with
        prominent nucleoli.
    3. Sialocele
        a. The fluid from this lesion contains large cells
            with small nuclei and bluish vacuolated cytoplasm
            with pinkish granules and varying numbers of
            nondegenerate neutrophils.
        b. Mucus appears as irregular patches of homogeneous
            pink-blue material in the background.
    4. Seroma. The fluid is of low cellularity and high in
        protein. Macrophages are the principal cell, and many
        are mesothelial cell-like in appearance. Erythrocytes
        and variable numbers of neutrophils and lymphocytes may
        be present.

C. Neoplasms
    1. Epithelial tumors
        a. Epithelial cells have large nuclei, 1 to 3
            prominent nucleoli, and abundant cytoplasm. They
            have tight cell junctions and are often arranged in
            groups or clusters. Identification of epithelial
            cells as neoplastic is difficult, but they should
            possess some of the characteristics listed in Table
            12.1.
        b. Epithelial tumors of the skin include squamous
            carcinoma, perianal adenoma, basal cell tumors
            (some tumors of this group may differentiate and
            produce keratin, causing confusion with epidermal
            cysts), and sweat and sebaceous gland tumors.
        c. From cytologic preparations one should be satisfied
            with an opinion of "possible epithelial tumor" and
            rely on histologic biopsy for an unequivocal
            diagnosis.

2. Round cell tumors. These include a variety of skin
    tumors composed of discrete round to oval cells of
    mesenchymal origin.
    a. Mast cell tumor
        (1) This tumor contains large numbers of cells
             with purple cytoplasmic granules. Nuclei stain
             poorly with Wright's stain.
        (2) Free granules from ruptured cells are
             scattered throughout the smear.
        (3) Varying numbers of eosinophils and neutrophils
             may be present. Lymphocytes may also be
             observed.
    b. Histiocytoma
        (1) Cells of this tumor have eccentric oval
             nuclei, granular chromatin, inconspicuous
             small nucleoli, and abundant bluish cytoplasm,
             which is usually nonvacuolated. Binucleated
             cells and nuclear clefts may be observed.
        (2) Fewer cells are aspirated than from other
             round cell tumors.
        (3) In contrast to macrophages of inflammation,
             vacuoles and phagocytized material are not
             found in these cells.
    c. Transmissible venereal tumor
        (1) This tumor has cells with round nuclei
             containing cordlike chromatin and prominent
             large blue nucleoli. Abundant cytoplasm with
             distinct plasma membranes contains several
             distinct vacuoles. Because of interdigitation
             of surface microvilli, these cells may be in
             close apposition. Mitoses are usually
             observed.
        (2) The tumor is usually located on the genitalia
             but may be found in other sites (e.g., nasal
             cavity).
    d. Cutaneous lymphosarcoma
        (1) This tumor is usually multiple and has a
             uniform population of lymphoid cells, which
             may vary in differentiation from case to case.
        (2) The cell has bluish cytoplasm and an oval
             nucleus with granular chromatin and 1 to 2
             nucleoli.
3. Spindle cell tumors
    a. This group of tumors is derived from connective
        tissue and composed of spindle, fusiform, sometimes
        polyhedral cells with oval nuclei and attenuated
        cytoplasm.
    b. Imprints and aspirations often yield very few
        intact cells because the network of reticular and
        collagenous fibers surrounding the cells prevents
        their detachment.
    c. This groups includes fibroblastic, melanotic,
        hemangiomatous, osteosarcomatous, and myxomomatous
        tumors. They are difficult to separate, unless
        identifying products are present (e.g., melanin).
    d. Usually only a cytologic opinion of "possible

connective tissue neoplasm" can be given.
Histologic biopsy is essential for confirmation.
4.   Lipoma. This well-demarcated lesion is similar to
     adipose tissue cytologically. It is characterized by
     large fat cells with small nuclei and abundant
     vacuolated cytoplasm. Free fat globules are usually
     numerous.
IV. Deep tissue lesions. A variety of solid lesions located in
     deep tissues or body cavities can be aspirated. As with skin
     lesions, they should be separated into inflammatory and non-
     inflammatory lesions. Neoplastic masses may be characterized as
     epithelial, spindle cell, or round cell tumors. A knowledge of
     the disease possibilities for the organ or area aspirated aids
     in formulating a diagnostic opinion.

REFERENCES

Allen SK, McKeever PJ: Skin biopsy techniques. Vet Clin North Am 4:269, 1974.
Bach LG, Ricketts SW: Paracentesis as an aid to the diagnosis of abdominal disease in the
     horse. Equine Vet J 6:116, 1974.
Barsanti JA, Prasse KW, Crowell WA, et al: Evaluation of various techniques for diagnosis
     of bacterial prostatitis in the dog. J Am Vet Med Assoc 183:219, 1983.
Barsanti JA, Shotts EB Jr, Prasse KW, et al: Evaluation of diagnostic techniques for
     canine prostatic diseases. J Am Vet Med Assoc 177:160, 1980.
Beech J: Cytology of transbronchial aspirates in horses. Vet Pathol 12:157, 1975.
Biberstein EL: Transudates, exudates, and miscellaneous fluids. In Cornelius CE, Kaneko JJ
     (eds): Clinical biochemistry of domestic animals. New York, Academic Press, 1963.
Bigner SH, Johnston WW: The cytopathology of cerebrospinal fluid. I. Nonneoplastic
     conditions, lymphoma and leukemia. Acta Cytol 25:335, 1981.
Broderick PA, Corvese N, Pierik MG, et al: Exfoliative cytology interpretation of
     synovial fluid in joint disease. J Bone Joint Surg 58A:396, 1976.
Brown NO, Noone KE, Kurzman ID: Alveolar lavage in dogs. Am J Vet Res 44:335, 1983.
Brownlow MA: Mononuclear phagocytes of peritoneal fluid. Equine Vet J 14:325, 1982.
Brownlow MA: Polymorphonuclear neutrophil leukocytes of peritoneal fluid. Equine Vet J
     15:22, 1983.
Brownlow MA, Hutchens DR, Johnston KG: Reference values for equine peritoneal fluid.
     Equine Vet J 13:127, 1981.
Brownlow MA, Hutchens DR, Johnston KG: Mesothelial cells of peritoneal fluid. Equine Vet J
     14:86, 1982.
Cantrell HD, Rebar AH, Allen AR: Pleural effusion in the dog: Principles for diagnosis. J
     Am Anim Hosp Assoc 19:227, 1983.
Christie DW, Bailey JB, Bell ET: Classification of cell types in vaginal smear during the
     canine oestrous cycle. Br Vet J 128:301, 1972.
Coffman JR: Peritoneal fluid. Vet Med Small Anim Clin 1:1285, 1980.
Coffman JR: Technique and interpretation of abdominal paracentesis. Mod Vet Pract 54:79,
     1973.
Coles EH: Cerebrospinal fluid. In Kaneko JJ (ed): Clinical biochemistry of domestic
     animals, 3rd ed. New York, Academic Press, 1980.
Coles EH: Veterinary clinical pathology, 3rd ed. Philadelphia, WB Saunders Co, 1980.
Creighton SR, Wilkins RJ: Transtracheal aspiration biopsy: Technique and cytologic
     evaluation. J Am Anim Hosp Assoc 10:219, 1974.
Creighton SR, Wilkins RJ: Bacteriologic and cytologic evaluation of animals with lower
     respiratory tract disease using transtracheal aspiration biopsy. J Am Anim Hosp Assoc
     10:227, 1974.
Creighton SR, Wilkins RJ: Thoracic effusions in the cat. Etiology and diagnostic feature.
     J Am Anim Hosp Assoc 11:66, 1975.
Creighton SR, Wilkins RJ: Pleural effusions. In Kirk RW (ed): Current veterinary therapy,
     7th ed. Philadelphia, WB Saunders Co, 1980.
Crowe DT, Crane SW: Diagnostic abdominal paracentesis and lavage in the evaluation of
     abdominal injuries in dogs and cats: Clinical and experimental investigations. J Am
     Vet Med Assoc 168:700, 1976.
Cutler RW, Spertell RB: Cerebrospinal fluid: A selective review. Ann Neurol 11:1, 1982.
deLahunta A: Veterinary neuroanatomy and clinical neurology. Philadelphia, WB Saunders,
     1977.
Duncan JR, Prasse KW: Cytologic examination of the skin and subcutis. Vet Clin North Am
     6:637, 1976.

Duncan JR, Prasse KW: Cytology of canine cutaneous round cell tumors. Mast cell tumor, histiocytoma, lymphosarcoma and transmissible venereal tumor. Vet Pathol 16:673, 1979.

Dyson S: Review of 30 cases of peritonitis in the horse. Equine Vet J 15:25, 1983.

Elkins AD, Green RA: Pleural effusion: Collection, examination, and laboratory diagnosis. Vet Med Small Anim Clin 552, 1983.

Feldman BF, Ruehl WW: Examination of body fluids. Mod Vet Pract 65:295, 1984.

Fernandez FR, Grindem CB, Lipowitz AJ, et al: Synovial fluid analysis: Preparation of smears for cytologic examination of canine synovial fluid. J Am Anim Hosp Assoc 19:727, 1983.

Greenlee PG, Roszel JF: Feline bronchial cytology: Histiologic/cytologic correlation in 22 cats. Vet Pathol 21:308, 1984.

Gruffydd-Jones TJ, Flecknell PA: The prognosis and treatment related to the gross appearance and laboratory characteristics of pathologic thoracic fluids in the cat. J Small Anim Pract 19:315, 1978.

Hoffman D, Spradbrow PB, Wilson BE: An evaluation of exfoliative cytology in the diagnosis of bovine ocular squamous carcinoma. J Comp Pathol 88:497, 1978.

Howard JR: Neurologic disease differentiation. J Am Vet Med Assoc 154:1174, 1969.

Jonas LD: Feline pyothorax: A retrospective study of twenty cases. J Am Anim Hosp Assoc 19:865, 1983.

Kagan KG, Stiff ME: Pleural diseases. In Kirk RW (ed): Current veterinary therapy VIII. Philadelphia, WB Saunders Co, 1983.

Kolata RJ: Diagnostic abdominal paracentesis and lavage: Experimental and clinical evaluations in the dog. J Am Vet Med Assoc 168:697, 1976.

Krum SH, Cardinet GH, Anderson BC, et al: Polymyositis and polyarthritis associated with systemic lupus erythematosus in a dog. J Am Vet Med Assoc 170:61, 1977.

Lavach JD, Thrall MA, Benjamin MM, et al: Cytology of normal and inflamed conjunctivas in dogs and cats. J Am Vet Med Assoc 170:722, 1977.

Legendre AM, Krahwinkel DJ, Carrig CB, et al: Ascites associated with intrahepatic arteriovenous fistula in a cat. J Am Vet Med Assoc 168:589, 1976.

Mayhew IG, Beal CR: Techniques of analysis of cerebrospinal fluid. Vet Clin North Am 10:155, 1980.

McIlwraith CW: Synovial fluid analysis in the diagnosis of equine joint disease. Equine Pract 2:44, 1980.

Miller JB, Perman V, Osborne CA, et al: Synovial fluid analysis in canine arthritis. J Am Anim Hosp Assoc 10:392, 1974.

Miller BH, Roudebush P, Ward HG: Pleural effusion as a sequela to aelurostrongylosis in a cat. J Am Vet Med Assoc 185:556, 1984.

Moise NS, Blue J: Bronchial washings in the cat: Procedure and cytologic evaluation. Compend Contin Educ Pract Vet 5:621, 1983.

Morris DD: Equine tracheobronchial aspirates: Correlation of cytologic and microbiologic findings. J Am Vet Med Assoc 184:340, 1984.

Nelson AW: Analysis of equine peritoneal fluid. Vet Clin North Am/Large Anim Pract 1:267, 1979.

Newton CD, Lipowitz AJ, Halliwell RE, et al: Rheumatoid arthritis in dogs. J Am Vet Med Assoc 168:113, 1976.

Olin DD: Examination of the aqueous humor as a diagnostic aid in anterior uveitis. J Am Vet Med Assoc 171:557, 1977.

Osweiler GD, Hurd JW: Determination of sodium content in serum and cerebrospinal fluid as an adjunct to diagnosis of water deprivation in swine. J Am Vet Med Assoc 165:165, 1974.

Pedersen NC: Synovial fluid collection and analysis. Vet Clin North Am 8:495, 1978.

Pedersen NC, Pool R: Canine joint disease. Vet Clin North Am 8:465, 1978.

Pedersen NC, Pool RC, Castles JJ, et al: Noninfectious canine arthritis: Rheumatoid arthritis. J Am Vet Med Assoc 169:295, 1976.

Pedersen NC, Weisner K, Castles JJ, et al: Noninfectious canine arthritis: The inflammatory nonerosive arthritides. J Am Vet Med Assoc 169:304, 1976.

Perman V: Synovial fluid. In Kaneko JJ (ed): Clinical biochemistry of domestic animals, 3rd ed. New York, Academic Press, 1980.

Perman V, Alsaker RD, Riis RC: Cytology of the dog an cat. South Bend, Ind, American Animal Hospital Assoc, 1979.

Perman V, Stevens JB, Alsaker R, et al: Lymph node biopsy. Vet Clin North Am 4:281, 1974.

Prasse KW, Duncan JR: Laboratory diagnosis of pleural and peritoneal effusions. Vet Clin North Am 6:625, 1976.

Rebar AH: Diagnostic cytology in veterinary practice: Current status and interpretive principles. In Kirk RW (ed): Current veterinary therapy VII. Philadelphia, WB Saunders Co, 1980.

Rebar AH: Handbook of veterinary cytology. St. Louis, Ralston Purina Co, 1980.

Rebar AH, DeNicola DB, Muggenburg BA: Bronchopulmonary lavage cytology in the dog: Normal findings. Vet Pathol 17:294, 1980.

Roszel JF: Membrane filtration of canine and feline cerebrospinal fluid for cytologic evaluation. J Am Vet Med Assoc 160:720, 1972.

Roszel JF, MacVean DW, Monlux AW: Use of cytology for tumor diagnosis in private
    veterinary practice. J Am Vet Med Assoc 173:1011, 1978.
Roudebush P: Percutaneous fine-needle aspiration biopsy of the lung in disseminated
    pulmonary disease. J Am Anim Hosp Assoc 17:109, 1981.
Schalm OW: Feline infectious peritonitis: Vital statistics and laboratory findings. Feline
    Pract 3(4):15, 1973.
Schutte AP: Canine vaginal cytology. I. Technique and cytological morphology. J Small Anim
    Pract 8:301, 1967.
Schutte AP: Canine vaginal cytology. II. Cyclic changes. J Small Anim Pract 8:307, 1967.
Smith BP: Pleuritis and pleural effusion in the horse: A study of 37 cases. J Am Vet Med
    Assoc 170:208, 1977.
Smith EM, Schmidt DA: Diagnostic cytology. In Medway W, Prier JE, Wilkinson JS (eds):
    Textbook of veterinary clinical pathology. Baltimore, Wilkins and Wilkins, 1969.
Soderstrom N: Fine needle aspiration biopsy. New York, Grune and Stratton, 1966.
Sorjonen DC, Warren JN, Schultz RD: Qualitative and quantitative determination of albumin,
    IgG, IgM and IgA in normal cerebrospinal fluid of dogs. J Am Anim Hosp Assoc 17:833,
    1981.
Stevens JB, Perman V, Osborne CA: Biopsy sample management, staining, and examination. Vet
    Clin North Am 4:233, 1974.
Swanick RA, Wilkinson VS: A clinical evaluation of abdominal paracentesis in the horse.
    Aust Vet J 52:109, 1976.
Tew WP: Synovial fluid particle analysis in equine joint disease. Mod Vet Pract 61:993,
    1980.
Tew WP, Hackett RP: Identification of cartilage and wear fragments in synovial fluid from
    equine joints. Arthritis Rheum 24:1419, 1981.
Thompson EJ: Fine needle aspiration cytology in the diagnosis of canine thyroid carcinoma.
    Can Vet J 21:186, 1980.
Thrall MA: Evaluation of thoracic effusions. Mod Vet Pract 64:288. 1983.
Vandevelde M, Spano JS: Cerebrospinal fluid cytology in canine neurologic disease. Am J
    Vet Res 38:1827, 1977.
Van Pelt RW: Interpretation of synovial fluid findings in the horse. J Am Vet Med Assoc
    165:91, 1974.
Van Pelt RW, Conner GH: Synovial fluid from the normal bovine tarsus. 1. Cellular
    constituents, volume, gross appearance. Am J Vet Res 24:112, 1963.
Wagner AE, Bennett DG: Analysis of equine thoracic fluid. Vet Clin Pathol 11(1):13, 1982.
Werner LL: Arthrocentesis and joint fluid analysis diagnostic applications in joint
    diseases of small animals. Compend Contin Educ Pract Vet 1:855, 1979.
Wilkie BN, Markham RJF: Bronchoalveolar washing cells and immunoglobulins of clinically
    normal calves. Am J Vet Res 42:241, 1981.
Wilson JW: Clinical application of cerebrospinal fluid creatine phosphokinase
    determination. J Am Vet Med Assoc 171:200, 1977.
Wilson JW, Stevens JB: Effects of blood contamination on cerebrospinal fluid analysis. J
    Am Vet Med Assoc 171:256, 1977.
Wright JA: Evaluation of cerebrospinal fluid in the dog. Vet Rec 103:48, 1978.

Reference Values

The term "reference value" has largely replaced "normal value" for semantic and scientific reasons in clinical laboratory medicine. The purpose of reference values is to provide a basis for comparison with values obtained from sick animals (i.e., to aid in identifying and characterizing the abnormal animal). They are derived from animals selected as "clinically normal" or "apparently healthy." Values are accumulated from at least 30 animals, and a standard deviation (SD) is calculated. Theoretically, a SD is only valid when the population values form a Gaussian distribution (a bell-shaped curve) when plotted. Although most biological data do not fit this distribution pattern, SD is still widely used to determine population normals. Tables of reference values usually list ±2 SD from the mean or average value. The average value is seldom listed and, in fact, has no interpretive importance. The reference range, then, represents an estimate within which values of 95% of the "clinically normal" individuals should be found. Wide reference value ranges are less useful than narrow ranges.

The ranges of values for normal and abnormal animals often overlap. Values for healthy animals that are within the abnormal limits are said to be "false-positive," whereas normal values for a sick animal (in which the test is usually abnormal) are said to be "false-negative." A careful taking of history, physical examination, and development of differential diagnosis before test selection greatly reduce the chances for false-positive or false-negative test findings.

Methods, techniques, instruments, and technicians vary among laboratories; therefore, each laboratory should establish its own set of reference values. Unfortunately, this is far easier said than done. The following two principles are essential to the preparation of a set of reference values.

1. The laboratory must be capable of obtaining reproducible results. Knowledge that reproducibility is accomplished is gained

through day-to-day use of control serums that have known values (available commercially). Laboratory values obtained by methods for which reproducibility is unknown or poor should not be used.

2. Selection of "clinically normal" individuals within a species must be done without introducing bias. Bias may be limited by consideration of:

(a) Breed, sex, and age distribution

(b) Subclinical disease(s) common to geographic location

(c) Influence of diet, weight, or nutritional status

(d) Sampling time or postabsorptive status

(e) Emotional state or level of excitement of the individual at sampling time

(f) Clear definition of the clinical parameters used to select a "clinically normal" individual

Comparison of the results derived in the practice laboratory with published reference values is valid if the following guidelines are understood and followed.

1. Confidence in the value derived in the practice laboratory is essential and obtained only through use of a simple, valid quality control program. Without confidence that the value is "in control," any comparison is useless.

2. Most hematological procedures are universal, and published values may be safely used for reference. Similarly, published electrolyte values may be used. Units of concentration (e.g., mEq/l vs mg/dl) must be identified for the comparison.

3. Most endpoint, colorimetric chemistries may be done by more than one method. Values from different methods vary, but there is not wide disparity. Published values may serve for reference even though methodologies might differ slightly (e.g., BUN, glucose, total protein, cholesterol, BSP, and creatinine).

4. Different methods for most enzyme tests and some endpoint, colorimetric chemistries yield widely disparate values (e.g., ALP, ALT, AST, SDH, CK, LDH, albumin, and globulin). Employment of identical methods is essential before the value derived in the practice laboratory can be compared with the published value. Furthermore, even when units appear identical [e.g., international units (I.U./l) or milliunits (mU/ml)], comparison is only valid when like substrates, pHs, and reaction temperatures are used.

Reference values for most routinely used laboratory tests are listed in Tables I.1 through I.5. These values may be used for comparison with those listed in the case studies in Appendix II.

REFERENCES

Butts WC, Lilje DJ: Clinically significant reference intervals. Am J Med Tech 48:587, 1982.
Bermes EW, Erviti V, Forman DT: Statistics, normal values, and quality control. In Tietz N (ed): Fundamentals of clinical chemistry, 2nd ed. Philadelphia, WB Saunders Co, 1976.
Copeland BE: Statistical tools in clinical pathology. In Davidsohn I, Henry JB (eds): Clinical diagnosis by laboratory methods, 15th ed. Philadelphia, WB Saunders Co, 1974.
Douglas TA: Standard international units. Vet Rec 100:28, 1977.

TABLE I.1. Hematology Values

	Canine	Feline	Bovine	Equine	Porcine	Ovine	Caprine
Hematocrit (PCV), %	37-55 (25-34)[a]	30-45 (24-34)[a]	24-46	32-48[b]	36-43(26-35)[a]	27-45	22-38
Hemoglobin (Hb), g/dl	12-18	8-15	8-15	10-18	9-13	9-15	8-12
Red blood cell count (RBC), n x 10^6/μl	5.5-8.5	5.0-10.0	5.0-10.0	6.0-12.0	5-7[d]	9-15	8-18
Reticulocyte count (Retic), %	0-1.5	0-1.0	0	0	0-12[d]	0	0
Mean corpuscular volume (MCV), fl	60-77	39-55	40-60	34-58	52-62[d]	28-40	16-25
Mean corpuscular Hb (MCH), pg	19.5-24.5	13.0-17.0	11.0-17.0	13.0-19.0	17-24	8-12	5.2-8.0
Mean corpuscular Hb conc. (MCHC), g/dl	32-36	30-36	30-36	31-37	29-34	31-34	30-36
Platelet count, n x 10^5/μl	2-9	3-7	1-8	1-6	2-5	2.5-7.5	3-6
White blood cell count (WBC), n/μl	6,000-17,000	5,500-19,500	4,000-12,000	6,000-12,000	11,000-22,000	4,000-12,000	4,000-13,000
Segmented neutrophil (seg), (%) n/μl	(60-77)3,000-11,400	(35-75)2,500-12,500	(15-45) 600-4,000	(30-75)3,000-6,000	(20-70)2,000-15,000	(10-50) 700-6,000	(30-48)1,200-7,200
Band neutrophil (band), (%) n/μl	(0-3) 0-300	(0-3) 0-300	(0-2) 0-120	(0-1) 0-100	(0-4) 0-800	0	0
Lymphocyte (lymph), (%) n/μl	(12-30) 1,000-4,800	(20-55) 1,500-7,000	(45-75)2,500-7,500	(25-60)1,500-5,000	(35-75)3,800-16,500	(40-75)2,000-9,000	(50-70)2,000-9,000
Monocyte (mono), (%) n/μl	(3-10) 150-1,350	(1-4) 0-850	(2-7) 25-850	(1-8) 0-600	(0-10) 0-1,000	(0-6) 0-750	(0-4) 0-550
Eosinophil (eos), (%) n/μl	(2-10) 100-750	(2-12) 0-750	(2-20) 0-2,400	(1-10) 0-800	(0-15) 0-1,500	(0-10) 0-1,000	(1-8) 50-650
Basophil (baso), (%) n/μl	Rare	Rare	(0-2) 0-200	(0-3) 0-300	(0-3) 0-500	(0-3) 0-300	(0-1) 0-120
Myeloid/erythroid ratio (M/E)	0.75-2.4/1.0	0.6-3.9/1.0	0.3-1.8/1.0	0.9-3.8/1.0[e]	1.2-2.2/1.0[e]	0.8-1.7/1.0	0.7-1.0/1.0
Plasma protein (PP), g/dl (refractometry)	6.0-7.5[e]	6.0-7.5[e]	6.0-8.0[e]	6.0-8.5[e]	6.0-8.0[e]	6.0-7.5	6.0-7.5
Plasma fibrinogen (fib), mg/dl (heat precipitation)	150-300	150-300	100-600	100-400	200-400	100-500	100-400
Serum iron (SI), μg/dl[f]	94-122	68-215	57-162	73-140	91-199	162-222	...
Unbound iron binding capacity (UIBC), μg/dl[f]	170-222	105-205	63-186	200-262	100-262	141±10	...

Source: Derived, with slight modification, from Schalm OW et al: Veterinary Hematology, 3rd ed, Philadelphia, Lea and Febiger, 1975; Leman AD et al: Diseases of Swine, 5th ed, Ames, Iowa State University Press, 1981; and Kaneko JJ: Clinical Biochemistry of Domestic Animals, 3rd ed, New York, Academic Press, 1980. See references for more precise age differences.

a. Parenthetic values: 5-to-6-wk-old pups; kittens; 3-to-45-day-old pigs.

b. Lower values in foals and cold-blooded horses.

c. Reticulocytes increase to maximum value about 3 wks old and decrease to less than 1% by 6 to 7 mos old.

d. MCV 59 to 73 in pigs from birth to 1 wk old.

e. Lower values in young.

f. Laboratories report SI and total iron binding capacity (TIBC); TIBC = SI + UIBC.

TABLE I.2. Hemostasis Values

	Canine	Feline	Bovine	Equine	Porcine	Ovine	Caprine
Bleeding times, min.	1-5	1-5	1-5	1-5	...	...	...
Clotting Time (Whole Blood):							
Lee-White, min.	3-13	3-8	4-15	4-15	3-4[a]	...	...
Activated clotting time (ACT), sec.	60-100	<65[b]	90-120	120-190	...	...	...
Clotting times (citrated plasma):							
partial thromboplastin time (APTT), sec. (Activated Thrombofax, Ortho Diagnostics, Raritan, NJ)	11-19	19-25	44-64	37-54	34-39[a]	...	40 ± 6[c]
Prothrombin time (OSPT), sec. (Simplastin, General Diagnostics, Morris Plains, NJ)	5-12	5-10	22-55	7-19	11-12[a]	...	11 ± 0.8[c]
Thrombin clotting time (TCT), sec. (Thrombin, Parke Davis, Morris Plains, NJ)	3-8	3-8	...	5-21	...	...	...
Fibrin degradation products (FDP)[d], ug/ml (Thrombo-Wellcotest, Wellcome Reagents Ltd, Beckenham, England)	<32	<8	<4	<16	<8	<4	...
Factor VIII activity, % of normal[e]	50-200	...	...	...	...	...	...
Factor VIII-related antigen, % of normal[e]	60-172	...	...	...	...	...	...

Source: UGA, College of Veterinary Medicine, Athens, Ga, unless otherwise noted.

a. Osweiler: Am J Vet Res 39:633, 1978.

b. Greene and Meriwether: Am J Vet Res 43:1473, 1982.

c. Dorner and Bass: Vet Med Small Anim Clin 69:647, 1974.

d. Concentration, μg/ml, = 2 times last positive dilution (e.g., +1:32 and -1:64 = 64 ug/ml).

e. Dodds, New York State Department of Health, Albany, NY.

TABLE I.3. Blood Gas, pH, Serum Electrolyte, and Osmolality Values

	Canine	Feline	Bovine	Equine	Porcine	Ovine	Caprine
Blood gas analysis:[a]							
Partial pressure of O_2 (PO_2), mmHg	85-95	85-95	92	94	...	...	...
pH	7.31-7.42	7.24-7.40	7.35-7.50	7.32-7.44	...	7.40-7.46[b]	...
Partial pressure of CO_2 (PCO_2), mmHg	29-42	29-42	35-44	38-46	...	38-46.2[b]	...
Bicarbonate (HCO_3^-), mEq/l[d]	17-24	17-24	20-30	24-30	...	22.8 ± 0.8[c]	...
Ion specific electrode:							
Total CO_2 Content, mEq/l	13-29	...	26-34	20-36	...	24.3 ± 0.9[c]	...
Sodium (Na^+), mEq/l	145-155	...	143-151	137-148	...	...	...
Potassium (K^+), mEq/l	2.7-5.0	...	4.1-5.3	2.8-5.1	...	...	...
Chloride (Cl^-), mEq/l	112-124	...	100-108	99-110	...	...	...
Flame photometry:[a]							
Sodium (Na^+), mEq/l	141-155	143-158	132-152	132-146	135-150[e]	139-152[e]	142-155[e]
Potassium (K^+), mEq/l	3.6-5.6	3.2-5.3	3.9-5.8	3.0-4.7	4.4-6.7[e]	3.9-5.4[e]	3.5-6.7[e]
Coulombmetric titration:							
Chloride (Cl^-), mEq/l[a]	96-122	108-128	97-111	99-109	94-106[e]	95-103[e]	99-110[e]
Colorimetry:[a]							
Calcium (Ca^{++}), mg/dl	9.8-12.0	8.6-10.8	9.4-12.2	9.0-13.0	7.1-11.6[e]	11.5-12.8[e]	8.9-11.7[e]
Phosphorus (P), mg/dl	2.5-5.0	4.0-7.0	2.3-9.6	3.0-7.0	5.3-9.6[e]	5.0-7.3[e]	3.8-17.6[f]
Magnesium (Mg^{++}), mg/dl	1.8-2.4	2.0-3.0	1.2-3.5	1.8-3.0	2.7-3.7[e]	2.2-2.8[e]	2.8-3.6[e]
Osmolality (freezing point),[a] mOsm/kg	280-305	280-305	270-300	270-300	...	...	...

a. Tasker, New York State Veterinary College, Ithaca, NY, unless otherwise noted.

b. Roller et al: Am J Vet Res 43:1068, 1982.

c. Lucus et al: J Am Vet Med Assoc 181:381, 1982.

d. UGA, College of Veterinary Medicine, Athens, Ga, unless otherwise noted.

e. Kaneko: Clinical Biochemistry of Domestic Animals, 3rd ed, New York, Academic Press, 1980.

f. Blackwell and Libby: Am J Vet Res 43:1060, 1982.

TABLE 1.4. Serum Biochemical Values

Biochemical and Method	Canine	Feline	Bovine	Equine	Porcine	Ovine	Caprine
Alanine aminotransferase (ALT, SGPT), mU/ml (30°C) (Gilford, Oberlin, Ohio)	4-66	1-64	...	...	...	...	...
Albumin, g/dl (Bromcresol Green, Worthington Biochemical Corp., Freehold, NJ)	2.3-4.3	1.9-3.8	2.5-3.5	2.5-3.5	(1.8-3.3)	(2.4-3.0)	(2.7-3.9)
Alkaline phosphatase (ALP), mU/ml (30°C) (p-Nitrophenylphosphate, Worthington Biochemical Corp., Freehold, NJ)	0-88	2.2-37.8	(0-488)	(143-395)	208 ± 55	(68-387)	(93-387)
Ammonia (NH_3), µg/dl (25°C) (Gilford, Oberlin, Ohio)	0-90	...	...	(13-108)	...	...	...
Amylase, U/1 (37°C) (Maltotetraose, Gilford, Oberlin, Ohio)	<1,450	...	...	...	...	...	...
Aspartate Aminotransferase, (AST, SGOT), mU/ml (30°C) (Gilford, Oberlin, Ohio)	0-40	0-20	0-150	0-150	(32-84)	(307 ± 43)	(167-513)
Bilirubin, total, mg/dl (Jendrassik bilirubin, Nosslin, modified, American Monitor Corp., Indianapolis, Ind)	0.1-0.6	0.15-0.3	0.01-1.0	0.2-5.0	(0-0.6)	(0.1-0.42)	(0-0.1)
Bilirubin, conjugated (direct), mg/dl (as above)	(0.06-0.12)	...	(0.04-0.44)	(0-0.4)	(0-0.3)	(0-0.27)	...
Cholesterol, mg/dl (Gilford, Oberlin, Ohio)	140-210	95-130	(80-120)	(75-150)	(36-54)	(52-76)	(80-130)
Cortisol: Baseline (resting), µg/dl	0.5-4.0[a]	<4.0[b]	...	3.0-6.5[c]	...	...	...
Post-ACTH, µg/dl	8.0-20.0 (2 hr)[a]	4.0-18.0 (1 hr)[b]	...	10.0-18.0 (2 hr)[c]	...	...	...
Post-dexamethasone, µg/dl (RIA)	1.0 (4 hr)[b]	...	...	1.0 (3 hr)[c]	...	...	...
Creatine phosphokinase (CK), mU/ml (30°C) (Gilford, Oberlin, Ohio)	8-60	< 75	< 200	< 200	(2-23)	(8-13)	(1-9)
Creatinine, mg/dl (Modified Jaffe, Kinetic Creatinine, Gilford, Oberlin, Ohio)	< 1.5	<1.5	0.5-2.0	0.5-2.0	(1-2.7)	(1.2-1.9)	(1.0-1.8)
Gamma glutamyltransferase (GGT), mU/ml (30°C) (Gilford, Oberlin, Ohio)	...	...	12-29	5-22	23 ± 7 (Sigma units)	44 ± 11[d]	...
Glucose, mg/dl (Hexokinase UV Glucose, Oberlin, Ohio)	71-115	53-120	40-80	60-100	(85-150)	(50-80)	(50-75)
Indocyanine green (ICG), k (%/min) and t½ (min) (Hynson, Westcott, Dunning, Baltimore, Md, 1.5 mg/kg dose)[e]	8.7 ± 2.2 %/min 8.4 ± 1.9 min	19.2 ± 4.5 %/min 3.8 ± 0.9 min	...	...	...	...	...
Insulin, uU/ml (RIA)	10-25[a]	...	...	...	...	...	...
Isocitrate dehydrogenase (ICD), mU/ml (30°C) (Sigma Chemical Co., St. Louis, Mo)	...	...	12-48	(4-18)	4.7 ± 3.5	...	...

232

TABLE I.4. (cont.)

Biochemical and Method	Canine	Feline	Bovine	Equine	Porcine	Ovine	Caprine
Lactic dehydrogenase (LDH), mU/ml (30°C) (Gilford, Oberlin, Ohio)	100	(63-273)	250	200	(380-634)	(238-440)	(123-392)
Lipase, Sigma Tietz U/ml (Sigma serum lipase, Sigma Chemical Co., St. Louis, Mo)	0-1.0	...	...	...	...	...	...
Lipase, U/l (25°C) (Triolein-turbidometric, UV, Boehringer Mannheim Diagnostics, Houston, Tex)	0-258	0-143	...	...	...	...	...
Protein, total serum, g/dl (Biuret, Worthington Biochemical Corp., Freehold, NJ)	5.3-7.8	5.8-7.8	6.7-7.5	5.0-7.9	(7.9-8.9)	(6.0-7.9)	(6.4-7.0)
Sorbitol dehydrogenase (SDH) mU/ml (30°C) (Sigma Chemical Co., St. Louis, Mo)	...	...	30-1,850	10-260	138 ± 88	...	...
Sulfobromophthalein (BSP) % retention (30 min) or t½ (min) (Davidsohn and Henry, Clinical Diagnosis by Laboratory Methods, Saunders, Philadelphia, Pa, 1969)	< 5%	< 5%	2.5-4.1 min	2.0-3.7 min	(2 min)	(2 ± 0.3 min)	...
Thyroxine (T4):							
Baseline (resting), ng/ml	10-40[b]	15-50[b]	...	(9-28)	...	...	...
Post-TSH, ng/ml	20-80 (4 hr)	...	...	...	...	...	...
(RIA)							
Urea nitrogen (BUN), mg/dl (30°C) (Urease UV, Gilford, Oberlin, Ohio)	5-28	14-32	10-20	10-20	(10-30)	(8-20)	(10-20)

Source: Values from UGA, College of Veterinary Medicine, Athens, Ga; parenthetic values from Kaneko, Clinical Biochemistry of Domestic Animals, 3rd ed, New York, Academic Press, 1980.

a. Values from Animal Health Diagnostic Laboratory, Lansing, Mich.

b. Johnston, Mather: Am J Vet Res 40:190, 1979.

c. Eiler et al: Am J Vet Res 41:430, 1980.

d. Braun et al: Res Vet Sci 25:37, 1978.

e. Center et al: Am J Vet Res 44:722, 727, 1983.

233

TABLE I.5. Serum Proteins

	Canine[a]	Feline[a]	Bovine[a]	Equine[a]	Porcine[b]	Ovine[b]	Caprine[b]
Protein, total serum, g/dl (Biuret, Worthington Biochemical Corp., Freehold, NJ)	5.3-7.8	5.8-7.8	6.7-7.5	5.0-7.9	7.9-8.9	6.0-7.9	6.4-7.0
Cellulose acetate electrophoresis:							
Albumin, g/dl	2.3-3.2	2.6-4.1	3.0-3.6	2.3-3.8	1.8-3.3	2.4-3.0	2.7-3.9
Alpha 1 globulin, g/dl	0.2-0.5	0.3-0.9	0.7-0.9	0.1-0.7	0.3-0.4	0.3-0.6	0.5-0.7
Alpha 2 globulin, g/dl	0.3-1.1	0.3-0.9	...	0.3-1.3	1.3-1.5	...	...
Beta 1 globulin, g/dl	0.6-1.2	0.4-0.9	0.8-1.2	0.4-1.6	0.1-0.3	0.7-1.2	0.7-1.2
Beta 2 globulin, g/dl	...	0.3-0.6	...	0.3-0.9	1.3-1.7	0.4-1.4	0.3-0.6
Gamma globulin, g/dl	0.5-1.8	1.7-2.7	1.7-2.3	0.6-1.9	2.2-2.5	0.2-1.1	0.9-3.0
Albumin/globulin ratio (A/G)[b]	0.6-1.1	0.5-1.2	0.8-0.9	0.6-1.5	0.4-0.5	0.4-0.8	0.6-1.3

a. UGA, College of Veterinary Medicine, Athens, Ga.
b. Kaneko: Clinical Biochemistry of Domestic Animals, 3rd ed, New York, Academic Press, 1980.

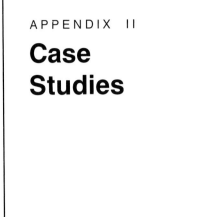

Case Studies

CASE **1** ACUTE HEMORRHAGIC ANEMIA (ANCYLOSTOMIASIS)

SUBJECT:
   Dog, pointer, male, 8 weeks old

PRESENTING PROBLEMS:
   Melena and pallor for several days

LABORATORY DATA:

Hematology		Other Tests
PCV	13 %	Fecal
Hb	3.9 g/dl	Ancylostoma sp. eggs
RBC	$1.59 \times 10^6/\mu l$	
MCV	81.7 fl	
MCH	24.5 pg	
MCHC	30.0 g/dl	
Polychromasia, anisocytosis		
Reticulocytes	16.6 %	
NRBC	3 /100 WBC	
Platelets increased		
Plasma clear, colorless		
Plasma protein	4.1 g/dl	

	$/\mu l$	%
WBC	17,500	
Seg. neutrophils	13,650	78
Band neutrophils	0	0
Lymphocytes	2,625	15
Monocytes	525	3
Eosinophils	700	4

PROBLEMS IDENTIFIED FROM LABORATORY DATA:

1. Hemorrhagic anemia. Regenerative anemia (reticulocytosis)

235

accompanied by hypoproteinemia and clinical signs of hemorrhage
indicate a blood loss mechanism. The high MCV value is caused by
the large reticulocytes. Although other tests would be necessary
to confirm, a panhypoproteinemia is expected to exist.
2. Thrombocythemia. Increase in platelet number is a response to
    blood loss.
3. Neutrophilic leukocytosis. Mild neutrophilia commonly accompanies
    acute hemorrhage.

SUMMARY:
    Hemorrhagic anemia in a young dog with ancylostomiasis suggested
    a causal relationship.

CASE 2 AUTOIMMUNE HEMOLYTIC ANEMIA AND THROMBOCYTOPENIA

SUBJECT:
    Dog, Spanish terrier, female, 5 years old

PRESENTING PROBLEMS:
    Anorexia
    Weakness
    Pale mucous membranes
    Grade II systolic murmur
    (The dog is on corticosteroid medication.)

LABORATORY DATA:

Hematology			Urinalysis (voided)	
PCV	24 %		Yellow, clear	
Hb	7.0 g/dl		Sp gr	1.046
RBC	$2.52 \times 10^6/\mu l$		pH	6.0
MCV	95.2 fl		Protein	1+
MCH	27.7 pg		Other chemistries negative	
MCHC	29.1 g/dl		No significant sediment	
Polychromasia, spherocytosis				
Reticulocytes	23 %		Other Tests	
NRBC	20 /100 WBC		Direct Coombs' antiglobulin	
Platelets	22,000 /μl		test	
Plasma protein	7.5 g/dl		Positive	
			LE cell test	
	/μl	%	Negative	
WBC	27,583	(corrected)		
Seg. neutrophils	21,239	77		
Band neutrophils	3,034	11		
Lymphocytes	276	1		
Monocytes	3,034	11		
Eosinophils	0	0		

PROBLEMS IDENTIFIED FROM LABORATORY DATA:

1. Hemolytic anemia. Regenerative anemia (particularly with a
    calculated reticulocyte production index greater than 3) occurring
    with normal plasma protein concentration and lack of clinical

signs of hemorrhage is characteristic of accelerated erythrocyte
destruction. An immune-mediated mechanism is indicated by spherocytosis and a positive antiglobulin test. Immune-mediated hemolytic anemia in an adult animal without history of transfusion is
most likely an autoimmune type.
2. Thrombocytopenia. Immune-mediated thrombocytopenia is often
    associated with autoimmune hemolytic anemia. A test for anti-
    platelet antibody will substantiate the mechanism.
3. Inflammatory leukogram. Neutrophilia and left shift is commonly
    associated with hemolytic disease and may be in response to
    erythrocyte breakdown products. Monocytosis frequently accompanies
    a need for phagocytic removal of abnormal erythrocytes and also
    may be a response to the corticosteroid medication. Lymphopenia is
    in response to the medication.
4. Mild proteinuria. A 1+ proteinuria in a very concentrated sample
    is of equivocal significance.

SUMMARY:
    Thrombocytopenia, autoimmune hemolytic anemia, and possible
    glomerulonephritis (proteinuria) indicated the possibility of
    canine lupus erythematosus. However, the LE cell test was
    negative.

CASE 3 ACUTE INTRAVASCULAR HEMOLYTIC ANEMIA (PHENOTHIAZINE TOXICITY)

SUBJECT:
    Horse, mixed breed, female, 4 years old

PRESENTING PROBLEMS:
    Weakness
    Depression
    Icterus
    Discolored urine
    Phenothiazine recently administered by owner

LABORATORY DATA:

Hematology		Urinalysis (voided)	
PCV	8.5 %	Port wine color, cloudy	
Hb	4.3 g/dl	Sp gr	1.020
RBC	$1.9 \times 10^6/\mu l$	pH	6.0
MCV	44.7 fl	Protein	4+
MCH	22.6 pg	Occult blood	4+
MCHC	50.5 g/dl	Other chemistries negative	
Heinz bodies present		Sediment	
Platelets adequate		0 to 1 RBC/HPF	
Plasma clear, reddish-yellow		3 to 4 WBC/HPF	
Plasma protein	8.1 g/dl		

	/μl	%
WBC	16,100	
Seg. neutrophils	13,846	86
Band neutrophils	161	1
Lymphocytes	1,288	8
Monocytes	805	5
Eosinophils	0	0

Serum Chemistry

BUN	28 mg/dl
Total bilirubin	10.5 mg/dl
Conjugated bilirubin	0.3 mg/dl

PROBLEMS IDENTIFIED FROM LABORATORY DATA:

1. Hemoglobinuria. Postive urine reactions for protein and occult
    blood, an absence of erythrocytes in the sediment, and the
    presence of hemoglobinemia (reddish plasma and high MCHC) indicate
    hemoglobinuria.
2. Intravascular hemolytic anemia. An anemia accompanied by a
    retention or hemolytic hyperbilirubinemia (conjugated bilirubin
    less than 25% of the total in the horse), hemoglobinemia, and
    hemoglobinuria is typical of intravascular hemolysis. The presence
    of Heinz bodies in erythrocytes suggests a chemical or plant
    toxicant as the etiology. Regenerative responses cannot be
    detected in the peripheral blood of the horse. Reticulocytes are
    not found in either health or anemia in this species.
3. Neutrophilic leukocytosis. The neutrophilia is most likely a
    response to hemoglobin breakdown products or systemic stress.

SUMMARY:
    An intravascular hemolytic anemia with Heinz bodies and a
history of phenothiazine therapy indicated a causal relationship.

CASE 4   ACUTE INFECTIOUS PANLEUKOPENIA

SUBJECT:
    Cat, domestic short hair, male, 10 months old

PRESENTING PROBLEMS:
    Repeated vomiting and profuse diarrhea for 18 hours
    Dehydration estimated to be 7%
    Pyrexia
    Anorexia
    Gingivitis
    Generalized slight enlargement of palpable lymph nodes

LABORATORY DATA:

Hematology

PCV	49 %
Hb	15.8 g/dl
RBC morphology normal	
Platelets adequate	
Plasma clear, colorless	
Plasma protein	8.4 g/dl

Serum Chemistry

BUN	46 mg/dl
Na^+	154 mEq/l
K^+	4.2 mEq/l
Cl^-	123 mEq/l
HCO_3^- (TCO_2)	10 mEq/l

	/μl	%
WBC	1,948	
Seg. neutrophils	39	2
Band neutrophils	58	3
Lymphocytes	468	24
Monocytes	1,383	71
Eosinophils	0	0

Urinalysis (voided)

Yellow, clear

Sp gr   1.065

pH   6.0

Other chemistries negative

No significant sediment

Other Tests

Bone marrow examination
  Hypocellular particles, M/E
  ratio = 0.6, erythroid
  series present in normal
  proportions, myeloid series
  all early stages, mega-
  karyocytes adequate
  Opinion: granulopoietic
  hypoplasia with evidence
  of recovery
Lymph node aspiration cytology
  Mixed lymphoid cell types
  observed, small lymphocytes
  most numerous, plasma cells
  common
  Opinion: Reactive hyperplasia
FeLV test
  Negative

PROBLEMS IDENTIFIED FROM LABORATORY DATA:

1. Neutropenia caused by granulopoietic hypoplasia. The virus of
   infectious panleukopenia causes destruction of all hematopoietic
   precursors, reducing the populations in metabolically active pools
   in 3 to 4 days after the onset of infection. The effect is most
   dramatic in the granulocytic series, and neutropenia is manifested
   at about the same time as the onset of clinical signs (as in this
   case). The bone marrow hematopoietic activity is in early recovery
   at this time, and if secondary bacterial enteritis and endotoxemia
   are not severe, neutrophil count recovery will follow. If endotoxemia is severe, neutropenia may persist. The viral effect on
   erythropoiesis and platelet production is less readily noticed on
   routine hematology of these cases.
2. Lymphopenia and monocytosis. Lymphopenia is a common finding in
   acute systemic infection, especially viral disease, whereby
   recirculating lymphocytes are entrapped within lymph nodes.
   Monocytosis is frequently associated with granulopoietic
   hypoplasia.
3. Dehydration, electrolyte deficit, and acidosis. Dehydration
   (estimated from the physical examination) is severe enough to have
   caused hemoconcentration, azotemia, and concentrated urine. Na^+
   has been lost in proportion with body water, leading to isotonic
   dehydration. Low HCO_3^- with high normal anion gap (25 mEq/l) and
   Cl^- denotes metabolic acidosis from secretion loss of HCO_3^--rich
   intestinal juices. No estimate of total body K^+ can be made from
   these data, but K^+ deficit is likely in cases of vomiting and
   diarrhea.
4. Prerenal azotemia. Mild increase in BUN concentration occurring
   with clinical and laboratory evidence of dehydration indicates
   reduced renal perfusion as the cause.
5. Reactive hyperplasia of lymph nodes. This reaction is most likely
   secondary to infection or some other antigenic stimulation.

SUMMARY:
    The diagnosis, infectious panleukopenia, was based on clinical
and laboratory findings. It was differentiated from the FeLV-
associated panleukopenia-like syndrome by the negative FeLV test.

CASE **5**   ACUTE SEPTIC MASTITIS

SUBJECT:
    Cow, Holstein, female, 6 years old

PRESENTING PROBLEMS:
    Hot swollen quarter with yellowish watery milk of less than
        12 hours duration
    Pyrexia
    Anorexia

LABORATORY DATA:

Hematology			Serum Chemistry	
PCV	37 %		BUN	21 mg/dl
Hb	12.4 g/dl		SDH (30°C)	25 mU/ml
RBC morphology normal			AST (30°C)	180 mU/ml
Platelets adequate			Glucose	222 mg/dl
Plasma protein	7.8 g/dl		Na^+	150.5 mEq/l
Plasma fibrinogen	1,400 mg/dl		K^+	4.2 mEq/l
			Cl^-	102 mEq/l
	/µl	%	HCO_3^- (TCO$_2$)	22 mEq/l
WBC	5,900			
Seg. neutrophils*	708	12		
Band neutrophils*	1,829	31		
Juv. neutrophils*	177	3		
Lymphocytes	2,891	49		
Monocytes	295	5		
*Toxic changes				

PROBLEMS IDENTIFIED FROM LABORATORY DATA:

1. Peracute purulent inflammatory disease and toxemia. Neutropenia
    with marked left shift and hyperfibrinogenemia reflect peracute
    purulent disease in the cow. A sequential leukogram revealing an
    increasing neutrophil count will indicate a favorable response to
    the tissue demand for phagocytes; whereas, persistent or intensi-
    fying neutropenia will denote a very poor prognosis. Toxic neutro-
    phils reflect severe bacterial disease and toxemia in this case.
2. Hyperglycemia. Hyperglycemia most likely indicates endogenous
    catecholamine release in the cow.
3. Liver disease. Hepatocellular disease, characterized by altered
    plasma membrane permeability, is denoted by the high serum
    activity of leakage enzymes (AST and SDH). SDH activity allows an
    interpretation of liver disease, since AST activity will increase
    with either liver or muscle disease.
4. High anion gap (30.7 mEq/l). This finding may denote lactic
    acidosis due to shock or ketosis; the latter could be excluded by

ketone assay of urine. The normal HCO_3^- with high anion gap may
indicate a mixed metabolic acidosis and alkalosis; the data are
not clear-cut. Cl^- is within normal limits. Repeated evaluations
as the disease continues may help define the acid base
abnormality.

SUMMARY:
    The laboratory data provided a basis for a guarded prognosis in
this case. Although electrolyte imbalance was not a problem at
that time, the calculated high anion gap reveals an otherwise
undetected acidosis.

CASE 6 ACUTE SALMONELLOSIS

SUBJECT:
    Horse, thoroughbred, gelding, 10 years old

PRESENTING PROBLEMS:
    Diarrhea of 24 hours duration
    Anorexia
    Weakness
    Pyrexia
    Dehydration estimated to be 7%
    Hyperpnea

LABORATORY DATA:

Hematology			Serum Chemistry	
PCV	51.5 %		BUN	51 mg/dl
Hb	17.1 g/dl		Na^+	112 mEq/l
RBC morphology normal			K^+	3.0 mEq/l
Platelets adequate			Cl^-	100 mEq/l
Plasma protein	8.5 g/dl			
Plasma fibrinogen	1,100 mg/dl		Other Tests	
			Blood gas analysis (venous)	
	/μl	%	HCO_3^-	6.1 mEq/l
WBC	4,200		PCO_2	20.5 mmHg
Seg. neutrophils*	882	21	pH	7.10
Band neutrophils*	2,310	55		
Lymphocytes	126	3		
Monocytes	882	21		
Eosinophils	0	0		
*Toxic changes				

PROBLEMS IDENTIFIED FROM LABORATORY DATA:

1. Peracute inflammatory disease. Neutropenia, marked left shift of
    neutrophils, and short duration of illness indicate overwhelming
    tissue demand for phagocytes. Endotoxemia is a likely cause.
    Extreme hyperfibrinogenemia substantiates the inflammatory
    character of the disease. These findings plus toxic changes in
    neutrophils and severe lymphopenia denote a guarded or poor

prognosis. Lymphopenia is caused by the acute infection or endotoxemia.

2. Dehydration and electrolyte deficit. The clinical estimate of dehydration is substantiated by the high PCV, plasma protein, and BUN values. The fibrinogen value is likewise affected, but a true fibrinogen increase exists, indicated by the low plasma protein/fibrinogen ratio (8.5 g/dl ÷ 1.1 g/dl = 7.7). Hyponatremia is particularly severe, indicating a disproportionately greater Na^+ loss than water loss, which is typical of acute diarrhea in horses. Although serum Cl^- is normal, total body Cl^- content is low (serum Cl^- × decreased ECF volume).

3. Metabolic acidosis. Severe metabolic acidosis is present. Although respiratory compensation is indicated by low PCO_2, the blood pH is dangerously low. Loss of HCO_3^--rich intestinal fluid (secretion acidosis) is indicated by the low anion gap (9 mEq/l) and normal Cl^- in the face of severe hyponatremia (relative hypochloridemia).

4. Probable K^+ depletion. The low normal K^+ in the face of marked acidemia caused by secretion acidosis is a probable indicator of severe K^+ depletion.

SUMMARY:
    Salmonellosis was diagnosed at necropsy.

CASE 7 DIROFILARIASIS

SUBJECT:
    Dog, coonhound, male, 6 years old

PRESENTING PROBLEMS:
    Cough when exercised
    Decreased endurance
    Ascites
    Enlarged heart on radiographic examination

LABORATORY DATA:

Hematology		Serum Chemistry	
PCV	37 %	BUN	27 mg/dl
Hb	12.0 g/dl	Total protein	6.7 g/dl
RBC morphology normal		Albumin	2.2 g/dl
Platelets adequate		ALT (30°C)	26 mU/ml
Plasma clear, colorless		ALP (30°C)	40 mU/ml
Plasma protein	7.0 g/dl	BSP retention	7.5 %
		Glucose	105 mg/dl

	/μl	%
WBC	15,300	
Seg. neutrophils	10,022	67.5
Band neutrophils	0	0
Lymphocytes*	2,065	13.5
Monocytes	229	1.5
Eosinophils	2,372	15.5
Basophils	306	2.0

*Immunocytes observed

Other Tests
Modified Knott's test
  D. immitis present
Abdominal fluid analysis
  Red and cloudy
  Protein 4.9 g/dl
  Nucleated cell count 1,249/μl
  Mesothelial cells, RBCs, and
      nondegenerate neutrophils
  Opinion: modified transudate

Urinalysis (voided)
Dark yellow, clear

Sp gr	1.024
pH	6.2
Protein	2+

Other chemistries negative
No significant sediment

PROBLEMS IDENTIFIED FROM LABORATORY DATA:

1. Eosinophilia and basophilia. Eosinophilia and basophilia are
    consistent with chronic parasitemia, and immunocytes denote
    probable parasitic antigenic stimulation in this case.
2. Cardiac insufficiency. The clinical signs and high protein
    ascites denote cardiac insufficiency consistent with chronic diro-
    filariasis. Liver disease is not in evidence in spite of the
    chronic passive congestion. BSP retention reflects the diminished
    hepatic blood flow of passive congestion. The BSP value may be
    diminished by the effect of expanded, protein-rich ECF volume.
    Also, low albumin concentration favors an enhanced BSP uptake by
    liver, further diminishing the BSP value.
3. Glomerular disease. Proteinuria in the absence of significant
    urine sediment and negative urine occult blood test (no hemoglo-
    binuria) denotes renal origin of the protein. However, renal
    functional integrity remains adequate (ability to concentrate
    urine and lack of azotemia).

SUMMARY:
     The major problems (cardiac and renal disease) were most likely
secondary to dirofilariasis.

CASE **8** PRELEUKEMIA

SUBJECT:
     Cat, domestic shorthair, female, 3 years old

PRESENTING PROBLEMS:
     Anorexia
     Depression of several days duration
     Pale mucous membranes

LABORATORY DATA:

Hematology			Other Tests
PCV	14 %		FeLV
Hb	4.5 g/dl		Positive
RBC	$2.80 \times 10^6/\mu l$		
MCV	50.0 fl		Bone marrow examination
MCH	16.1 pg		Hypercellular particles, M/E
MCHC	32.1 g/dl		ratio of 11:1, 6% erythroid,
RBC morphology normal			66% myeloid with marked
Reticulocytes	0 %		shift toward more immature
Platelets adequate			forms, 28% lymphocytes and
Plasma clear, colorless			plasma cells (normal mor-
Plasma protein	6.8 g/dl		phology), megakaryocytes
			adequate
	$/\mu l$	%	Opinion: granulocytic
WBC	2,789		leukemia, granulocytic
Seg. neutrophils	83	3	hyperplasia, or early
Band neutrophils	223	8	recovery from granulocytic
Lymphocytes	2,314	83	hypoplasia
Monocytes	167	6	
Eosinophils	0	0	

PROBLEMS IDENTIFIED FROM LABORATORY DATA:

1. Bone marrow disease, neutropenia, and granulopoietic hyperplasia.
    A nonregenerative anemia associated with neutropenia in the cat
    indicates bone marrow disease. The differential diagnosis is
    feline infectious panleukopenia, FeLV panleukopenia-like syndrome,
    overwhelming bacterial infection, and preleukemia (subleukemic
    granulocytic leukemia).

    Infectious panleukopenia and FeLV panleukopenia-like syndrome
    are characterized by hypocellular bone marrow and a near normal
    M/E ratio because both series are affected. The FeLV test dif-
    ferentiates between the two diseases.

    Preleukemia is characterized by hypercellular bone marrow with a
    high M/E ratio, increased proportion of early granulocytic precur-
    sors, and abnormal myeloid maturation. Cats with overwhelming
    bacterial infection (and neutropenia) and early recovery stages of
    infectious panleukopenia (still neutropenic) may also be found to
    have granulopoietic hyperplasia in the bone marrow.

SUMMARY:

    The diagnosis was determined by sequential studies that revealed
    persistent neutropenia and granulopoietic hyperplasia with abnor-
    mal maturation forms. The FeLV test also served in differentia-
    tion. The hyperplastic myeloid marrow with abnormal maturation
    occurring concomitant with persistent neutropenia indicates faulty
    marrow release and suggests the possibility of neoplasia. These
    cases may or may not develop into a full-blown granulocytic
    leukemia, therefore the term preleukemia. Increased numbers of
    lymphocytes may be found in the bone marrow of FeLV-positive cats.

CASE **9** LYMPHOSARCOMA AND PSEUDOHYPERPARATHYROIDISM

SUBJECT:
  Dog, Saint Bernard, male, 4 years old

PRESENTING PROBLEMS:
  Bilateral enlargement of mandibular, prescapular, and
    axillary lymph nodes

LABORATORY DATA:

Hematology			Serum Chemistry	
PCV	31 %		BUN	61 mg/dl
Hb	10.0 g/dl		Total protein	6.9 g/dl
RBC	$4.22 \times 10^6/\mu l$		ALT (30^oC)	9 mU/ml
MCV	73.4 fl		ALP (30^oC)	29 mU/ml
MCH	23.6 pg		Glucose	98 mg/dl
MCHC	32.2 g/dl		Ca^{++}	19.1 mg/dl
RBC morphology normal			P	4.5 mg/dl
Reticulocytes	0 %		Na^+	153 mEq/l
Platelets adequate			K^+	5.0 mEq/l
Plasma protein	7.1 g/dl		Cl^-	117 mEq/l
			HCO_3^- (TCO_2)	22 mEq/l

	$/\mu l$	%
WBC	23,400	
Seg. neutrophils	19,539	83.5
Band neutrophils	0	0
Lymphocytes*	1,053	4.5
Monocytes	2,691	11.5
Eosinophils	117	0.5

  *Some are immature

Other Tests

Bone marrow examination
  Particles of normal cellular-
    ity, M/E ratio of 3:1,
    slight shift to maturity in
    erythroid series, normal
    myeloid series and megakar-
    yocytes, 7% lymphocytes of
    normal morphology.
  Opinion: erythroid hypoplasia
Lymph node aspiration cytology
  Monomorphic population of
    lymphoblasts.
  Opinion: lymphosarcoma

  Urinalysis (voided)
Yellow and cloudy
Sp gr   1.011
pH   6.0
Protein   trace
Other chemistries negative
Sediment
  1 to 3 granular casts/HPF
  0 to 2 WBC/HPF

PROBLEMS IDENTIFIED FROM LABORATORY DATA:

1. Lymphosarcoma. The diagnosis is evident from clinical signs and
    cytology of the lymph node aspirate. The leukogram manifests
    endogenous stress but an overt leukemic blood picture does not
    exist. The bone marrow is apparently not involved.
2. Anemia secondary to chronic disease (lymphosarcoma). Nonregenera-
    tive anemia with a slightly high M/E ratio is consistent with
    erythropoietic hypoplasia. A bone marrow lesion creating
    myelophthisis is not evident.
3. Pseudohyperparathyroidism. Hypercalcemia is indirect evidence of
    the presence of this syndrome that is a sequela to lymphosarcoma

and perhaps other tumors. Low serum phosphorus, expected in this syndrome, is not present because of secondary renal disease.

4. Renal disease. Renal disease is suspected because of the urine sp gr value within the isosthenuric range, azotemia, and casts.

SUMMARY:

Calcium nephrosis is a common sequela to persistent hypercalcemia.

CASE 10   RENAL ABSCESS WITH SECONDARY DISSEMINATED INTRAVASCULAR COAGULATION

SUBJECT:

Dog, English bulldog, spayed female, 2 years old

PRESENTING PROBLEMS:

Epistaxis of less than 48 hours duration
Ecchymotic hemorrhage of oral mucosa
Signs of abdominal pain for several days
Abnormal mass palpable in the abdomen
(Dexamethasone was administered within the past 24 hours.)

LABORATORY DATA:

Hematology			Serum Chemistry		
PCV	25 %		BUN	10 mg/dl	
Hb	8.3 g/dl		Total protein	8.3 g/dl	
RBC	$3.88 \times 10^6/\mu l$		Albumin	2.6 g/dl	
MCV	64 fl		ALT (30°C)	20 mU/ml	
MCH	21 pg		ALP (30°C)	45 mU/ml	
MCHC	33 g/dl		Glucose	83 mg/dl	
Fragmented erythrocytes					
Reticulocytes	0.8 %		Other Tests		
Platelets	83,000 /μl		Modified Knott's test		
Plasma protein	8.5 g/dl		Negative		
Plasma fibrinogen	50 mg/dl		Hemostasis profile		
			Bleeding time	11.0 min	
	/μl	%	TCT	18.2 sec	
WBC	35,300		APTT	42.2 sec	
Seg. neutrophils	23,827	67.5	OSPT	19.1 sec	
Band neutrophils	7,060	20.0	Fibrin degradation		
Juv. neutrophils	529	1.5	products	128 μg/ml	
Lymphocytes	706	2.0			
Monocytes	3,001	8.5			
Eosinophils	176	0.5			

Urinalysis (voided)
Yellow and cloudy
Sp gr   1.005
pH   6.0
Other chemistries negative
Sediment
  1 to 4 RBC/HPF
  3 to 5 WBC/HPF
  Rare epithelial cells
  Amorphous crystals

PROBLEMS IDENTIFIED FROM LABORATORY DATA:

1. Anemia secondary to chronic disease. Preexisting subclinical
    secondary anemia is suspected because the anemia is non-
    regenerative and moderately severe. Chronic disease is suspected
    (abdominal mass). Hemorrhagic anemia, prior to the onset of
    reticulocytosis, is possible although hypoproteinemia is not
    evident. Tests to substantiate the above interpretation would be
    serum iron (low), total iron binding capacity (normal to low), and
    iron stain of bone marrow smears (positive). Fragmented erythro-
    cytes suggest a hemolytic component.
2. Purulent inflammatory disease. The leukogram has features
    consistent with dexamethasone therapy (absolute lymphopenia), but
    the magnitude of neutrophilic left shift clearly indicates a
    tissue demand for phagocytes. Monocytosis is consistent with
    either a demand for phagocytes or a response to dexamethasone.
3. Disseminated intravascular coagulation (DIC). Abnormal hemostasis
    consistent with the DIC syndrome is indicated by thrombocytopenia
    (insufficiently severe to cause hemorrhage by itself), hypo-
    fibrinogenemia (prolonged TCT), coagulation factor deficiency
    (prolonged APTT and OSPT), and a high FDP concentration.
    Fragmented erythrocytes are caused by trauma from intravascular
    fibrin strands.
4. Hyperglobulinemia. The difference between total protein and
    albumin concentrations indicates a high serum globulin
    concentration. Protein electrophoresis is necessary to charac-
    terize the nature of globulin alteration (increased immunoglobulin
    concentration is most likely).

SUMMARY:
    A unilateral renal abscess (diagnosed by laparotomy) caused
chronic secondary anemia and disseminated intravascular coagulation. Serum chemistry and urinalysis did not reveal renal disease
in this case because unilateral lesions are insufficient to cause
signs of renal failure (i.e., azotemia and loss of concentrating
ability). Exudate from the abscess was not accessible to patent
nephrons, since pyuria was not present.

CASE 11   CHRONIC CHOLANGIOHEPATITIS

SUBJECT:
    Cat, Persian, male, 1 year old

PRESENTING PROBLEMS:
    Poor appetite for several weeks
    Emaciation developed over several weeks
    Dehydration estimated to be 5%
    Hepatomegaly
    Icterus

LABORATORY DATA:

Hematology			Serum Chemistry		
PCV	27 %		BUN	36	mg/dl
Hb	9.2 g/dl		Total protein	7.8	g/dl
RBC morphology normal			Albumin	3.3	g/dl
Reticulocytes	0 %		ALT (30°C)	398	mU/ml
Platelets adequate			ALP (30°C)	104	mU/ml
Plasma icteric			Total bilirubin	3.5	mg/dl
			Conjugated bilirubin	2.1	mg/dl
	/μl	%	Glucose	83	mg/dl
WBC	6,533		Na^+	151	mEq/l
Seg. neutrophils	3,887	59.5	K^+	4.1	mEq/l
Band neutrophils	621	9.5	Cl^-	118	mEq/l
Lymphocytes	1,731	26.5	HCO_3^- (TCO_2)	19.5	mEq/l
Monocytes	98	1.5			
Eosinophils	196	3.0			

Urinalysis (voided)
Amber and clear
Sp gr   1.045
pH   5.0
Bilirubin   2+
Other chemistries negative
Sediment
    0 to 1 RBC/HPF
    Bilirubin and amorphous crystals
    Fat

PROBLEMS IDENTIFIED FROM LABORATORY DATA:

1. Anemia secondary to chronic disease. The PCV is within normal
    limits, but dehydration obscures the probable true lower value.
    Lack of reticulocytes and the chronic inflammatory nature of the
    disease indicates secondary anemia.
2. Inflammatory disease. Inflammation is suspected because of a
    significant left shift of neutrophils. The neutrophilic response
    must be considered an inappropriate response (normal WBC count
    with a significant left shift) to tissue demand at this stage. If
    the response is found to be either stable or increasing in magni-
    tude on sequential leukograms, the tissue demand is considered
    being met.

3. Hepatocellular and cholestatic liver disease. Hepatocellular
    permeability alteration is evidenced by high activity of the
    leakage enzyme, ALT. Marked cholestasis is indicated by combined
    retention and regurgitation hyperbilirubinemia (conjugated
    bilirubin about 60% of the total bilirubin), high ALP activity,
    and bilirubinuria.
4. Dehydration and electrolyte deficit. Azotemia and urine
    concentration reflect effects of dehydration (estimated from
    physical inspection of the patient). Serum electrolyte concen-
    trations are within normal limits, and since dehydration is
    evident, total body water and electrolyte deficits are probably
    proportional.

SUMMARY:
    The diagnosis, chronic cholangiohepatitis, was based on needle
    biopsy of the liver and histopathologic examination.

CASE 12 PORTAL CAVAL VENOUS SHUNT

SUBJECT:
    Dog, mixed breed, male, 10 months old

PRESENTING PROBLEMS:
    Abdominal distention by ascites for past 3 weeks
    Excessive panting
    Weight loss

LABORATORY DATA:

Hematology			Serum Chemistry	
PCV	41 %		BUN	5.5 mg/dl
Hb	13.2 g/dl		Total protein	5.6 g/dl
RBC morphology normal			Albumin	1.1 g/dl
Platelets adequate			ALT (30°C)	11 mU/ml
Plasma protein	6.1 g/dl		ALP (30°C)	16 mU/ml
			BSP (retention)	13.5 %
	/µl	%	Glucose	77 mg/dl
WBC	14,200		Ca^{++}	8.9 mg/dl
Seg. neutrophils	10,366	73	P	4.0 mg/dl
Band neutrophils	0	0	Na^+	146 mEq/l
Lymphocytes	3,408	24	K^+	4.7 mEq/l
Monocytes	426	3	Cl^-	107 mEq/l
Eosinophils	0	0		

Urinalysis (voided)

Yellow, slightly cloudy

Sp gr	1.017
pH	6.5

Other chemistries negative

Sediment

NH_4^+ biurate crystals

Other Tests

Fasting NH_3	140 ug/dl

Modified Knott's Test

  Negative

Abdominal fluid analysis

  Clear and colorless

Protein	1.8 g/dl
Nucleated cell count	210/μl

  Rare nondegenerate neutrophils
    and mesothelial cells

  Opinion: pure transudate

Blood gas analysis (venous)

HCO_3^-	18.2 mEq/l
PCO_2	24.4 mmHg
pH	7.49

PROBLEMS IDENTIFIED FROM LABORATORY DATA:

1. Reduced functional hepatic mass. Evidence for this lesion includes BSP retention (in the absence of apparent cardiac insufficiency disease and diminished hepatic blood flow), hypoproteinemia, hyperammonemia, and low BUN concentration. Normal ALP and ALT values indicate an absence of cholestasis or altered hepatocellular permeability. Since BSP uptake by hepatocytes is more efficient in hypoalbuminemic states, the BSP value in this case may be an underestimate of the degree of reduced functional mass.

2. Hypoproteinemia, hypoalbuminemia, and ascites. Analysis of the ascitic fluid is consistent with a pure transudate secondary to hypoalbuminemia. Causes of hypoproteinemia (hypoalbuminemia) may be nutritional inadequacy, malabsorption, diminished synthesis by the liver, or prolonged proteinuria. The latter is ruled out by urinalysis, but the former possibilities require further evaluation. The other laboratory findings indicate that diminished hepatic synthesis is the most likely cause.

3. Respiratory alkalosis. The blood gas data indicate uncompensated respiratory alkalosis typical of a panting or hyperventilating dog. The cause of panting may be a manifestation of hepatic encephalopathy or a related mechanism in this case.

4. Increased total body Na^+. Normonatremia and high ECF volume indicates high total body Na^+.

5. Hypocalcemia. The low calcium level is most likely caused by hypoalbuminemia. Normocalcemia (9.9 mg/dl) is calculated using the formula for dogs to adjust the Ca^{++} concentration to rule out functional hypocalcemia.

SUMMARY:

Portal caval venous shunting of blood was confirmed by radiography. The liver was greatly reduced in size and hepatic atrophy was found histologically. No hepatocellular degeneration was evident.

CASE **13** MUSCLE DISEASE, MYOGLOBINURIC NEPHROSIS

SUBJECT:
   Horse, quarterhorse, female, 5 years old

PRESENTING PROBLEMS:
   Profuse sweating
   Pyrexia
   Stiffness
   Pain on palpation of firm gluteal muscles
   Oliguria

LABORATORY DATA:

Hematology			Serum Chemistry	
PCV	37 %		BUN	70 mg/dl
Hb	13 g/dl		Creatinine	4.7 mg/dl
RBC morphology normal			Total protein	6.6 g/dl
Platelets adequate			Albumin	2.9 g/dl
Plasma clear, colorless			AST (30°C)	1,420 mU/ml
			CK (30°C)	320 mU/ml
	/μl	%	Glucose	90 mg/dl
WBC	16,100		Ca^{++}	7.3 mg/dl
Seg. neutrophils	11,914	74	P	5.4 mg/dl
Band neutrophils	483	3		
Lymphocytes	2,415	15		
Monocytes	1,288	8		
Eosinophils	0	0		

Urinalysis (catheterized)
Brown, cloudy
Sp gr	1.031
pH	7.5
Protein	4+
Occult blood	4+

Other chemistries negative
Sediment
   0 to 1 RBC/HPF
   4 to 5 WBC/HPF
   2 to 3 granular casts/HPF
   Calcium carbonate crystals
   Mucus

PROBLEMS IDENTIFIED FROM LABORATORY DATA:

1. Myoglobinuria. Brownish urine with positive reactions for protein
   and occult blood, an absence of erythrocytes in the sediment, and
   normal plasma color indicate myoglobinuria.
2. Muscle disease. Increased AST and CK activity coupled with
   myoglobinuria indicate muscle disease. Sequential CK determinations will reveal if the disorder is persistent or diminishing.
3. Renal disease. Azotemia, hyperphosphatemia, and urinary granular
   casts are indicative of renal disease. Calcium carbonate crystals
   and mucus are normal in horse urine.

4. Inflammatory leukogram. Neutrophilia with significant left shift and monocytosis denotes a tissue demand for phagocytes.

SUMMARY:

    The history, clinical signs, and laboratory findings support a diagnosis of azotemia and/or myositis (inflammatory leukogram). Nephrosis can be sequel to myoglobinuria.

CASE 14   END-STAGE RENAL DISEASE

SUBJECT:

    Dog, beagle, spayed female, 8 years old

PRESENTING PROBLEMS:
    Emaciation
    Gingival ulcers
    Vomiting
    Polyuria, polydipsia
    Small kidneys on palpation

LABORATORY DATA:

Hematology				Serum Chemistry	
PCV	24.5 %			BUN	288 mg/dl
Hb	8.0 g/dl			Creatinine	9.5 mg/dl
RBC	$3.7 \times 10^6/\mu l$			Total protein	7.2 g/dl
MCV	66.2 fl			Albumin	3.5 g/dl
MCH	21.6 pg			ALT (30°C)	46 mU/ml
MCHC	32.6 g/dl			ALP (30°C)	150 mU/ml
RBC morphology normal				Glucose	109 mg/dl
Reticulocytes	0 %			Ca^{++}	10.1 mg/dl
Platelets adequate				P	16.0 mg/dl
				Na^+	152.5 mEq/l
	$/\mu l$	%		K^+	5.5 mEq/l
WBC	5,834			Cl^-	121 mEq/l
Seg. neutrophils	5,134	88			
Band neutrophils	0	0		Other Tests	
Lymphocytes	234	4		Blood gas analysis (venous)	
Monocytes	408	7		HCO_3^-	13.8 mEq/l
Eosinophils	58	1		PCO_2	22.4 mmHg
				pH	7.409

Urinalysis (voided)
Amber, clear
Sp gr   1.012
pH   5.5
Protein   1+
Other chemistries negative
No significant sediment

PROBLEMS IDENTIFIED FROM LABORATORY DATA:

1. Renal failure. Azotemia, isosthenuria (urine sp gr 1.008 to filtration.

1.012), hyperphosphatemia, and clinical signs of uremia indicate renal failure.
2. Anemia secondary to renal disease. A nonregenerative anemia associated with renal failure indicates this mechanism as the cause. Lymphopenia may reflect associated systemic stress.
3. Secondary hyperparathyroidism. The high serum phosphorus value associated with increased ALP activity and normal serum calcium value may indicate a compensating secondary hyperparathyroidism. Since ALT activity is normal, liver disease is probably not the cause of increased ALP activity.
4. Partially compensated metabolic acidosis. HCO_3^- concentration is moderately low. Respiratory compensation (low PCO_2) has brought blood pH within normal limits. The anion gap (23 mEq/l) is in the normal range, making titration acidosis unlikely. A possible cause of secretion loss of HCO_3^- is renal tubular acidosis.

SUMMARY:
    Renal failure associated with nonregenerative anemia and small kidneys indicated that the disease was chronic, and the renal lesions were most likely irreversible.

CASE **15** RENAL AMYLOIDOSIS, NEPHROTIC SYNDROME

SUMMARY:
    Dog, pointer, male, 7 years old

PRESENTING PROBLEMS:
    Lethargy
    Depression
    Subcutaneous edema, ascites

LABORATORY DATA:

Hematology			Serum Chemistry	
PCV	18.5 %		BUN	133 mg/dl
Hb	5.9 g/dl		Creatinine	4.1 mg/dl
RBC	2.60×10^6/μl		Total protein	3.3 g/dl
MCV	71.2 fl		Albumin	0.7 g/dl
MCH	22.6 pg		ALT (30°C)	26 mU/ml
MCHC	31.8 g/dl		ALP (30°C)	16 mU/ml
RBC morphology normal			Cholesterol	530 mg/dl
Reticulocytes	0 %		Ca^{++}	8.4 mg/dl
Platelets adequate			P	6.9 mg/dl
			Na^+	151 mEq/l
	/μl	%	K^+	5.4 mEq/l
WBC	20,100		Cl^-	124 mEq/l
Seg. neutrophils	18,894	94.0	HCO_3^- (TCO$_2$)	17 mEq/l
Lymphocytes	704	3.5		
Monocytes	301	1.5		
Eosinophils	201	1.0		

    Urinalysis (voided)
Yellow, cloudy
Sp gr   1.016
Protein   3+
Other chemistries negative
Sediment
    1 to 2 RBC/HPF
    2 to 5 WBC/HPF
    Rare granular cast
    Amorphous crystals

PROBLEMS IDENTIFIED FROM LABORATORY DATA:

1. Renal proteinuria. Proteinuria without significant cellular
    sediment and with a negative reaction for occult blood (rules out
    hematuria, hemoglobinuria, and myoglobinuria) denotes protein of
    renal origin.
2. Renal failure. Azotemia, reduced urine concentration, and an
    absence of signs of urinary tract obstruction suggest renal
    disease. Prerenal azotemia is unlikely because of the low sp gr
    and lack of evidence for dehydration and cardiac disease. Hyper-
    phosphatemia indicates decreased glomerular filtration.
3. Glomerulotubular imbalance. Renal azotemia accompanied by some
    concentrating ability of the tubules and renal proteinuria
    indicates a primary glomerular lesion. This pattern may be
    described as glomerulotubular imbalance, since isosthenuria
    usually precedes azotemia in renal disease in the dog if the
    glomerulus is not the primary site.
4. Anemia secondary to renal disease. Nonregenerative anemia
    accompanying renal azotemia is a consequence of chronic renal
    disease.
5. Hypoproteinemia and hypocalcemia. Renal loss is the most likely
    cause of hypoproteinemia. Normocalcemia (10.4 mg/dl) is calculated
    using the canine formula to adjust serum Ca^{++} level for hypoalbu-
    minemic effect.
6. Stress leukogram. Lymphopenia and neutrophilia without a left
    shift are characteristic of systemic stress.
7. High total body Na^+. This is based on finding normonatremia and
    expanded ECF volume (edema, ascites).

SUMMARY:
    The tetrad of edema, hypoproteinemia, proteinuria, and
    hypercholesterolemia characterizes the nephrotic syndrome. The
    laboratory data indicated a glomerular lesion that was diagnosed
    as amyloidosis by percutaneous renal biopsy.

CASE **16** FELINE UROLOGIC SYNDROME

SUBJECT:
    Cat, domestic shorthair, male, 3 years old

PRESENTING PROBLEMS:
    Vomiting
    Anorexia, depression
    Unable to urinate
    Tense enlarged bladder
    (An obstruction was removed by catheterization.)

LABORATORY DATA:

Hematology			Serum Chemistry	
PCV	39 %		BUN	169 mg/dl
Hb	12.6 g/dl		Creatinine	13.6 mg/dl
RBC morphology normal			Total protein	6.9 g/dl
Platelets adequate			Albumin	2.9 g/dl
			ALT (30°C)	16 mU/ml
	/μl	%	ALP (30°C)	17 mU/ml
WBC	18,400		Glucose	175 mg/dl
Seg. neutrophils	16,928	92	Ca^{++}	10.1 mg/dl
Band neutrophils	0	0	P	11.2 mg/dl
Lymphocytes	1,452	8	Na^+	138 mEq/l
Monocytes	0	0	K^+	7.9 mEq/l
Eosinophils	0	0	Cl^-	102 mEq/l
			HCO_3^- (TCO$_2$)	13 mEq/l

Urinalysis (catheterized)
Reddish-brown, cloudy
Sp gr   1.031
pH   7.2
Protein   3+
Occult blood   4+
Other chemistries negative
Sediment
    Innumerable RBCs
    15 to 20 WBC/HPF
    Triple phosphate crystals
    3+ bacteria

PROBLEMS IDENTIFIED FROM LABORATORY DATA:

1. Hemorrhagic cystitis. Positive reactions for urine protein and
    occult blood associated with significant erythrocytes in the
    sediment indicate hemorrhage, which is the result of trauma and/or
    inflammation in the urinary tract. Catheterization eliminates the
    genital tract as a possible source of hemorrhage. Bacteria of this
    number in a catheterized sample are probably of etiologic signifi-
    cance, but contamination may occur in a catheterized sample.
2. Postrenal azotemia. Azotemia, concentrated urine, and clinical
    evidence of urinary obstruction indicate a postrenal azotemia.
    Hyperphosphatemia is further evidence of reduced glomerular

3. Metabolic acidosis and hyperkalemia. Acidosis often accompanies
    renal and postrenal azotemia. The elevated K^+ is a sequel to
    acidosis and anuria. The mechanism of acidosis is most likely
    titration (organic acid excess) from uremic acids, which is
    further indicated by a high anion gap (30.9 mEq/l).
4. Low total body Na^+. Hyponatremia with clinically apparent, normal
    hydration indicates a low total body Na^+ content.
5. Systemic stress. Lymphopenia, eosinopenia, neutrophilia without
    significant left shift, and hyperglycemia denote endogenous
    corticosteroid release (painful disorder).

SUMMARY:

Serum K^+ evaluation is very important in this syndrome because in
high concentrations it may reach life threatening levels early in
the clinical course.

CASE **17** PANCREATIC EXOCRINE INSUFFICIENCY AND DIABETES MELLITUS

SUBJECT:

Dog, Cairn terrier, castrated male, 8 years old

PRESENTING PROBLEMS:

Depression
Weight loss for the past 6 weeks
Occasional vomiting
Voluminous soft pale feces
Polyuria

LABORATORY DATA:

Hematology		Urinalysis (voided)	
PCV	39 %	Yellow and clear	
Hb	13.0 g/dl	Sp gr	1.034
RBC morphology normal		pH	6.0
Platelets adequate		Glucose	4+
Plasma clear, colorless		Ketone	2+
Plasma protein	5.8 g/dl	Other chemistries negative	
		No significant sediment	

	/μl	%
WBC	13,200	
Seg. neutrophils	10,824	82
Band neutrophils	0	0
Lymphocytes	2,112	16
Monocytes	132	1
Eosinophils	132	1

Serum Chemistry

BUN	10 mg/dl
Total protein	5.1 g/dl
Albumin	2.0 g/dl
ALT (30°C)	86 mU/ml
ALP (30°C)	90 mU/ml
Glucose	320 mg/dl
Cholesterol	250 mg/dl
Amylase	425 Caraway U.
Na^+	142 mEq/l
K^+	5.8 mEq/l
Cl^-	104 mEq/l
HCO_3^- (TCO_2)	19.5 mEq/l

Other Tests

Plasma osmolality	294 mOsm/kg
Fecal digestion tests	
Proteases (trypsin)	absent
Starch	present
Muscle	present
Fat	present

Fecal flotation
  Ascarid eggs
Fat absorption

Prefeeding	plasma clear
1 hr postfeeding	plasma clear
2 hr postfeeding	plasma clear

Fat absorption after digestion
  with pancreatic enzymes

Prefeeding	plasma clear
1 hr postfeeding	plasma turbid
2 hr postfeeding	plasma turbid

PROBLEMS IDENTIFIED FROM LABORATORY DATA:

1. Diabetes mellitus. Hyperglycemia, glycosuria (causing osmotic diuresis and polyuria), ketonuria, and hypercholesterolemia are features of diabetes mellitus.
2. Pancreatic exocrine insufficiency. Steatorrhea, creatorrhea, and a lack of fecal protease (trypsin) activity (should be confirmed by repeated analysis) indicate a deficiency of digestive enzymes. Hypoproteinemia is consistent with nutritional inadequacy created by abnormal digestion. Results of the fat absorption tests confirm pancreatic exocrine insufficiency and rule out disease charac-terized by intestinal malabsorption. Pancreatic necrosis and inflammation are not evident (normal leukogram and amylase value).
3. Liver disease. Hepatocellular fatty change secondary to diabetes mellitus is the most likely cause of the mild ALT and ALP abnormalities.

SUMMARY:
    The diagnosis remained unclarified with respect to the primary lesion of the pancreas but was most likely a consequence of chronic progressive pancreatitis.

CASE **18** INTESTINAL MALABSORPTION AND PROTEIN-LOSING ENTEROPATHY

SUBJECT:
    Dog, mixed breed, female, 4 years old

PRESENTING PROBLEMS:
    Diarrhea of 2 months duration
    Weight loss
    Subcutaneous edema, ascites, and pleural effusion

LABORATORY DATA:

Hematology			Other Tests	
PCV	41 %		Fat absorption:	
Hb	13.4 g/dl		Prefeeding	plasma clear
RBC morphology normal			1 hr postfeeding	plasma clear
Platelets adequate			2 hr postfeeding	plasma clear
		D-xylose absorption	
/μl	%	Prefeeding plasma level	1.2 mg/dl
WBC	12,400		1/2 hr postfeeding	
Seg. neutrophils	11,408	92	level	22.0 mg/dl
Band neutrophils	248	2	1 hr postfeeding level	29.4 mg/dl
Lymphocytes	620	5	2 hr postfeeding level	24.0 mg/dl
Monocytes	124	1	3 hr postfeeding level	17.8 mg/dl
Eosinophils	0	0	Fecal flotation	
		Negative	
Urinalysis (voided)			Fecal examination	
Yellow, clear			Protease (trypsin)	present
Sp gr	1.027		Fat	present
pH	6.5		Muscle	absent
Other chemistries negative			Starch	absent
No significant sediment			Abdominal fluid analysis	
		Colorless, clear	
Serum Chemistry			Protein less than	1.0 g/dl
BUN	19 mg/dl		Nucleated cell count	152/μl
Total protein	2.6 g/dl		Mesothelial cells and	
Albumin	0.9 g/dl		nondegenerate neutrophils	
Alpha globulin	0.7 g/dl		Opinion: pure transudate	
Beta globulin	0.8 g/dl			
Gamma globulin	0.2 g/dl			
ALT (30°C)	9 mU/ml			
ALP (30°C)	2 mU/ml			
BSP (retention)	1.5 %			
Glucose	108 mg/dl			
Cholesterol	83 mg/dl			
Ca^{++}	7.1 mg/dl			

PROBLEMS IDENTIFIED FROM LABORATORY DATA:

1. Steatorrhea caused by intestinal malabsorption. The presence of
    fecal protease (trypsin) activity indicates adequate pancreatic
    exocrine function. In the absence of a high fat diet or bile
    stasis (normal ALP and absence of icterus), the most likely cause
    is intestinal malabsorption. This is confirmed by a relatively

flat xylose absorption curve (peak under 45 mg/dl) and the lack of plasma turbidity following oral fat feeding. Low serum cholesterol can accompany lipid malabsorption.

2. Hypoproteinemia and protein-losing enteropathy. Panhypoproteinemia with a lack of evidence for hemorrhage, proteinuria, or liver disease indicates possible intestinal protein loss.

3. Hypocalcemia. Hypoproteinemia can be accompanied by a decrease in protein bound calcium. Biologically active ionized calcium is probably normal, since signs of neuromuscular disease are absent. The correction formula to rule out functional hypocalcemia in hypoalbuminemic dogs yields 9.4 mg/dl.

4. Lymphopenia. Intestinal lymph loss and lymphopenia often accompany protein-losing enteric disease.

5. Transudative effusion. Hypocellular peritoneal effusion with low protein content is characteristically associated with hypoproteinemia, particularly if the serum albumin is below 1.0 g/dl.

SUMMARY:

Protein loss was demonstrated by increased ^{51}Cr excretion in the feces following ^{51}Cr-albumin administration intravenously. A jejunal biopsy revealed intestinal lymphangiectasia.

CASE 19 ACUTE PANCREATIC NECROSIS

SUBJECT:
Canine, miniature poodle, female, 5 years old

PRESENTING PROBLEMS:
Tense, painful abdomen of short duration
Vomiting noted once by owner
Anorexia
Dehydration not apparent

LABORATORY DATA:

Hematology			Serum Chemistry	
PCV	42 %		BUN	17 mg/dl
Hb	13.9 g/dl		Total protein	6.7 g/dl
RBC morphology normal			Albumin	3.1 g/dl
Platelets adequate			ALT (30°C)	78 mU/ml
Plasma lipemic			ALP (30°C)	101 mU/ml
			Glucose	83 mg/dl
	/μl	%	Lipase	6.2 Sigma Tietz U.
WBC	27,300		Amylase	2,802 Caraway U.
Seg. neutrophils*	21,294	78	Ca^{++}	10.2 mg/dl
Band neutrophils*	4,914	18	P	3.8 mg/dl
Lymphocytes	546	2	Na^{+}	137.5 mEq/l
Monocytes	546	2	K^{+}	3.3 mEq/l
Eosinophils	0	0	Cl^{-}	115 mEq/l
*Toxic changes			HCO$_3^{-}$ (TCO$_2$)	23 mEq/l

  Urinalysis (voided)
Yellow, clear
Sp gr   1.030
pH   6.5
Other chemistries negative
Sediment
  3 to 4 RBC/HPF
  1 to 2 WBC/HPF
  Triple phosphate crystals

PROBLEMS IDENTIFIED FROM LABORATORY DATA:

1. Pancreatic necrosis. Hyperlipasemia and hyperamylasemia in the
    absence of azotemia denote pancreatic acinar cell release of these
    enzymes. Increased plasma lipid concentration, to the point of
    turbidity, may be observed with pancreatic necrosis even in the
    absence of diabetes mellitus.
2. Inflammatory leukogram. Neutrophilia with a left shift indicates
    an appropriate response to a tissue demand for neutrophils in
    response to fat necrosis caused by spillage of pancreatic enzymes
    into the peritoneal cavity. The lymphopenia and eosinopenia are a
    reflection of systemic stress (a painful disorder).
3. Hyponatremia and Hypokalemia. Na^+ and K^+ measured by flame
    photometry (as done in this case) will often be factitiously low
    when the sample is lipemic. Cl^- and TCO_2 may be affected in a
    similar way.

SUMMARY:
    Extensive pancreatic necrosis was observed at necropsy.

CASE **20** HYPERADRENOCORTICISM

SUBJECT:
    Dog, dachshund, spayed female, 4 years old

PRESENTING PROBLEMS:
    Abdominal enlargement
    Polyuria, polydipsia
    Obesity
    Generalized alopecia

LABORATORY DATA:

Hematology			Serum Chemistry	
PCV	44 %		BUN	21 mg/dl
Hb	14.4 g/dl		Total protein	6.4 g/dl
RBC morphology normal			Albumin	3.4 g/dl
Platelets adequate			ALT (30°C)	178 mU/ml
Plasma protein	8.0 g/dl		ALP (30°C)	6,811 mU/ml
			Glucose	147 mg/dl
	/μl	%	Cholesterol	296 mg/dl
WBC	37,500		Ca^{++}	9.8 mg/dl
Seg. neutrophils	30,375	81	Na^+	157 mEq/l
Band neutrophils	375	1	K^+	3.3 mEq/l
Lymphocytes	750	2	Cl^-	115 mEq/l
Monocytes	6,000	16	HCO_3^- (TCO_2)	22 mEq/l
Eosinophils	0	0		

Urinalysis (cystocentesis)		Other Tests	
Gold, cloudy		Plasma cortisol (day 1)	
Sp gr	1.012	Resting	6.7 μg/dl
pH	6.5	Postdex (low-dose)	6.8 μg/dl
Other chemistries negative		Plasma cortisol (day 8)	
Sediment		Resting	8.3 μg/dl
Triple phosphate crystals		Postdex (high-dose)	3.9 μg/dl
Fat		Post-ACTH	144 μg/dl
		Plasma T4 (day 3)	
		Resting	1.9 ng/ml
		Post-TSH	14.9 ng/ml

PROBLEMS IDENTIFIED FROM LABORATORY DATA:

1. Pituitary dependent hyperadrenocorticism. Although resting plasma
   cortisol values are within normal limits, failure to suppress with
   low-dose dexamethasone and exaggerated response with ACTH stimulation tests confirm hyperadrenocorticism. Suppression of plasma
   cortisol after the high-dose dexamethasone stimulation test
   confirms that the hyperadrenocorticism is pituitary dependent and
   excludes adrenal-dependent types.
     Neutrophilia without a significant left shift, lymphopenia,
   monocytosis, eosinopenia, hyperglycemia, and hypercholesterolemia
   reflect altered metabolism secondary to the effects of corticosteroids.
     High ALP value reflects apparent release of a hepatic isoenzyme
   to the plasma caused by corticosteroid. If cholestasis was the
   cause, bilirubinuria would be expected. Corticosteroids in dogs
   cause hepatic ALP induction and a reversible hepatopathy; the
   increased ALT activity is consistent with the problem.
     Renal disease (low sp gr and polyuria) cannot be absolutely
   ruled out without the water deprivation test. The gradual test is
   indicated because polyuria may have caused medullary washout and
   reduced medullary tonicity.
2. Euthyroid low resting plasma T4. Although resting plasma T4 was
   low, adequate thyroid activity is indicated by the marked response
   to TSH stimulation. Low resting plasma T4 may occur during
   concurrent disease such as hyperadrenocorticism.

SUMMARY:
   The dog improved clinically with medical treatment.

CASE **21** ABOMASAL DISPLACEMENT

SUBJECT:
   Cow, Jersey, female, 2-1/2 years old

PRESENTING PROBLEMS:
   Decreased milk production
   Anorexia
   Ruminal and intestinal atony
   Decreased respiratory rate

LABORATORY DATA:

Hematology			Serum Chemistry	
PCV	38 %		Glucose	220 mg/dl
Hb	12.4 g/dl		Na^+	141 mEq/l
RBC morphology normal			K^+	3.0 mEq/l
Platelets adequate			Cl^-	87 mEq/l
Plasma protein	7.5 g/dl		HCO_3^- (TCO_2)	39.8 mEq/l

	/μl	%	Other Tests	
WBC	9,330		Blood gas analysis (venous)	
Seg. neutrophils	5,318	57	HCO_3^-	38.4 mEq/l
Band neutrophils	0	0	PCO_2	52.6 mmHg
Lymphocytes	3,359	36	pH	7.492
Monocytes	466	5		
Eosinophils	187	2		

Urinalysis (voided)
Pale yellow, clear
Sp gr   1.012
pH   5.0
Glucose   2+
Other chemistries negative
No significant sediment

PROBLEMS IDENTIFIED FROM LABORATORY DATA:

1. Hyperglycemia and glucosuria. Most hyperglycemias in cattle are
   transient, induced by catecholamine or corticosteroid, and commonly exceed the renal threshold in nondiabetic bovine conditions.
2. Hypokalemia. Anorexic herbivores often have negative K^+ balance
   due to decreased oral intake and continued renal loss. Also, loss
   of gastric and intestinal fluids to absorption, as in abomasal
   displacement, represents an additional change in external K^+
   balance. Internal shift in K^+, in which ECF K^+ exchanges with ICF
   H^+ during alkalosis, is thought to be a minor cause of
   hypokalemia.
3. Metabolic alkalosis, hypochloridemia, and paradoxical aciduria.
   Abomasal displacement causes sequestration and loss of gastric HCl
   to absorption, net gain in HCO_3^- (alkalosis), and hypochloridemia.
   Normally renal correction of metabolic alkalosis should be
   secretion of excess HCO_3^- and retention of H^+ ions to restore the

HCO_3^-/H_2CO_3 ratio to 20:1 ($HCO_3^-/.03 \times PCO_2$ = 32:1 in this case). Because Cl^- and K^+ are deficient in the plasma and glomerular filtrate and because the kidney is reabsorbing Na^+ to restore body water, HCO_3^- is reabsorbed instead of Cl^- and H^+ is secreted instead of K^+, alkalosis is potentiated, and paradoxical aciduria occurs. The anion gap is approximately 18 mEq/l, a normal value that excludes complicating acidosis in this case.

SUMMARY:
    The diagnosis, right side displacement of the abomasum, was confirmed by laparotomy and surgically corrected.

CASE 22 FELINE INFECTIOUS PERITONITIS

SUBJECT:
    Cat, Siamese, castrated male, 4 years old

PRESENTING PROBLEMS:
    Enlargement of the abdomen of 1 to 2 weeks duration
    Lethargy
    Hemorrhage in iris
    Anorexia
    Emaciation

LABORATORY DATA:

Hematology

PCV	29 %	
Hb	8.3 g/dl	
RBC morphology normal		
Platelets adequate		

	/µl	%
WBC	20,600	
Seg. neutrophils	15,769	76.5
Band neutrophils	1,236	6.0
Lymphocytes	3,090	15.0
Monocytes	515	2.5
Eosinophils	0	0

Urinalysis (voided)

Yellow, clear	
Sp gr	1.035
pH	6.0
Other chemistries negative	
Sediment	
Amorphous crystals	

Serum Chemistry

Total protein	9.3	g/dl
Albumin	1.9	g/dl
Alpha globulin	0.5	g/dl
Beta globulin	0.5	g/dl
Gamma globulin	6.4	g/dl

Other Tests

Abdominal fluid analysis
  Yellow-green, cloudy, viscid
  Nucleated cell count 5,008/µl
  Nondegenerate neutrophils,
    macrophages, and granular
    background precipitate

Protein	6.0	g/dl
Albumin	1.5	g/dl
Alpha globulin	0.2	g/dl
Beta globulin	0.3	g/dl
Gamma globulin	4.0	g/dl

Opinion: Exudate consistent
  with feline infectious
  peritonitis

PROBLEMS IDENTIFIED FROM LABORATORY DATA:

1. Inflammatory leukocyte response. Neutrophilia with a significant
   left shift indicates an intense but appropriate response to a
   tissue demand for phagocytes. A purulent effusion with moderate to
   low cell count containing a high concentration of globulin
   (represented by granular precipitate on the smear) is characteristic of feline infectious peritonitis. The effusion protein
   concentration and electrophoretic pattern more closely approaches
   serum protein values in this disease than in other exudative
   effusions.
2. Hypergammaglobulinemia. Very high concentration of immunoglobulins
   is characteristic of feline infectious peritonitis.

SUMMARY:
    Diagnosis was confirmed at necropsy.

CASE 23 NEPHROSIS, PERIRENAL HEMORRHAGE

SUBJECT:
    Cow, Hereford, female, 12 years old

PRESENTING PROBLEMS:
    Hematuria
    Dehydration estimated to be 8%

LABORATORY DATA:

Hematology

PCV	30	%
Hb	11	g/dl
RBC morphology normal		
Platelets increased		
Plasma protein	9.4	g/dl
Plasma fibrinogen	1,500	mg/dl

	/μl	%
WBC	9,338	
Seg. neutrophils	7,097	76
Band neutrophils	373	4
Lymphocytes	1,307	14
Monocytes	373	4
Eosinophils	93	1
Basophils	93	1

Serum Chemistry

BUN	161	mg/dl
Creatinine	10.5	mg/dl
Total protein	8.2	g/dl
Albumin	3.1	g/dl
AST (30°C)	126	mU/ml
GGT (30°C)	12	mU/ml
Glucose	498	mg/dl
Ca^{++}	7.3	mg/dl
P	13.8	mg/dl
Na^{+}	115	mEq/l
K^{+}	2.2	mEq/l
Cl^{-}	50	mEq/l
HCO_3^{-} (TCO_2)	28.3	mEq/l

Other Tests

Blood gas analysis (venous)

HCO_3^{-}	27.1	mEq/l
PCO_2	37.7	mmHg
pH	7.483	

Urinalysis (voided)

Red, cloudy
Sp gr (over 3 days)   1.018
pH   7.0
Protein   3+
Occult blood   4+
Glucose   2+
Other chemistries negative
Sediment
  Numerous RBC/HPF
  1 to 2 granular casts/HPF

PROBLEMS IDENTIFIED FROM LABORATORY DATA:

1. Renal disease. Renal azotemia (low urine sp gr with 8%
    dehydration), isosthenuria, hyperphosphatemia, and granular casts
    indicate renal disease. Proteinuria and hematuria may be
    associated with a renal lesion or lower urinary tract problem.
2. Mixed metabolic alkalosis and acidosis with hypochloridemia. High
    plasma HCO_3^- concentration (metabolic alkalosis) and hypochlori-
    demia are common in bovine renal disease due to upper gastro-
    intestinal stasis and functional loss of gastric HCl. Metabolic
    acidosis caused by titration against the plasma buffer systems
    with uremic acids, phosphatic acids (high P concentration), and
    perhaps lactic acid (shock) is detected only by calculation of
    the anion gap, which is about 40 mEq/l in this case.
3. Hyponatremic dehydration and hypokalemia. Bovine renal disease
    causes urinary loss of Na^+ and water in excess of intake. Total
    body Na^+ content is very low. Hypokalemia is most likely secondary
    to change in external K^+ balance (i.e., decreased oral intake and
    kaliuresis).
4. General systemic stress. Hyperglycemia with glucosuria,
    neutrophilia, and lymphopenia indicates catecholamine and
    glucocorticoid stimulation.
5. Hyperfibrinogenemia. The change may indicate inflammation, but no
    other evidence (leukogram) is present. Very high fibrinogen
    measured by the heat precipitation test is common in bovine renal
    disease.

SUMMARY:
    At necropsy, unilateral perirenal and renal hemorrhage and
    bilateral nephrosis were the primary lesions. The cause remained
    unknown.

CASE 24 COUMARIN TOXICOSIS

SUBJECT:
    Dog, German shepherd, male, 6 months old

PRESENTING PROBLEMS:
    Lameness in rear leg
    Hyphema
    Hematuria
    (A female littermate died with pulmonary hemorrhage.)

Hematology		
PCV	30 %	
Hb	9.9 g/dl	
Polychromasia, anisocytosis		
Reticulocytes	4.5 %	
Platelets adequate		
Plasma protein	6.0 g/dl	

	/μl	%
WBC	25,600	
Seg. neutrophils	19,712	77
Band neutrophils	0	0
Lymphocytes	1,792	7
Monocytes	4,096	16
Eosinophils	0	0

Serum Chemistry	
BUN	21 mg/dl
Total protein	5.8 g/dl
Albumin	3.5 g/dl
ALT (30°C)	17 mU/ml
ALP (30°C)	71 mU/ml

Other Tests

Hemostasis profile

Platelets	279,000 /μl
Fibrinogen	256 mg/dl
ACT	4 min 50 sec
APTT	35.7 sec
OSPT	30.2 sec
TCT	5.2 sec
Fibrin degradation products	32 μg/ml

Synovial fluid analysis
Red, cloudy, reduced viscosity
Mucin clot quality poor
Nucleated cell count 1,300/μl
RBCs numerous, 20% neutro-
  phils and 80% monocytes
  (erythrophagia) and
  lymphocytes
Opinion: Traumatic joint
  disease

PROBLEMS IDENTIFIED FROM LABORATORY DATA:

1. Hemorrhagic anemia. Regenerative anemia, hypoproteinemia, and
   clinical signs indicate hemorrhagic anemia. Neutrophilia and
   monocytosis also are consistent with hemorrhage.
2. Coagulation factor deficiency, most likely vitamin K-dependent
   factor deficiency. Hemophilia A or B and von Willebrand's disease,
   the most common hereditary bleeding disorders, are excluded
   because both APTT and OSPT are prolonged; only APTT would be
   prolonged in the hereditary problems. Normal platelet count, TCT,
   and FDP concomitant with the prolonged clotting times tend to
   rule out disseminated intravascular coagulation syndrome.
   Prolonged ACT and citrated plasma clotting tests (APTT and OSPT)
   are consistent with acquired deficiency of vitamin K-dependent
   factors; liver disease as a cause is unlikely because ALT and ALP
   are normal.

SUMMARY:
    Possible exposure to coumarin-type rat poison was confirmed by
the owner. The dog was successfully treated.

CASE **25** ACUTE PULMONARY HEMORRHAGE AND EDEMA

SUBJECT:
   Dog, German shepherd, female, 2 years old

PRESENTING PROBLEMS:
   Known exposure to paraquat followed by severe vomiting
   Rapid, deep, painful (groaning) respiration
   (Continuous intravenous lactated Ringer's solution, 4700 ml total
      volume, spiked with KCl totalling 39 mEq, were given over 20
      hours prior to obtaining the sample for the following laboratory
      data.)

LABORATORY DATA:

Hematology		Other Tests	
PCV	52.5 %	Blood gas analysis (arterial)	
WBC	16,800 /μl	HCO_3^-	25.5 mEq/l
		PCO_2	32.8 mmHg
Urinalysis (catheterized)		pH	7.515
Sp gr	1.015	PO_2	52.0 mmHg

Serum Chemistry

BUN	58 mg/dl
Glucose	120 mg/dl
Na^+	127 mEq/l
K^+	2.8 mEq/l
Cl^-	78 mEq/l
HCO_3^- (TCO_2)	26.8 mEq/l

PROBLEMS IDENTIFIED FROM LABORATORY DATA:

1. Azemia and low urine specific gravity. These findings indicate
   possible renal failure, although the high PCV in spite of fluid
   therapy suggests dehydration and therefore prerenal azotemia. The
   low urine sp gr may represent diuresis secondary to fluid therapy.
2. Hyponatremia, hypokalemia, and hypochloridemia. Since dehydration
   was not clinically apparent at the time of sampling, ECF volume
   may be presumed to be normal or increased (possible pulmonary
   edema). This indicates that Na^+ content of fluids given may have
   been inadequate, and overhydration may have developed. Hypokalemia
   is a common consequence of prolonged fluid therapy, especially
   with alkalinizing fluid, during which K^+ shifts to the ICF.
   Hypochloridemia parallels hyponatremia. Diuresis may produce
   kaliuresis.
3. Hypoxemia. Low arterial PO_2 concomitant with rapid respiration and
   normal PCO_2 indicates a perfusion/diffusion abnormality as with
   pneumonia, pulmonary edema, or pulmonary thrombosis.
4. Mixed respiratory and metabolic alkalosis. The marked increase in
   blood pH is due to a combination of mild metabolic alkalosis and
   lack of respiratory compensation. The hypoxemia is maintaining the
   respiratory drive and preventing hypoventilation needed to
   increase PCO_2 to compensate for metabolic alkalosis.

SUMMARY:
   Necropsy revealed nephrosis and pulmonary hemorrhage and edema.

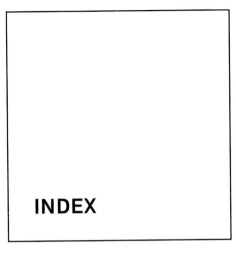

INDEX

Polyuria, causes, 155
Porphyria, 3
Portal vein obstruction, effusion in, 206
Portal venous-systemic venous shunt, 122-23
  case example, 249-50
  causative lesions, 137
  effect
    on amino acid ratio, 135
    on ammonia, 134
    on BSP, 132
  laboratory findings, 141
Potassium, 95-97. See also Hyper-kalemia; Hypokalemia
  in CSF, 211
  effect, of lipemia, 110
  methods, 91-92
  reference values, 231
Pregnancy toxemia, glucose changes, 116
Preleukemia, 68
  case example, 243-44
Proestrus, cytology, 215
Progranulocyte, 32
  occurrence in blood, 41
Promyelocyte. See Progranulocyte
Prostacyclin, 73
Protein. See also Albumin; Globulin
  abnormalities, 108-9
  acute phase reactants, 108
  Bence-Jones, 66
  colostral, 106
  in CSF, 210
  in dehydration, 87
  effects of hemorrhage, 109
  in effusions, 201
  electrophoresis, 106-7
  functions, 105
  means of measurement, 105-6
  monoclonal gammopathy, 66-67, 108-9
  origins, 105
  plasma protein/fibrinogen ratio, 108
  polyclonal gammopathy, 108
  reference values, 229, 233-34
Protein-losing enteropathy
  case example, 258-59
  protein changes, 109
Proteinuria, 156-57
  Bence-Jones, 66
  in diabetes mellitus, 193
  in glomerular disease, case

  examples, 242-43, 253-54
Prothrombin, 76
  deficiency, hereditary, breeds affected, 84
Prothrombin time. See One-stage prothrombin time
Pseudochylous effusion, 206-7
Pseudohyperparathyroidism, 184, 187. See also Hyper-parathyroidism
  case example, 245-46
Pseudo-Pelger-Huet anomaly, 41
Puerpural tetany, 186
Pyometra, leukocyte response, 48

Red blood cell count, 8
  reference values, 229
Reference values, 229-34
Renal disease. See also Azotemia; Urine
  calcinosis in, 182
  case examples, 251-54
  effects, on calcium and phos-phorus, 185-87
  function tests in, 164-67
  miscellaneous alterations, 171
  mixed alkalosis and acidosis, 100
  potassium changes, 96
  protein changes, 109
  sodium changes, 94
  urine concentration tests in, 166-67
Renal secondary hyperparathyroid-ism, ALP changes, 126. See also Hyperparathyroidism
Renal tubular acidosis, 98
  case example, 252-53
Respiratory acidosis, 101
  blood gas analysis, 92
  mixed with metabolic acidosis or alkalosis, 102
Respiratory alkalosis, 102
  blood gas analysis, 92
  mixed with metabolic alkalosis or acidosis, 102
  case example, 267
  in portal caval venous shunt, case example, 249-50
Reticulocyte, 5-6, 13-15, 18
  absolute count, 14
  feline, 14
  interpretation, 14-15
  percentage, 14
  production index, 14